The Diagnosis and Management of Paediatric Respiratory Disease

The Diagnosis and Management of Paediatric Respiratory Disease

Robert Dinwiddie
Consultant Paediatrician, Respiratory Unit,
The Hospitals for Sick Children,
Great Ormond Street, London
Honorary Senior Lecturer, Institute
of Child Health, University of London

CHURCHILL LIVINGSTONE
EDINBURGH LONDON MELBOURNE AND NEW YORK 1990

CHURCHILL LIVINGSTONE
Medical Division of Longman Group UK Limited

Distributed in the United States of America by Churchill
Livingstone Inc., 1560 Broadway, New York, N.Y. 10036,
and by associated companies, branches and representatives
throughout the world.

First published 1990
  Reprinted 1991 (twice)

ISBN 0-443-02744-7

British Library Cataloguing in Publication Data
Dinwiddie, Robert
    The diagnosis and management of paediatric
    respiratory disease.
    1. Children. Respiratory system. Diseases
    I. Title
    618.92′2

Library of Congress Cataloging-in-Publication Data
Dinwiddie, R.
    The diagnosis and management of paediatric respiratory disease/
    Robert Dinwiddie.
        p.   cm.
    1. Pediatric respiratory diseases.   I. Title.
    [DNLM: 1. Respiratory Tract Diseases — in infancy & childhood.   WS
200 D587d]
    RJ431.D56   1990
    618.92′2 — dc20
    DNLM/DLC   89–22107
    for Library of Congress   CIP

Produced by Longman Singapore Publishers (Pte) Ltd.
Printed in Singapore

Preface

Diseases of the respiratory system are the most frequently encountered problem in the childhood years. Paediatric Respiratory Medicine is a rapidly growing field and one in which there is now a constant flow of new investigative techniques and treatments available even for the smallest of patients. Examples of this include rapid techniques for viral or bacterial diagnosis, increasingly sophisticated and less invasive methods for measuring pulmonary function and for imaging of the respiratory system, new antibiotics for serious infections and the availability of improved prenatal diagnosis by chronic villous sampling, amniocentesis or ultrasound for an increasing number of respiratory conditions including cystic fibrosis.

This textbook is designed to give a basic overview of the subject, to highlight areas of recent advance and to point the reader to appropriate references and recommended reading if he or she wishes to deepen their knowledge further in any particular area. It is aimed primarily at those who have recently entered the field, interested General Practitioners and particularly those who are preparing for the MRCP. It is hoped that it may also be of interest to others such as paediatric nurses and physiotherapists who frequently deal with children in hospital because of their respiratory problems.

London, 1990   RD

To: Mary, Robert and Jane

Acknowledgements

I would like to acknowledge the input of my colleagues at the Hospitals for Sick Children, Great Ormond Street — for their stimulating and helpful discussion of the clinical problems which exercise us day to day. I am particularly indebted to Dr Duncan Matthew and Dr Peter Helms for their constant support in the management of our patients; this review of our practice would not be possible without their help. Dr Isky Gordon is an invaluable member of the team and his expertise in imaging of the respiratory system is greatly appreciated.

Chapters 3, 5 and 14 have been written by colleagues with special expertise in their field. These include Dr Paul McMahon, Dr Ilya Kovar, Mr John Evans, Mr Robert Black and Dr Edward Sumner. Their contributions are specially acknowledged and their support for this book particularly valued.

Other colleagues at Great Ormond Street and the Institute of Child Health who have been helpful in their advice and review of individual chapters include Dr Alison Hislop (chapter 1), Dr Janet Stocks (chapter 2), Dr Stephan Strobel (chapter 7), and Drs Helen Holzel and Shelley Heard (chapter 11). The nursing support of Sister Sue Madge and the physiotherapy advice of Miss Ammani Prasad have been invaluable.

A number of paediatric colleagues and medical publishers have been kind enough to allow the use of their material in the figures. They are acknowledged individually in the text but their help in this publication is much appreciated. The work of Magpie Reprographics, London, and the Department of Medical Illustration at the hospital in preparation of the figures has been invaluable.

Beverley Walker, Leigh Stanger, Paula Smith and Vickie Grace have shared the typing of the manuscript and are especially thanked.

Contributors

Robert J Black MB BS (Qld) FRACS FRCS(Ed)
Formerly Senior Ear, Nose and Throat Registrar, The Hospitals for Sick
Children, Great Ormond Street, London, UK; Consultant Ear, Nose and
Throat Surgeon, Mater Childrens Hospital and Mater Adults Hospital,
Brisbane, Australia

John N G Evans MB BS DLO FRCS(Eng)
Consultant Ear, Nose and Throat Surgeon, The Hospitals for Sick
Children, Great Ormond Street, and St Thomas's Hospital, London, UK

Ilya Z Kovar MB MRCP FRCP(C) FAAP
Senior Lecturer in Child Health, Charing Cross and Westminster
Medical School, Consultant Paediatrician, Charing Cross Hospital,
London, UK

Paul MacMahon MB MRCP(I) MRCP(UK) DCH
Consultant Paediatrician, Waterford Regional Hospital, Ardkeen,
Waterford, Eire

Edward Sumner MA BM BCh FFARCS
Consultant Anaesthetist, The Hospitals for Sick Children, Great Ormond
Street; Chairman, Department of Anaesthetics; Director, Cardiac Intensive
Care Unit; Honorary Senior Lecturer, Institute of Child Health, London,
UK

Contents

1. Development of the lungs

Although it is some time before the fetus reaches a stage of development at which life can be supported independently, the lungs are already at a relatively advanced stage of maturation. This is an extremely complex process and begins very early in fetal life, probably just before 28 days of gestation. Lung development in utero is then classically divided into four periods (Nomina Embryologica 1974, Inselman & Mellins 1981):

1. Embryonic period: 3rd to 5th week.
2. Pseudoglandular period: 6th to 16th week.
3. Canalicular period: 17th to 24th week.
4. Alveolar sac period: from 24 weeks to term.

EMBRYONIC PERIOD (3–5 weeks)

The embryonic period includes the time in which the initial lung bud appears as an endodermal outgrowth of the fetal foregut (Fraser 1940); this consists of epithelial cells forming a single tube which soon branches into two components representing the major bronchi. The process of cell division then continues burying into the surrounding mesoderm with which there is an important interaction if further normal branching is to occur (Wessells 1970). It is at this stage that collagen fibres are also first seen and these too increasingly influence the structure of the branching lung buds (Wessells & Cohen 1968). By the end of this period the major lung branches are already formed although there is as yet no significant development of the pulmonary circulation.

PSEUDOGLANDULAR PERIOD (6–16 weeks)

The next stage is the pseudoglandular period, extending up to the end of the 16th week. During this time the airways grow by dichotomous branching and become lined with tall columnar or cuboidal epithelial cells in close association with the adjacent mesenchyme. By the end of this period all conducting generations of the airway from trachea down to the terminal bronchioles are formed. This portion of the airway is known as the pre-acinus and includes all structures from the trachea down to and including

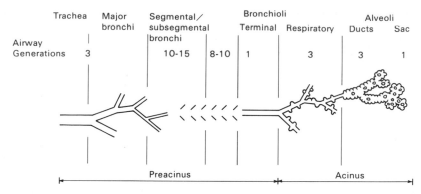

Fig. 1.1 Anatomy of the tracheobronchial tree.

the terminal bronchioles themselves. Three further generations of respiratory bronchioles develop later (Fig. 1.1). Cartilage and lymphatic formation also occurs from 10 weeks onwards (Avery & Fletcher 1974, Yu 1986). Cilia too make their appearance at this gestation and have spread peripherally by 13 weeks.

The pulmonary arterial and venous systems also develop rapidly. The arteries begin from the sixth branchial arches, the main pulmonary artery arising from the sixth left arch which subsequently subdivides to form the right and left pulmonary arteries. A right-sided aortic arch is also present at this time but most of it subsequently disappears; the dorsal portion persists as the ductus arteriosus leaving the pulmonary artery in direct connection with the aorta.

CANALICULAR PERIOD (17–24 weeks)

During this period the lung develops its more conventional architecture. The airways become longer and the epithelial cells adopt a more cuboidal shape in the lower airway generations. The mesodermal tissue thins out and the microcirculation matures rapidly.

The lung capillaries are now in close approximation to the simultaneously developing last three airway generations, the respiratory bronchioles, and the alveolar ducts. The peripheral epithelial cells thin out further in preparation for future gas exchange (Woods & Dalton 1958). This distal portion of the lung which will soon form the gas exchanging unit is called the acinus; it comprises the respiratory bronchioles, alveolar ducts and the alveoli themselves (Figs 1.1 and 1.2).

The peripheral pulmonary arterial system develops alongside the preacinus (Hislop & Reid 1981). The pulmonary venous system also

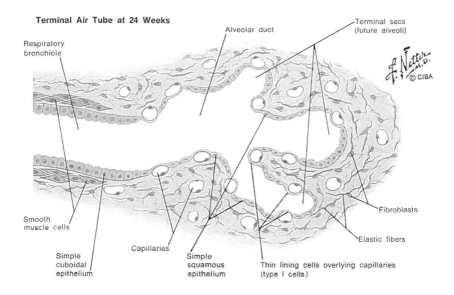

Fig. 1.2 Terminal air tube at 24 weeks. From CIBA Clinical Symposia number 4, volume 27, 1975. Reproduced by courtesy of CIBA-GIEGY Ltd, Basle, Switzerland. All rights reserved.

develops rapidly from the left atrium at this time. By 20 weeks all the preacinar veins have developed in parallel with the capillary and arterial systems but the more peripheral veins develop later (Yu 1986).

Surfactant synthesis is also beginning. The most peripheral epithelial cells which will ultimately become the alveolar lining cells begin to subdivide themselves into two major types — type I and type II pneumocytes which are identifiable by 24 weeks (Campiche et al 1963). The lung starts to fill with fluid which ultimately reaches a volume of 30 ml/kg in the term infant which is similar to the functional residual capacity after breathing is established (Nelson 1966, Olver et al 1973).

TERMINAL SAC PERIOD (24 weeks to term)

The terminal sac period takes place from 24 weeks to term. During this time the lung becomes capable of supporting extrauterine life. The more mature the fetus the greater the chances of survival. At 24 weeks birth weight may be only 600 g, however a small but significant number of babies have survived even at this gestation.

This last stage of fetal lung development comprises the further differentiation of epithelial cells into type I and type II alveolar lining cells (Kuhn 1982) and the establishment of the final intimate inter-relationship of the capillary membrane to the epithelial lining surface. The final three bronchiolar generations, the respiratory bronchioles, give off further subdivisions or saccules which subdivide to form the alveoli. The alveoli are lined by two distinct types of cells, type I and type II pneumocytes. The type I pneumocyte covers the majority of the alveolar surface, about 96%, and performs the function of gas exchange within the lung. Their average thickness is 0.1–0.01 μm. The second cell in the alveolus, the type II cell, has a diameter of 10 μm and, although only covering 5–10% of the lung surface, has a vital role in the metabolic activity of the lung (Strang 1977). Its principal role is the production of pulmonary surfactant which is vital to the normal expansion and contraction of alveoli and prevention of alveolar collapse during spontaneous breathing. These type II cells contain osmiophilic granular inclusion bodies which are thought to be the source of the surfactant material. Surfactant consists of a number of important substances which function together to stabilise surface tension. The major components are shown in Table 1.1.

Although small quantities of surfactant may be detected at 23–24 weeks, it is not found in physiologically large amounts until 30 weeks or more (Gluck & Kulovich 1973). Birth itself and the onset of air breathing accelerate the maturation of surfactant production (Gluck et al 1967). The major pathway of surfactant lipid synthesis is via choline phosphorylation utilising choline kinase. This is then attached to a diglyceride molecule to produce phosphatidyl choline (Kennedy & Weiss 1956). The completed substance along with the other components is then secreted onto the alveolar surface by degranulation from the type II cell. The half life of surfactant within the lung is 10–14 hours and it is cleared by upward movement on the ciliary escalator of the bronchial tree and by direct absorption across the alveolar membrane and into alveolar macrophages.

The pulmonary circulation continues to develop. The muscle coat around the pulmonary arterioles at this stage is thicker than in later life (Hislop & Reid 1973). This allows for intense vasoconstriction during times of intrauterine stress but can contribute to pulmonary hypertensive syndromes in the early neonatal period. In the normal child, this proportionately thickened muscle diminishes very rapidly after birth.

After birth, at which time the alveoli are multilocular, there is progressive increase in alveolar size and numbers and outbudding from the saccule. There is a wide variation in the number of alveoli present at term in the newborn human lung, an average figure would be 150 million (Hislop et al 1986). The adult number of 300–400 million may be reached by the age of

Table 1.1   Composition of surfactant

Phospholipids	78%
Phophatidylcholine	66%
Phosphatidylglycerol	4%
Phosphatidylethanolamine	5%
Sphingomyelin	3%
Cholesterol and glycerides	12%
Protein	9%
Fatty acids	1%

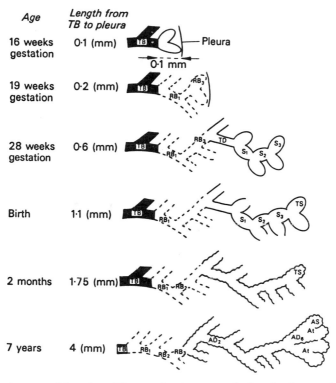

Fig. 1.3 Development of the acinus. Diagram showing stages of acinar development in fetal and postnatal life. TB=terminal bronchiole; RB=respiratory bronchiole; TD=terminal duct; S=saccule; AD=alveolar duct; At=atrium; AS=alveolar sac. From Hislop & Reid, 1974, reproduced with permission.

3–4 years. A large proportion of this number appear in the first year of life (Dunhill 1962) although alveolar growth continues for the first 7 years.

During the early years there is also a significant increase in diameter of the large airways and remodelling of the acinus (Hislop & Reid 1974) (Fig. 1.3). The alveoli continue to multiply. There is also expansion of existing lung units, a process which continues particularly after alveolar budding is complete. The lung then continues to increase in size but not in alveolar numbers until physical growth is complete. The dynamic volumes are shown in Chapter 2. Alveolar surface area increases from 4 m^2 at birth (Hislop et al 1986) to 12.2 m^2 at 1 year and 75 m^2 in the adult (Dunhill 1962).

FACTORS AFFECTING LUNG GROWTH

A number of factors are known to influence normal lung growth and development, either before or after birth. Lung growth in utero is known to be accelerated by the presence of glucocorticoids, thyroid hormone, prolactin and oestradiol. Extrinsic agents such as aminophylline, heroin and beta adrenergic stimulants accelerate surfactant production. Phenobarbitone or excess insulin inhibit maturation. Congenital malformation within one part of a lung may have profound effects on the growth and development of the system as a whole. This is best illustrated in the case of diaphragmatic hernia. If this is present during the pseudoglandular period when airway multiplication is at its maximum it can result in a significant reduction in the number of conducting airway generations in both lungs (Hislop & Reid 1976). Other abnormalities which can produce a similar effect include cystic adenomatoid malformation, bronchogenic cyst, lobar sequestration and unilateral pulmonary agenesis. Diseases such as intrauterine haemolytic disease, bilateral renal agenesis or renal hypoplasia lead to a decreased number of airway generations and alveoli. Changes in amniotic fluid volume either involving oligohydramnios, polyhadramnios or persistent fluid leak can diminish alveolar numbers (Inselman & Mellins 1981). Alveolar growth is also inhibited in utero by chest wall defects such as asphyxiating thoracic dystrophy (Finegold et al 1971).

Postnatal insult can also cause permanent impairment of lung growth. This may occur in severe respiratory tract infection such as with adenovirus or when there is bronchiectasis. Prolonged oxygen therapy can lead to a reduction in alveolar numbers (Bartlett 1970), as can artificial ventilation (Hislop et al 1987) — this is particularly relevant in infants with bronchopulmonary dysplasia where it is just one of several factors adversely affecting the lungs. Therapeutic irradiation for other conditions significantly affects lung function (Wohl et al 1975) and is thought to alter acinar growth but not the preacinar portion of the lung. Cardiac malformations can produce a wide range of changes within the pulmonary vascular bed and these may be seen either pre- or postnatally.

The growth and development of the lungs is thus seen to be a continuous process from early fetal life to adulthood but with the most important changes occurring before birth and in early childhood. It is at these times that other events can have the most profound effects on the future structure and function of this important organ system.

REFERENCES

Avery M E, Fletcher B D (eds) 1974 Lung development. In: The lung and its disorders in the newborn infant. Saunders, Philadelphia. pp 1–21
Bartlett D 1970 Postnatal growth of the mammalian lung: influence of low and high oxygen tensions. Respiratory Physiology 9: 58–64
Bucher U, Reid L 1961 Development of the intrasegmental bronchial tree. The pattern of branching and development of cartilage at various stages of intrauterine life. Thorax 16: 207–218
Campiche M A, Gautier A, Hemandeg E I, Raymond A 1963 An electron microscope study of the fetal development of the human lung. Pediatrics 32: 967–994
Crelin E S 1975 Development of the lower respiratory system. In: Shapter R K (ed) Clinical symposia. Ciba Geigy, New Jersey, vol 27, pp 3–28

Dunhill M S 1962 Postnatal growth of the lung. Thorax 17: 329–333

Fraser J E (ed) 1940 Manual of embryology. Ballière Tindall and Cox, London, pp 353–368

Finegold M J, Katzew H, Genieser N B, Becker M H 1971 Lung structure in thoracic dystrophy. American Journal of Disease of Childhood 122: 153–159

Gluck L, Motoyama E K, Smits H L, Kulovich M V 1967 The biochemical development of the surface activity in the mammalian lung 1. Pediatric Research 1: 237–246

Gluck L, Kulovich M V 1973 L/S ratios in amniotic fluid and abnormal pregnancies. American Journal of Obstetrics and Gynecology 115: 539–552

Hislop A, Reid L 1973 Pulmonary arterial development during childhood: branching pattern and structures. Thorax 28: 129–135

Hislop A, Reid L 1974 Development of the acinus in the human lung. Thorax 29: 90–94

Hislop A, Reid L 1976 Persistent hypoplasia of the lung after repair of congenital diaphragmatic hernia. Thorax 31: 450–455

Hislop A, Reid L 1981 Growth and development of the respiratory system. Anatomical Development. In: Davis J A, Dobbing J (eds) Scientific foundations of paediatrics. Heinemann, London, p 390

Hislop A, Wigglesworth J S, Desai R 1986 Alveolar development in the human fetus and infant. Early Human Development 13: 1–11

Hislop A, Wigglesworth J S, Desai R, Aber V 1987 The effects of preterm delivery and mechanical ventilation on human lung growth. Early Human Development 15: 147–164

Inselman L S, Mellins R B 1981 Growth and development of the lung. Journal of Pediatrics 98: 1–15

Kennedy E P, Weiss S B 1956 The function of cytidine coenzymes in the biosynthesis of phospholipids. Journal of Biological Chemistry 222: 193–214

Kuhn C 1982 The cytology of the lung. In: Farrell P M (ed) Lung development: biological and clinical perspectives. Academic Press, New York, vol 1, p 13

Nelson N M 1966 Neonatal pulmonary function. Pediatric Clinics of North America. 1. The Newborn 13: 769–799

Nomina Embryologica 1974 International Anatomical Nomenclature Committee: Federation of American Societies for Experimental Biology, FASEB, Bethesda, Maryland

Olver R E, Reynolds E O R, Strang L B 1973 Fetal lung liquid. In: Foetal and neonatal physiology, proceedings of the Joseph Barcroft centenary symposium. Cambridge University Press, Cambridge, pp 186–207

Strang L B 1977 Morphology of lung development. In: Neonatal respiration, physiological and clinical studies. Blackwell Scientific, Oxford, pp 1–19

Wessells N K, Cohen J H 1968 Effects of collagenase on developing epithelia in vitro.

Wessells N K 1970 Mammalian lung development: interactions in formation and morphogenesis of lung buds. Journal of Experimental Zoology 175: 455–466

Wohl M E B, Griscom M T, Traggis D G, Jaffe N 1975 Effects of therapeutic irradiation delivered in early childhood upon subsequent lung function. Pediatrics 55: 507–516

Woods de G L, Dalton A J 1958 The ultrastructure of lung tissue for newborn and embryo mice. Journal of Ultrastructure Research 2: 28–54

Yu V Y H (ed) 1986 Development of the lung. In: Respiratory disorders of the newborn. Churchill Livingstone, Edinburgh, pp 1–7

2. Physiology of breathing

The physiology of breathing is intimately integrated with the maintenance of acid–base balance in the body which is vital for survival. Before birth, the fetus maintains this balance via the placenta. Fetal breathing movements occur in utero but these are minimal compared to those seen after birth (Platt & Manning 1980, Yu 1986). Major changes occur at the time of birth when breathing is first established. The fluid filled lungs must be emptied and aerated satisfactorily in order for respiration to be established. At the same moment in time, major circulatory changes are occurring since in fetal life 90% of the cardiac output is shunted away from the lungs and this must be redistributed to the pulmonary vascular bed in order to facilitate the uptake of oxygen as breathing begins (Rudolph & Heymann 1974). These processes are under the control of the respiratory centres in the brain reacting to incoming afferent stimuli from chemoreceptors and baroreceptors within the circulation and mechanoreceptors in the airways. These controlling systems must be intact if satisfactory respiration is to be established at birth. Further details of these important changes are reviewed in Chapter 3. During life the lungs grow and develop new alveoli up to about 7 years of age; it is particularly important to protect them from damage during this early growing phase if normal function is to be maintained in the longer term.

Increasing interest is also being paid to the effects of paediatric disease on adult lung function and disorders of the lungs in later life. As more infants survive after ventilation in the neonatal period, it will be interesting to learn of their longterm outcome, particularly for those who have had early damage to the lungs, such as bronchopulmonary dysplasia (Smyth et al 1981, Samuels & Warner 1987). Increasing public health measures will also reduce the damage to the lungs caused by smoking directly, or — more commonly in childhood — by so-called passive smoking secondary to smoking by parents or other relatives in the home.

LUNG VOLUMES AND MECHANICS

The lungs function by expansion and relaxation to their resting volume at specific rates determined by cerebral control of breathing and by their own intrinsic elastic and viscous resistive properties. The volume changes

9

are proportional to the negative pressure applied across the pleural cavity by the rib cage and to the natural resistance of the airways and lung tissues to the passage of air. The lungs may be divided into a number of basic divisions or volumes for the purposes of measurement (Fig. 2.1). The volumes measured are represented by the following values:

Tidal volume (Vt) is the volume per breath, beginning at functional residual capacity.

Functional residual capacity (FRC) is the volume of air left in the lungs which is in direct contact with the airways at the end of a normal breath.

Thoracic gas volume (TGV) is the volume of all the air in the lungs at the end of a normal breath; this includes FRC plus any air which is trapped behind closed airways. In a normally functioning lung, FRC and TGV are approximately equal, but in the presence of airway disease causing obstruction a significant volume of trapped gas may be present.

Measurements of FRC and TGV require complicated apparatus. FRC is most frequently measured using a spirometer with a helium dilution technique. This only measures gas in direct communication with the airways. TGV requires the use of a whole body plethysmograph and measures total gas within the chest including FRC and all trapped gas (Godfrey 1979). TGV is particularly likely to be abnormal in those who have chronic airway obstruction, for example in asthma or cystic fibrosis. Another reflection of this gas trapping can be obtained by assessment of the residual volume to total lung capacity (RV/TLC) ratio which is usually below 30% in healthy children.

Residual volume (RV) is the volume of air left in the lungs after a maximal expiration. This occurs due to closure of the small airways at low lung volumes which leaves some gas trapped behind them.

Vital capacity (VC) or *forced vital capacity* (FVC) is the volume of air expired during forced expiration from total lung capacity (TLC) down to residual volume (RV). It is measured by spirometry and expressed as a volume in ml or litres. It is also quoted as a percentage of predicted normal

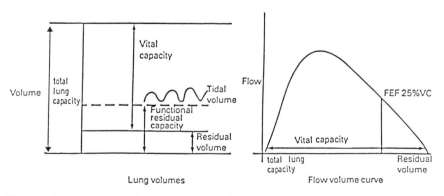

Fig. 2.1   Lung volumes and the expiratory flow volume curve (FEF 25%VC = Forced Expiratory Flow at 25% of Vital Capacity).

for sex and height. Values below 75% predicted indicate a significant reduction in VC.

The *forced expiratory volume in 1 second* (FEV$_1$) is the volume of air which can be expired from TLC in 1 second. It is often expressed as a ratio of FVC (FEV$_1$/FVC ratio). It is also expressed as a percentage of the predicted normal for sex and height. Values of less than 75% predicted indicate airway obstruction especially of the larger airways.

Peak expiratory flow rate (PEFR) is the maximum flow achieved on expiration from TLC. It is easily measured using a peak flow meter. It is the most useful simple test of airway obstruction and can be used to monitor day to day treatment in the home if necessary. One disadvantage is that it is effort dependant. Values are expressed as litres/min or as a percentage of the predicted normal for sex and height. Levels below 75% indicate significant airway obstruction.

Total lung capacity (TLC) represents vital capacity plus residual volume.

Normal values for these parameters are shown in Fig. 2.2, Tables 2.1 and 2.2.

The measurement of flow at various lung volumes is represented by the expiratory flow volume curve (Fig. 2.1). A vital capacity manoeuvre is performed from TLC and air expired maximally down to residual volume. This allows measurement of the peak expiratory flow rate and also the relative flow at different proportions of lung volume. A commonly quoted level being forced expiratory flow at 25% vital capacity (FEF 25% VC). This may be a useful measure of small airway obstruction (Zapletal et al 1971).

The volume of the lungs is also dependant on the balance between the expansive forces of the chest wall and rib cage and the elastic recoil of the lungs away from them. This balance is affected in patients who have neuromuscular disease or abnormalities of the rib cage such as rickets. A

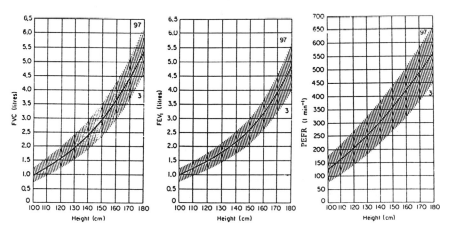

Fig. 2.2 Forced vital capacity (FVC), forced expiratory volume in 1 second (FEV$_1$), and peak expiratory flow rate (PEFR) in healthy boys and girls. (Adapted from Godfrey 1979, with permission.)

Table 2.1   Respiratory function mean value for height

Height	Forced vital capacity (FVC) Litres		Forced expiratory volume in 1 sec (FEV1) Litres		Peak expiratory flow rate (PEFR) Litres/min
	Boys	Girls	Boys	Girls	Boys and Girls
100 cm	0.92	0.92	0.84	0.84	110
110 cm	1.24	1.22	1.13	1.12	150
120 cm	1.57	1.53	1.44	1.43	205
130 cm	1.94	1.86	1.76	1.71	250
140 cm	2.35	2.27	2.13	2.11	300
150 cm	2.81	2.74	2.51	2.51	350
160 cm	3.40	3.31	3.00	3.00	410
170 cm	4.04	3.91	3.57	3.52	480

Adapted from Cogswell 1975a, b, Polgar & Promadhat 1971 and Godfrey et al 1970. Results are usually expressed as absolute values and as percent predicted for height.

measure of elastic recoil is made using static pressure volume curves as shown in Fig. 2.3. These measurements are complicated and have not been easy to perform in children (Zapletal et al 1976).

Lung compliance (Cl) is a measure of the volume of air inspired per unit change of pressure in the lung at points of no flow. It is the inverse of

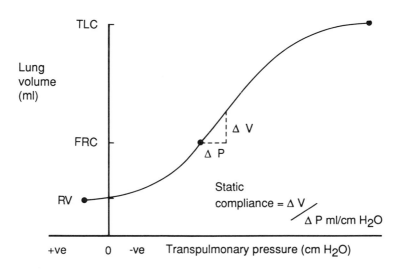

Fig. 2.3   Schematic representation of static lung compliance. Δ = unit change in volume or pressure under resting conditions.

elastance and is a measure of lung distensibility. Lung compliance may be divided into two types, static and dynamic. Static compliance (Cstat) is measured at different lung volumes while the breath is being held (Godfrey 1979), whereas dynamic compliance (Cdyn) is measured at points of no flow during continuous natural breathing (Clutario 1975). Recent techniques using a face mask and airway occlusion have enabled non-invasive measurements of total respiratory compliance (chest wall plus lung) to be made in infants (Heaf et al 1987, Stocks et al 1987).

The resistance to air flow through the airways is measured as airway resistance (Raw); this is a measure of pressure divided by flow. Its reciprocal, flow divided by pressure, is airway conductance (Gaw). Raw is measured in a body plethysmograph by assessing the change in mouth pressure to alveolar pressure and relating this to flow. The points of maximum airway resistance occur at different levels in the respiratory system. The nasal passages account for 50% of airway resistance and a significant proportion of the remainder occurs at the level of the larynx and the large airways in the chest. As the airways subdivide the total cross sectional area increases rapidly although the size of the individual airway is decreasing. The relationship of airway resistance to lung volume is measured by the ratio of Gaw to TGV (specific conductance) and remains fairly constant throughout life at 0.23 cmH$_2$O/l/s/lTGV (Godfrey 1979). One exception to this is the preterm infant who has a higher value because of the immaturity of the lungs (Stocks & Godfrey 1977).

The basic lung function tests described so far are most frequently performed on children over the age of 4 or 5 who can cooperate and who understand the requirements of the tests. The most commonly measured values are VC, FEV$_1$, PEFR and the flow volume curve. The peak flow rate measurements are useful for seeking evidence of large airway obstruction, whereas the flow volume (FEF 25% VC) measurements are more helpful in conditions where there is early small airway closure due to increased resistance as in asthma or cystic fibrosis (Zapletal et al 1971). The shape of the flow volume curve may also be helpful in determining the level at which obstruction is occurring.

EXERCISE TESTING

Exercise testing of children is also useful and typical results are shown in Fig. 2.4 (Godfrey 1979). In its simplest form this involves free running along a corridor for a period of six minutes. The pulse rate should rise to over 180/min and peak flow or FEV$_1$ measurements are made throughout the study. There is usually an initial increase in peak flow or FEV$_1$ during the exercise but this is followed by a rapid fall over the next 3–10 minutes indicating bronchial lability (Kuzemko & Bedford 1980). This is particularly seen in asthmatic children and a fall of greater than 15% over baseline is thought to be significant. Should a large fall in peak flow or FEV$_1$ occur, usually within two to three minutes of completion of the exercise, a

Table 2.2   Lung function at different ages

Lung function	Neonate		Child aged 7		Adult		Units
	/kg	Average (3.5 kg)	/kg	Average (25 kg)	/kg	Average (70 kg)	
Vital capacity (VC)	35	120	65	1600	54	3800	ml
Forced expiratory volume 1 second (FEV_1)	—	—	60	1500	51	3600	ml
Peak expiratory flow rate (PEFR)	2.5	9	8	200	7	300–700	l/min
Tidal volume (Vt)	7	25	7	175	7	500	ml/breath
Respiratory rate	—	40	—	20	—	15	breaths/min
Residual volume (RV)	23	80	18	460	16	1120	ml
Functional residual capacity (FRC)	28	100	30	750	30	2100	ml
Thoracic gas volume (TGV)	32	110	30	750	30	2100	ml
Total lung capacity (TLC)	65	230	75	1900	80	5600	ml
RV/TLC %	—	35	—	25	—	20–30	%
Lung compliance (Cl)	1.7	6	2.4	60	2.8	200	ml/cmH_2O
Specific lung compliance Cl/FRC	—	0.05	—	0.05	—	0.05	$ml/cmH_2O/ml$
Airway resistance (Raw)	—	35	—	0.05–2.0	—	0.05–2.0	$cmH_2O/1/sec$
Specific conductance (SGaw)	—	0.3	—	0.23	—	0.25	$cmH_2O/1/sec/$ lFRC
Work of breathing	430	1500	480	12 000	490	16 000–50 000	g.cm/min
Maximum inspiratory pressure	—	100	—	120	—	125	cmH_2O
Maximum expiratory pressure	—	150	—	200	—	250	cmH_2O

Table 2.2 Cont.

Lung function	Neonate		Child aged 7		Adult		Units
	/kg	Average (3.5 kg)	/kg	Average (25 kg)	/kg	Average (70 kg)	
Oxygen uptake	6	20	4	100	5	350	mlO_2/min
CO diffusion capacity DLCO	—	2.4	—	20	—	30	$mlCO/min/mmHg$

bronchodilator such as salbutamol may be given by nebuliser or inhaler and there will usually be a rapid response to this, indicating reversibility of airway obstruction. Exercise testing (Fig. 2.4) is quite useful where one is attempting to assess airway lability in the asymptomatic child. Exercise induced asthma (EIA) may occur in as many as 80% of asthmatic children. This is discussed in more detail in Chapter 8.

A further method of assessing bronchial lability is by the inhalation of standardised doses of pharmacological agents such as histamine or

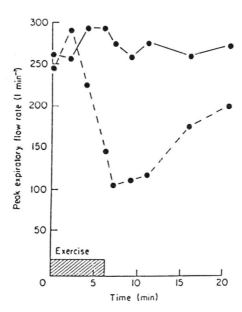

Fig. 2.4 Typical exercise induced asthma as a result of 6 minutes running in an asthmatic boy (broken line; expected PEFR=285 l/min) contrasted with result in a normal girl (solid line; expected PEFR=270 l/min) of similar size. (From Godfrey 1979, with permission.)

methacholine (Silverman & Wilson 1985) (See Ch. 8). Hyperventilation and cold air challenge or direct antigen inhalation (bronchial provocation test) have also been used in specialised laboratories.

DIFFUSION

At the alveolar level gas exchange takes place across the alveolar membrane. This is the process of diffusion which may be measured by techniques involving the use of carbon monoxide (Stahlman 1957). Diffusion may be disturbed in patients who have alveolar wall disease such as interstitial pneumonitis. Oxygen diffuses less readily than carbon dioxide and in the initial stage of these illnesses hypoxia occurs as the first blood gas abnormality.

VENTILATION/PERFUSION ABNORMALITY

The availability of the radioisotopes Krypton 81 (half-life 13 secs) and Technetium 99 (half-life 6 hours) has led to the development of lung scan techniques for the measurement of regional lung function. These enable one to measure ventilation and perfusion (V/Q) to each area of the lung almost simultaneously and allow direct evaluation of matched or unmatched ventilation/perfusion defects. Although requiring complex equipment these scans are relatively simple to perform and the radiation dose is no greater than 1.5 minutes of screening (Gordon et al 1987). The use of these techniques is described in more detail in Chapter 13.

ARTERIAL BLOOD GASES

The final common pathway of ventilation is the arterial blood gases. Nowadays these may be measured easily on small samples of blood, via an intra-arterial oxygen electrode, through the skin by heated transcutaneous oxygen and carbon dioxide electrodes or with a fibreoptic oxygen saturation device. End tidal carbon dioxide may be measured in infants and children who have a relatively slower respiratory rate so allowing for equilibration with the machine at the end of each breath. This is a useful reflection of arterial carbon dioxide providing there is even distribution of ventilation and no major diffusion abnormality.

Oxygen

Direct measurements of arterial oxygen, (Pa_{O_2}), carbon dioxide, (Pa_{CO_2}), and pH indicate the efficacy of respiration at any individual point in time. It is vital to record the inspired oxygen concentration when the measurement is made as without it interpretation of the oxygen level is valueless. Capillary blood samples are helpful in assessing carbon dioxide and pH levels but are unreliable for P_{O_2}. Oxygen saturation measurements are be-

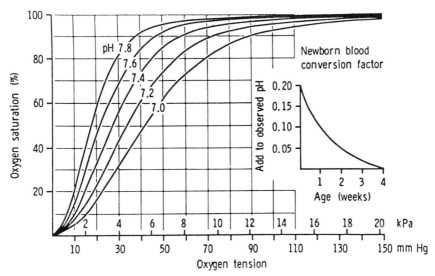

Fig. 2.5   The oxygen dissociation curve. The inset shows the shift due to fetal blood in terms of the equivalent pH change. (From Godfrey 1979, with permission.)

coming increasingly popular as noninvasive fibre optic saturation probes become available. The interpretation of the results obtained must be related to the oxygen saturation curve (Fig. 2.5) which is also dependent on type of haemoglobin, temperature and pH.

Saturation levels of over 100% indicate Pa_{O_2} in excess of 13.3 kPa (100 mmHg). It is not possible to quantify oxygen levels by saturation above this level. Low levels of oxygen saturation, less than 85%, indicate oxygen tensions under 6.7 kPa (50 mmHg) at a pH of 7.4. Great caution must therefore be used in applying these techniques since extremely low oxygen tensions may be encountered if saturation results are interpreted incorrectly. Tissue delivery of oxygen is also dependent on adequate haemoglobin levels and tissue release factors which may be abnormal in cases of severe acid base disturbance. Patients with severe pulmonary hypertension will also have low Pa_{O_2} secondary to right to left shunting. This shunt may be within the lung itself through areas of unmatched perfusion and ventilation or through an associated cardiac abnormality such as a ventricular septal defect or patent ductus arteriosus.

Carbon dioxide

Arterial carbon dioxide (Pa_{CO_2}) reflects lung function almost directly and is a measure of gas exchange at alveolar level. Any rise in Pa_{CO_2} is an acute stimulant to breathing in the normal child and results in an increased respiratory rate and tidal volume in an attempt to correct the situation. Elevated CO_2 levels indicate respiratory failure which can be brought about by disturbed lung function, loss of central control of breathing, or a combination of both. Occasionally, low carbon dioxide levels are found, due to causes such as anxiety with overbreathing, as compensation for a primary metabolic acidosis or in the initial stages of interstitial pneumonitis where there is a diffusion block causing hypoxia which itself stimulates breathing. Carbon dioxide levels directly affect cerebral blood flow and an increase in Pa_{CO_2} results in cerebral vasodilation causing headache and bounding pulses. Reduced Pa_{CO_2} results in cerebral vasoconstriction and decreased cerebral blood flow. This is used therapeutically in patients with cerebral oedema to reduce intracranial pressure. The Pa_{CO_2} level should not however be reduced below 3.3 kPa (25 mmHg), for example by artificial ventilation, as the reduction in cerebral perfusion this causes could be dangerous to cerebral function.

CENTRAL CONTROL OF BREATHING

The areas controlling respiration principally lie within the brainstem (Strang 1977). These are under the influence of various afferent stimuli, particularly blood gas changes, but also pressure changes in the circulation, mechanical changes in the lungs and alterations in cerebral pH. As has already been mentioned, the respiratory centres are acutely sensitive to changes in carbon dioxide which is one of the most potent stimuli to the onset of breathing. Hypoxia also stimulates breathing. These effects are mediated through chemoreceptor nerve endings at various sites within the body, particularly in the carotid bodies and in the aortic arch. Carbon dioxide also has a direct effect on CSF pH. Patients who have chronic respiratory failure may have a blunted carbon dioxide response and live mainly on their hypoxic drive. It is important not to give them high concentrations of oxygen suddenly as this may worsen their respiratory failure (Godfrey 1979). The respiratory centres are under the influence of many reflexes from the nerves and muscles of the rib cage and the pleural lining itself, for example the Hering-Breuer reflex. Thermal stimulation is important in the neonate.

Accurate control of breathing thus requires an intact cerebral circulation and brainstem function and diseases which damage these areas will have profound effects on the respiratory system.

REFERENCES

Clutario B C 1975 Clinical pulmonary function. In: Scarpelli E M, Auld P M (eds) Pulmonary physiology in the fetus, newborn and child. Lea and Febiger, Philadelphia, pp 299–324
Cogswell J J, Hull D, Milner A D, Norman A P, Taylor B 1975a Lung function in childhood. I The forced expiratory volumes in healthy children using a spirometer and reverse plethysmograph. British Journal of Diseases of the Chest 69: 40–50
Cogswell J J, Hull D, Milner A D, Norman A P, Taylor B 1975b Lung function in childhood. III Measurement of airflow resistance in healthy children. British Journal of Diseases of the Chest 69: 177–187

Godfrey S 1979 Respiration. In: Godfrey S, Baum J D (eds) Clinical paediatric physiology. Blackwell Scientific, Oxford, pp 240–283

Godfrey S, Kamburoff P L, Naim J R 1970 Spirometry, lung volumes and airway resistance in normal children aged 5–18 years. British Journal of Diseases of the Chest 64: 15–25

Gordon I, Matthew D, Dinwiddie R 1987 Respiratory System. In: Gordon I (ed) Diagnostic imaging in paediatrics. Chapman and Hall, London, pp 27–57

Heaf D P, Turner H, Stocks J, Helms P 1987 Comparison of the occlusion and inflation techniques for measuring total respiratory compliance in sick intubated infants. Pediatric Pulmonology 3: 78–82

Kuzemko J A, Bedford S 1980 Lung function tests and their interpretation. In: Kuzemko J A (ed) Asthma in children. Pitman Medical, Tunbridge Wells, pp 36–43

Platt L D, Manning F A 1980 Fetal breathing movements: an update. Clinics in Perinatology 7: 423–433

Polgar G, Promadhat V (eds) 1971 Pulmonary function testing in children: techniques and standards. Saunders, Philadelphia

Rudolph A M, Heymann M A 1974 Fetal and neonatal circulation and respiration. American Review of Physiology 36: 187–207

Samuels M P, Warner J O 1987 Bronchopulmonary dysplasia: the outcome. Archives of Disease in Childhood 62: 1099–1101

Silverman M, Wilson N 1985 Bronchial responsiveness in children: a clinical view. In: Milner A D, Martin R J (eds) Neonatal and pediatric respiratory medicine. Butterworths, London, pp 161–189

Smyth J A, Tabachnik E, Duncan W J, Reilly B, Levison H 1981 Pulmonary function and bronchial hyperreactivity in long term survivors of bronchopulmonary dysplasia. Journal of Pediatrics 68: 336–340

Stahlman M T 1957 Pulmonary ventilation and diffusion in the human newborn infant. Journal of Clinical Investigation 36: 1081–1091

Stocks J, Godfrey S 1977 Specific airway conductance in relation to postconceptual age during infancy. Journal of Applied Physiology 43: 144

Stocks J, Nothen U, Sutherland P, Hatch D, Helms P 1987 Improved accuracy of the occlusion technique for assessing total respiratory compliance in infants. Pediatric Pulmonology 3: 71–77

Strang L B (ed) 1977 Onset of breathing and its control in the neonatal period. In: Neonatal respiration physiological and clinical studies. Blackwell Scientific, Oxford, pp 47–65

Yu V Y H (ed) 1986 Perinatal respiratory physiology. In: Respiratory disorders of the newborn. Churchill Livingstone, Edinburgh, pp 8–17

Zapletal A, Motoyama E K, Gibson L E, Bouhuys A 1971 Pulmonary mechanics in asthma and cystic fibrosis. Pediatrics 48: 64–72

Zapletal A, Paul T, Samanek M 1976 Pulmonary elasticity in children and adolescents. Journal of Applied Physiology 40: 953–961

RECOMMENDED READING

Silverman M 1983 Respiratory function testing in infancy and childhood. In: Laszlo G, Swedlow M E (eds) Measurement in clinical respiratory physiology. Academic Press, New York, pp 293–328

3. Neonatal respiratory disorders

Paul MacMahon and Ilya Z. Kovar

The complex cardio-respiratory changes necessary for the transition from intrauterine to extrauterine life make the newborn particularly vulnerable to respiratory disorders. The establishment of breathing and the adaptation of the neonatal circulation are two of the most important events which occur throughout life. These physiological changes are mediated via local and systemic factors which are ultimately under the neurological control of a number of important centres situated in the brainstem. Most of the problems relating to the respiratory system in the neonatal period are due either to disturbances of these natural processes or congenital malformations.

FETAL PHYSIOLOGY

In utero the lungs are fluid filled and gas exchange takes place across the placenta. Several factors influence oxygen transport through this important organ.

1. Fetal haemoglobin (HbF) has a higher affinity for oxygen than adult haemoglobin, the blood leaving the placenta with a Pao_2 of 4 kPa (30 mmHg) is 68% saturated. The oxygen saturation of the maternal blood at this tension is 6–8% lower.

2. Fetal blood also has a high haemoglobin concentration (mean 18 g per 100 ml) which results in a further increase in oxygen carrying capacity. The combined effect of these two mechanisms is that fetal blood carries 60% more oxygen per unit volume than maternal blood (Strang 1977a).

3. When fetal blood gives up carbon dioxide, the change this produces in pH increases its oxygen affinity (the Bohr effect). Carbon dioxide itself is less efficiently carried in fetal blood because of a relative deficiency of carbonic anhydrase. These biochemical factors are not however the critical determinants of placental gas transfer. The major factors are those which control regional blood flow within the placenta itself. Arteriovenous anastomoses are also abundant so there is a considerable reserve capacity for dealing with hypoxic stress.

Fetal circulation

The fetal circulation is chiefly involved in supplying a large blood flow to the placenta as well as to the fetus itself. During fetal life the pulmonary vascular resistance is very high and only 10% of the cardiac output actually passes through the fetal lung (Dawes et al 1953). This vascular resistance is maintained by the compressive effects of the lung fluid and the relative hypoxia of fetal blood. The right side of the heart receives the blood returning from the placenta and functions in equal partnership with and at virtually the same systemic pressure as the left ventricle. Thus in utero the right and left ventricles are of equal size and muscle thickness. Oxygenated blood returns to the fetal heart via the umbilical vein, ductus venosus and the inferior vena cava (IVC). As it enters the heart it is streamed in two directions by a tissue flap called the crista dividens which extends across the right atrium into the IVC. One stream is passed into the right atrium and the other into the left atrium through the foramen ovale. The foramen ovale is covered by a membrane which is held open during fetal life by the positive pressure difference between the IVC and the left atrium. The rest of the right atrial blood from the IVC together with the desaturated blood from the superior vena cava and coronary sinuses, passes directly through the right ventricle into the pulmonary artery. The bulk of this flows through the ductus arteriosus into the descending aorta down towards the umbilical arteries (Rudolph & Heymann 1974).

At birth the fetal circulation changes rapidly. The onset of breathing which aerates the lungs causes a large fall in pulmonary vascular resistance and in pulmonary artery pressure. There is then a rapid rise in pulmonary blood flow. The foramen ovale closes due to the increased pressure in the left atrium consequent on the higher venous return from the lungs via the pulmonary veins and the fall in IVC pressure resulting from the clamping of the umbilical cord. The ductus arteriosus closes by contraction of the ductal muscle which is stimulated by the rise in the level of oxygen in the blood flowing through it, possibly by increasing ATP production in the ductal muscle. Local mechanical factors also play a part. The ductus is sensitive to locally acting prostaglandins. Prostaglandin $F_{2\alpha}$ constricts the ductus and prostaglandin E_1 dilates it; this latter response is overridden by the raised arterial oxygen tension of the blood after birth.

The pulmonary vascular bed of the fetus and newborn is extremely sensitive to change in oxygen and carbon dioxide. A fall in oxygen or a rise in carbon dioxide produces intense vasoconstriction. The vasoconstrictor response to hypoxia is enhanced in the presence of a low pH. This sensitivity is thought to occur because there is a thicker muscle coat around the arterioles at this age than later in life. These reflexes are probably mediated locally within the lung itself because they persist even when the nerve supply is cut. They are very important in determining the response to perinatal asphyxia and in those who subsequently show pathological persistence of the fetal circulation (PFC).

SURFACE ACTIVE MATERIAL

In order for gas exchange to take place in the lung there must be an adequate surface area available within the alveoli. As these reduce in size during expiration their surface area decreases and the surface tension increases (La Place's Law). If this occurs unopposed then there is a risk that the alveoli will collapse completely at the end of a breath and subsequently require a large amount of energy to re-expand them at the beginning of the next breath. The lung overcomes this problem by the secretion of surface active agents — surfactants which stabilise alveolar surface tension during expiration (Pattle 1955).

The alveoli are lined by two types of cells called pneumocytes. Type I pneumocytes provide the surface across which gas exchange takes place. They cover 96% of the alveolus and have a cell thickness of 0.1–0.01 μm. The type II pneumocytes are the source of the surfactant materials, and it is in these cells that they are stored and ultimately secreted onto the alveolar surface. The surfactant is stored in the lamellar bodies within the cells and released by fusion of the lamellar body membrane with the cell wall. The surfactant materials are seen as osmiophilic granules (Strang 1977b). The composition of surfactant is largely lipid in nature, particularly dipalmitoyl-phosphatidyl-choline (PC), phosphatidyl-glycerol (PG) and phosphatidyl-inositol (PI) (Ten Centre Study Group 1987) (See Table 1.1).

The major biochemical pathway for the synthesis of phosphatidyl-choline is via the choline phosphorylation pathway, utilising choline-kinase (Kennedy & Weiss 1956). A second pathway utilising the methylation of phosphatidyl-ethanolamine is also known to exist, but is not a major contributor to surfactant production in comparison to the choline phosphorylation pathway. Phosphatidyl-choline is by far the most important surface tension reducing agent, but functions most efficiently when it is present in the correct ratio to the other lipids, particularly PG and PI. The degree of saturation of the PC is also important   the higher the degree of saturation the more efficient it is in lowering surface tension. At least 60% of the PC is saturated in term infants, but considerably less in the pre-term (Yu 1986a).

Surfactant is found in the fetal lung as early as 24 weeks gestation, but it is only delivered in significant amounts to the alveolar surface from 30–32 weeks gestation onwards. Animal studies suggest that there is a net outflow of surfactant material from the lungs into the amniotic fluid at a rate of 2–4 ml/kg/hour, most of which is swallowed. The concentration of surfactant material in the amniotic fluid can be measured utilising the ratio of lecithin to sphingomyelin — L/S ratio (Gluck & Kulovitch 1973) (Table 3.1).

Surfactant production is also reduced by a number of extrinsic factors. Some of these have particular relevance clinically, especially pre-term delivery and birth asphyxia. Surfactant production is reduced in the presence of hypothermia, hypoxia and acidosis, particularly if

Table 3.1   L/S ratio and risk of RDS (adapted from Kelnar & Harvey 1987)

L/S ratio	% incidence of RDS	% mortality from RDS
>2.0	2	0.1
1.5–2.0	40	4
<1.5	75	14

the infant's core temperature is less than 35°C or arterial pH less than 7.25.

The use of glucocorticoids such as betamethasone has been shown to accelerate surfactant production in pre-term infants, particularly at 30–34 weeks gestation. This must however be given more than 24 hours before delivery and the effect appears to last up to 7 days after administration (Collaborative Group 1981, Howie & Patel 1984). Intrauterine stress such as premature rupture of the membranes, maternal hypertension or intrauterine growth retardation can stimulate surfactant production possibly because of the release of endogenous steroid from the fetal adrenal glands. Various chemical substances including theophylline, heroin, beta adrenergic stimulants such as terbutaline or salbutamol and endogenous substances such as oestrogen, prolactin and particularly thyroid hormone are also known to accelerate surfactant production. One trial (Ballard 1984) has shown an additive affect of prenatal administration of steroids in conjunction with thyroid hormone to stimulate surfactant synthesis in the fetal lung. Schönberger et al (1981) also demonstrated improved survival in infants with RDS treated with thyroxine. Once breathing is established and the lungs are inflated surfactant production and release is also accelerated. The half life in the lungs is about 10–14 hours.

Much of the surfactant is reabsorbed by the type II pneumocytes and recycled back into the alveoli and the remainder is washed upwards into the bronchial tree by the normal ciliary movement, broken down by local tissue enzymes or absorbed by alveolar macrophages. Very high oxygen concentrations and overventilation of the lungs cause accelerated breakdown. Positive end expiratory pressure which stabilises lung volume helps to preserve surfactant levels.

ADAPTATION TO EXTRAUTERINE LIFE

The three major components of adaptation to extrauterine life are: aeration of the lungs, perfusion of the lungs and central control of breathing.

Aeration of the lungs

Immediately after birth the lungs fill with air and regular breathing commences. The critical first breath is provoked by a number of stimuli which act on the baby during and immediately after birth. The lungs in utero contain a liquid volume of 20–30 ml/kg which is similar to the functional residual capacity after birth. The chest is compressed as it passes through the birth canal and intrathoracic pressures of up to 50 cmH$_2$O have been recorded at this time (Karlberg et al 1962). These pressures result in the expression through the mouth of about 10 ml/kg of lung fluid during birth. As the chest emerges from the birth canal the rib cage demonstrates elastic recoil and this contributes to the initial aeration of the lungs.

A number of other factors stimulate breathing at this time, including thermal and tactile stimulation, intravascular pressure changes consequent on clamping of the umbilical cord and the biochemical changes of hypoxia and hypercapnia which this produces (Yu 1986a). The remaining two-thirds of the lung fluid are absorbed via the pulmonary lymphatics and across the pulmonary capillary membranes in roughly equivalent amounts. An opening pressure of 20 cmH$_2$O is thought to be required to expand the alveoli, based on the anatomy and surface tension properties of the lung. Actual data of first breath mechanics obtained by measuring intrathoracic pressure with an oesophageal balloon and air movement into the lungs with a pneumotacho-graph suggests that few normal term infants have evidence of an opening pressure greater than 10 cmH$_2$O (Milner & Vyas 1982). Initial peak inspiratory pressures do however vary considerably and may be in excess of 30 cmH$_2$O. Some infants expand their lungs completely with less than half these pressures. Mechanical events during labour are also important in the clearance of lung fluid as shown by the fact that term infants delivered by Caesarean section have a reduced crying vital capacity indicating increased residual lung liquid in the first few hours of life (Milner et al 1978). Catecholamines may also be important in lung liquid absorption (Walters & Olver 1978) and in the enhancement of surfactant secretion.

Perfusion of the lungs

Simultaneously with the onset of major respiratory movement, there is a dramatic fall in pulmonary vascular resistance which results in a massive increase in pulmonary blood flow. In utero only 10% of the cardiac output flows through the lungs (Rudolph 1977). This increase in pulmonary blood flow causes a rise in Pao$_2$ which in itself stimulates pulmonary vasodilation. There is also a mild metabolic acidosis at birth even in normal infants but as the pH rises there is further reduction in pulmonary vascular resistance and an increase in pulmonary blood flow (Dawes et al 1966). The acute intravascular pressure changes associated with clamping of the umbilical cord cause a marked reduction in right atrial and right ventricular pressure. This encourages closure of the flap-like foramen ovale and contributes to ultimate closure of the ductus arteriosus. The ductus itself probably closes under the influence of the marked rise in Pao$_2$ and inhibition of locally acting prostaglandins E$_1$ and E$_2$. Mechanical factors affecting the position of the ductus in relation to the adjacent major blood vessels also play a role in ductal closure.

Central control of breathing

The third major component in the onset of respiration is the control of breathing which is mediated by afferent chemoreceptor input and by neurological input from pulmonary stretch receptors (mechanoreceptors) (Haddad & Mellins 1977).

The fetus demonstrates breathing movements in utero from as early as 11 weeks of gestation (Platt & Manning 1980). As gestation increases the movements become more prolonged, but even by term are occurring less than 50% of the time. The fetal Pao_2 is less than 4 kPa (30 mmHg), a level at which intense respiratory effort would be made after birth, thus the chemoreceptors are very insensitive in utero. The fetal breathing movements are associated with REM sleep periods and are relatively inactive during non-REM sleep.

At the moment of birth vigorous stimulation occurs which promotes the initiation of respiration. The levels of Pao_2 and $Paco_2$ required for initiation of breathing appear to be of the order of 0.6 kPa (5 mmHg) Pao_2 in the presence of $Paco_2$ of 5.5 kPa (45 mmHg) rising to a Pao_2 of 2.5–3 kPa (17–22.5 mmHg) in the presence of a $Paco_2$ greater than 13.3 kPa (100 mmHg). The chemoreceptors are thus heavily inhibited in utero, but since blood gas changes at these levels occur rapidly on clamping of the umbilical cord this appears to be the most important stimulus to the onset of breathing (Pagtakhan et al 1971).

After birth the term newborn shows a response of hyperventilation to relative hypoxia (12% oxygen) in the thermoneutral environment. This is achieved by increasing tidal volume and respiratory rate for 1–2 minutes at the onset of the stimulus; after this period the term infant hypoventilates. The pre-term infant hyperventilates by an increase in tidal volume only but after the first 2 minutes begins to have a periodic breathing pattern. If the environment is relatively cold both term and pre-term infants hypoventilate in response to hypoxia. This paradoxical response appears to persist during the first week of life after which hypoxia produces the more normal generalised stimulus to breathing. Hyperoxia — achieved by breathing 100% oxygen for up to one minute — causes a relative decrease in ventilation in all neonates possibly leading to apnoea in the pre-term infant. It is thought that this effect is mediated through the carotid body (Roberton 1986).

The response to carbon dioxide by the chemoreceptors appears to be very active in term infants, but is blunted in pre-term infants who are suffering from recurrent apnoea.

Mechanoreceptors are mainly found in the muscles of respiration and supply afferent stimuli chiefly through the vagal nerve to the respiratory centres which have an important influence on respiratory function after birth. The major reflexes involved in these mechanisms are the Hering-Breuer reflex and Head's paradoxical reflex.

The Hering-Breuer inspiratory reflex initiates inhibition of breathing after lung inflation. This is important in term and particularly in pre-term infants in the control of respiratory rate and volume. Doubt exists as to whether the Hering-Breuer deflation reflex (increased ventilation on reducing lung volume) is actually of importance in the pre-term infant. The sensitivity of this reflex is markedly reduced during REM sleep.

Head's paradoxical reflex occurs as an extra voluntary inspiratory effort after an inflation pressure is rapidly applied to the lung. It is present particularly during the first few days of life and is important in the establishment of breathing after birth.

A different type of chest wall reflex responds to mechanical distortion of the chest wall particularly during REM sleep. Increased mechanical distortion results in a short inspiratory time — this is mediated through the phrenic nerve and is particularly seen in pre-term infants.

Upper airway reflexes are also important. Cold stimuli on the face (diving reflex) are powerful stimuli to breathing; also the presence of certain liquids in the pharynx which would be unfamiliar to the fetus can result in apnoea. This suggests that there are receptors in the pharyngeal area which are sensitive to these substances.

BIRTH ASPHYXIA

Asphyxia is the simultaneous occurrence of hypoxia, hypercapnia and acidosis. Intrapartum placental insufficiency and failure to establish adequate breathing at birth are the major causes of this complication. The incidence of severe perinatal asphyxia is in excess of 1% of all deliveries (Primhak et al 1984). A number of factors may be associated with an increased risk of birth asphyxia and these are shown in Table 3.2. They may be divided into three major groups — maternal, placental and fetal.

Our current understanding of birth asphyxia owes much to the work of Dawes (1968). Studies of acute asphyxia in rhesus monkeys revealed a standard pattern of response (Fig. 3.1). Vigorous respiratory gasping efforts

Table 3.2 Causes of birth asphyxia

Maternal	Fetal	Placental
Maternal hypertension	Abnormal presentation	Abruptio placentae
Hypertension of pregnancy	Cephalopelvic	Placental malformation
Extremes of maternal age	disproportion	Placenta praevia
Underlying chronic illness	Multiple birth	Cord prolapse
Cardiac disease	Intrauterine growth	Fetomaternal haemorrhage
Pulmonary insufficiency	retardation	Twin to twin transfusion
Renal failure	Rhesus immunisation —	Slipped cord clamp
Maternal diabetes	hydrops	
Hypotension, haemorrhage	Congenital malformation	
or epidural analgesia	Preterm delivery	
Excess sedation	Postmaturity	
	Recurrent intrauterine	
	stress	

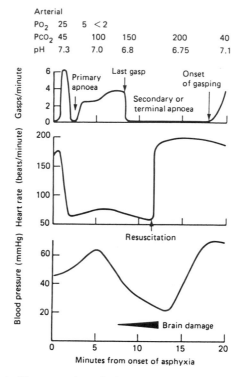

Fig. 3.1 Changes in Rhesus monkeys during asphyxia and on resuscitation by positive-pressure ventilation. Brain damage was assessed by histological examination some weeks or months later. (From Dawes 1968 with kind permission from Year Book Medical Publishers, Chicago.)

are followed by a short period of apnoea called primary apnoea, blue asphyxia or asphyxia livida, lasting approximately one minute. This is followed by intermittent gasping for about 5 minutes, after which the last gasp occurs and there is complete cessation of breathing. This is called terminal or secondary apnoea, white asphyxia or asphyxia pallida. Spontaneous breathing can usually be initiated in primary apnoea by external stimulation such as rubbing the baby dry or giving facial oxygen. When terminal apnoea occurs, the lungs must be artificially inflated or death will occur.

Cardiovascular and biochemical changes

During asphyxia efforts are made to maintain cerebral blood flow at the expense of other organs such as the lungs and kidneys. These changes support oxygenation and perfusion of vital centres in the presence of critical oxygen deprivation. These circulatory adjustments are similar to the diving reflex seen in whales and seals which enables them to withstand oxygen lack when diving under water. During any asphyxial episode hypoxia and hypotension can lead to the onset of cerebral oedema and an associated increase in intracranial pressure. These changes are thought to be very important in the induction of cerebral damage during perinatal asphyxia (Lou et al 1979). Cerebral ischaemia is therefore a common complication of birth asphyxia, the watershed regions at the borders of the anterior, middle and posterior cerebral arteries are particularly vulnerable. These areas may infarct and go on to form porencephalic cysts with associated cerebral atrophy.

Resuscitation

The delivery of a potentially compromised infant can often be anticipated from the obstetric history, early gestation, fetal monitoring abnormalities or the expectation of a complicated birth (Primhak et al 1984). Deliveries in which there is a high risk should be attended by a paediatrician as a matter of course. These include infants of less than 35 weeks gestation, fetal distress, meconium staining of the amniotic fluid, cord prolapse, malpresentation such as breech, Caesarean section, antepartum haemorrhage, multiple births, severe maternal hypertension, maternal diabetes, complicated instrumental deliveries, rhesus disease, previous history of neonatal death and infants known to have congenital malformations.

At birth the infant should be placed under a radiant heater, dried and generally assessed using the Apgar score, at 1 and 5 minutes (Table 3.3). If severe asphyxia is thought to have occurred a more accurate assessment can be made by obtaining a sample of umbilical arterial or venous blood (Sykes et al 1982, O'Souya et al 1983); this must not however interfere with the acute resuscitation process. The sequence of events which occurs in an asphyxiated infant is shown in Fig. 3.1. A baby who is apnoeic at birth may be in primary or secondary apnoea depending on the events preceding the asphyxial episode. Infants in primary apnoea will usually start to gasp and develop more regular breathing if placed under a radiant heater, dried and stimulated generally or when they are given an intramuscular injection such as naloxone to reverse the effects of maternal sedation or vitamin K. In a less asphyxiated baby there is commonly an initial period of gasping followed by primary apnoea in which there is a decrease of heart rate but maintenance of blood pressure and circulation associated with hypoxaemia and acidosis.

Table 3.3 Apgar score

	0	1	2
Heart rate	Absent	Below 100	Above 100
Respiratory effort	Absent	Slow, irregular	Regular, crying
Muscle tone	Flaccid	Some flexion of extremities	Active motion
Reflex irritability	No response	Grimace	Cough or sneeze
Colour	Blue, pale	Peripheral cyanosis	Completely pink

If the breathing pattern is irregular or shallow then further stimulation is needed with the administration of oxygen or the use of bag and mask ventilation after careful suction of the airways, particularly the nose, with a soft catheter. Bag and mask ventilation is effective if carried out properly (Field et al 1986, Hoskyns et al 1987). It is important to ensure that the mask has a proper seal on the baby's face and that the chest is moving adequately in response to this stimulus. If the baby does not respond immediately to this manoeuvre then intubation and positive pressure ventilation of the lungs is required. This is especially important for the preterm infant (Drew 1982). If the baby is in terminal apnoea then it is vital to intubate and to inflate the lungs under positive pressure immediately. During intubation the vocal cords should be carefully inspected for the presence of meconium which should be sucked out from above the pharynx before intubation and through the endotracheal tube once it is in situ. With any form of mechanical inflation of the lungs during resuscitation it is advisable to prolong the inspiratory time of the first breath for 3–5 seconds since this has been shown to result in better lung inflation and the establishment of more regular respiration (Vyas et al 1981). Positive pressure ventilation should be performed at a rate of 30–40 breaths/min ensuring that the maximum pressure does not exceed 30 cmH$_2$O. Most standard resuscitation equipment now has a blow-off valve inserted in the circuit to prevent this happening. The most efficient bag and mask systems are the Ambu or the Laerdal bag, each of which is capable of generating considerably higher pressures than 30 cmH$_2$O if maximally squeezed. It is important that these are therefore used by experienced staff and the safe pressure only exceeded where there are particular circumstances, such as in a baby with hydrops fetalis who has bilateral pleural effusions and where higher pressures may be needed initially to achieve adequate inflation.

Infants with severe asphyxia often develop significant bradycardia. The heart rate is commonly less than 100/min, but if this drops below 60/min then external cardiac massage is indicated. The infant's chest should be squeezed with the hand round the thorax and the sternum depressed vigorously with the thumb — this will ensure an adequate cardiac output. The chest should be squeezed for 5 beats between each manual breath. An umbilical or peripheral venous infusion should be commenced and the infant given 3 mmol/kg of sodium bicarbonate in conjunction with 10 ml of 10% dextrose/kg and 1 ml of 10% calcium gluconate/kg estimated birth weight. These measures are intended to decrease the associated metabolic acidosis and hypoglycaemia and calcium gluconate will cause stimulation of the myocardium. If this does not produce the desired effect then adrenaline should be given, either intravenously or via the endotracheal tube (Greenberg et al 1981); it is seldom necessary to give direct intracardiac adrenaline. Naloxone 0.01 mg/kg should be given to reverse the effects of pethidine. The infant's condition is routinely assessed by the Apgar score at 1 and 5 minutes and at 10 minutes or later if still depressed (see Table 3.3).

The maintenance of core temperature in the neutrothermal zone is vital for a number of reasons, particularly to minimize oxygen consumption and to reduce the risk of developing hyaline membrane disease. Oxygen consumption varies from 4.5–7.5 ml/kg/min in the first 4 weeks of life. This is minimised when the environment of the baby places the least thermal stress upon him (Hey & Katz 1970, Cashore & Stern 1984). Heat production in the neonatal period is mainly by non-shivering thermogenesis through the metabolism of brown fat. This particular type of adipose tissue is found posteriorly in the paravertebral areas from the nape of the neck down to the lumbar region and around the adrenal glands. It is capable of metabolising rapidly in the presence of oxygen, releasing 10.5 kJ/g (2.5 calories/g) brown fat as thermal energy per minute and this is a valuable way of producing heat quickly during periods of thermal stress. The baby's oxygen consumption can easily double in an environment in which the ambient temperature drops from 34°C to 26°C. It is known that surfactant production is inhibited if there is hypothermia and that this is associated with an increase in respiratory distress syndrome and neonatal mortality, especially in infants under 1.5 kg (Stanley & Alberman 1978). Maintenance of body temperature in the delivery room with the use of an overhead radiant heater is therefore just as vital as an adequate ambient temperature in the incubator after transfer to the Special Care Unit.

Some asphyxiated babies may be suffering from shock as a result of hypovolaemia secondary to massive haemorrhage. This may be due to such conditions as feto-maternal or twin to twin transfusion, acute placental haemorrhage or to a slipped cord clamp. These babies require urgent transfusion with appropriate blood products. The possibility of other complications such as pneumothorax or diaphragmatic hernia should also be considered in those who fail to respond to normal resuscitative measures. If there is no response at all to active resuscitation then a decision has to be made as to how long to continue. The exact duration of terminal apnoea that the human newborn can tolerate without long term damage is not known but probably varies considerably from one individual to another (Yu 1986b).

Those who suffer from severe asphyxia, but who are successfully resuscitated may require intensive support over the next few days, including control of acid–base balance, maintenance of blood pressure and circulation, treatment of cerebral oedema, control of renal failure, and anticonvulsant therapy for seizures secondary to hypoxia, hypoglycaemia or cerebral oedema (Whitelaw 1989). Severe birth asphyxia remains a major cause of death in the neonatal period and although there is a significant incidence of cerebral palsy and mental retardation among the survivors a surprising number turn out to be normal (Thompson et al 1977).

Infants who recover quickly from asphyxia who have not had evidence of severe prenatal stress or major acidosis after birth should be given to the mother as soon as practical after resuscitation. It is only necessary to admit infants to Special Care who have shown evidence of severe asphyxia and who are likely to have continuing problems either with the maintenance of respiration or who are at risk of developing cerebral oedema, hypoglycaemia or fits.

RESPIRATORY DISTRESS SYNDROME (RDS)

Respiratory distress syndrome is the commonest cause of respiratory difficulty in the neonatal period. It is manifested clinically by dyspnoea, rapid respiratory rate, recession, cyanosis and expiratory grunting. Hyaline membrane disease (HMD) is the most common cause of RDS and is seen in its most severe form in infants who weigh less than 1.5 kg at birth and whose gestation is less than 32 weeks. RDS may occur due to a number of conditions which are shown in Table 3.4.

Hyaline membrane disease

Aetiology

Hyaline membrane disease or classical RDS is primarily due to surfactant deficiency (Avery & Mead 1959). Surfactant is released from type II alveolar lining cells whose function is impaired due to immaturity of the lungs exacerbated by stress such as perinatal asphyxia or hypothermia. The underdeveloped muscles of respiration and the soft compliant chest wall of the very pre-term infant also reduce the potential to compensate for pulmonary dysfunction by an increased respiratory effort. The infant usually shows signs of respiratory difficulty within the first 2 hours of life. Apart from increased work of breathing demonstrated by marked indrawing of the chest and use of accessory muscles of respiration there is an expiratory grunt, a mechanism used by the infant to maintain oxygen levels (Harrison et al 1968). The chest X-ray typically shows a ground glass appearance secondary to alveolar hypoventilation and an air bronchogram due to maintenance of large airway patency by its cartilage content. As the respiratory effort fails to maintain adequate Paco$_2$ and Pao$_2$, the pH begins to fall. This results in pulmonary vasoconstriction leading to increased right to left shunting at the intrapulmonary and extrapulmonary (foramen ovale and ductus arteriosus) level.

Table 3.4   Causes of respiratory distress syndrome

Upper airway obstruction	Lung cysts
Hyaline membrane disease	Pleural effusion
Transient tachypnoea of the newborn	Persistent fetal circulation
Aspiration syndrome especially meconium	Heart failure
Pneumonia	Diaphragmatic hernia
Pneumothorax	Neuromuscular disease: chest wall or
Pulmonary hypoplasia	diaphragm weakness
Pulmonary haemorrhage	Failure of central control of breathing

Treatment

Despite optimal antenatal care the majority of preterm births still cannot be prevented. When infants at high risk of developing HMD are seen in labour between 28 and 32 weeks gestation, there may be a place for the administration of antenatal steroids to accelerate pulmonary maturation. These substances work if they are given between 24 hours and 7 days before delivery (Collaborative Group 1981). These agents however are thought to be of relatively little value in infants less than 28 weeks gestation (Roberton 1982). The mode of delivery may also be important and there is evidence to suggest that preterm babies, especially breech presentations delivered by Caesarean section, have a lower incidence of birth asphyxia and subsequent developmental delay than those delivered vaginally (Ingemarsson et al 1978).

Intraventricular haemorrhage is also reported to be lower in the preterm infant delivered by Caesarean section (Lamont et al 1983). It must however be borne in mind that at less than 28 weeks gestation the lower segment of the uterus is not fully formed and a classical Caesarean section may be required which carries an increased risk for the mother. This is particularly important in those with a gestation of 24 to 28 weeks (Howie & Patel 1984). The major pathophysiological processes which occur in HMD are shown in Fig. 3.2. Current therapy is directed towards correcting each of these abnormalities wherever possible. Specific management is shown in Table 3.5.

Adequate resuscitation is vital as birth asphyxia impairs the synthesis of surfactant by the type II lining cell and also results in pulmonary vasoconstriction. Elective intubation of babies less than 30 weeks gestation improves lung expansion and decreases the incidence of perinatal asphyxia and its associated mortality (Drew 1982).

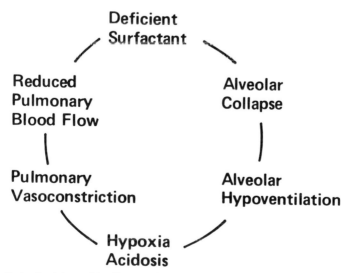

Fig. 3.2 Pathophysiology of hyaline membrane disease.

Table 3.5 Management of hyaline membrane disease

Prevention and treatment of birth asphyxia

Surfactant replacement

Neutral thermal environment

Increased Fio_2 — maintain Pao_2 8–12 kPa (60–90 mmHg)

Correction of acid–base imbalance

Adequate fluid, electrolyte and glucose intake

Artificial ventilation

Positive end expiratory pressure

Continuous positive airway pressure

Pulmonary vasodilator — tolazoline

Paralysis (selected cases)

Antibiotics for Group B streptococci

Surfactant replacement

Surfactant replacement also has a role in the treatment of the baby with RDS. Various studies have shown benefit from this therapy (Fujiwara et al 1980, Morley 1984). The Ten Centre Study Group (1987) utilised a protein-free synthetic surfactant 'artificial lung expanding compound' ('ALEC') composed of phosphatidyl-choline and phosphatidyl-glycerol in a double blind prospective randomised trial of 328 babies between 25 and 29 weeks gestation.

Treated babies received 100 mg of artificial surfactant and further doses if they continued to be intubated during the first 24 hours after birth. The artificial surfactant group had a significantly lower mortality (27% vs 14%) and fewer babies died while in the Neonatal Intensive Care Unit (19% of the treated babies vs 30% of the controls). In the first 10 days babies treated with artificial surfactant who survived averaged 19 hours less treatment in 30% oxygen, 20 hours less ventilation and 17 hours less supplemented oxygen. Overall parenchymal brain haemorrhage was reduced from 24% to 16% (P = 0.07). Artificial surfactant had no effect on the overall incidence of pneumothorax and pulmonary interstitial emphysema (28%), patent ductus arteriosus (25%) or post-natal infections (22%). Thus artificial surfactant has a place in the treatment of RDS in very pre-term babies, but its role will be as an adjunct to rather than as a replacement for other conventional management.

A chest X-ray (Fig. 3.3) should be taken in all cases where significant early signs of respiratory distress persist. Supplemental oxygen to maintain the Pao_2 levels between 8 and 12 kPa (60–90 mmHg) produces optimum tissue oxygenation and avoids the risks of acidosis from hypoxaemia and retrolental fibroplasia from hyperoxia. It is desirable to monitor blood gas levels continuously by transcutaneous oximetry, saturation monitor (90–

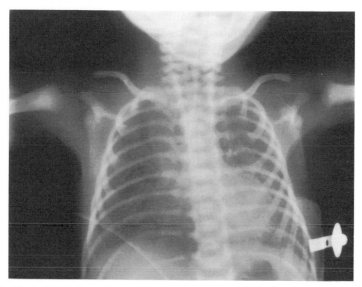

Fig. 3.3 Typical chest X-ray of hyaline membrane disease showing generalised 'ground glass appearance'.

95%) or indwelling arterial electrode. This must always be reinforced by the use of frequent arterial blood gas analysis obtained through an indwelling arterial line in all pre-term infants who require oxygen. The arterial line may be placed in the umbilical artery, radial or posterior tibial artery all of which are associated with a low level of complications. Capillary blood gases do not reliably detect hypoxaemia or hyperoxia although they give a reasonable approximation of arterial pH and carbon dioxide level.

Intermittent positive pressure ventilation (IPPV)

The main indications for the use of ventilation in RDS including HMD are:

1. Infants who never establish adequate respiration and who require intubation and assisted breathing from the moment of birth.
2. Infants who show sudden deterioration with apnoeic attacks or irregular gasping respiration indicating exhaustion.
3. Deteriorating blood gases. Pao_2 less than 8 kPa (60 mmHg) in an inspired oxygen concentration of 60% (Fio_2 0.6). $Paco_2$ greater than 8 kPa (60 mmHg).

In all of these situations the baby's general condition must also be considered before starting ventilation. As staff in neonatal units have become more skilled in the use of these machines, their earlier introduction has become common practice and this has reduced the incidence of severe episodes of acidosis and hypercapnia which are known to be associated with an increased incidence of intraventricular haemorrhage. Intubation is by the oral or nasal route and each unit has its own preferred method of introduction and attachment to the baby. Most neonatal ventilators available at present are pressure limited, time cycled, constant flow generators which produce a square wave input and have independently variable settings for peak inspiratory pressure, inspiratory time, respiratory rate, percent inspired oxygen, inspiratory/expiratory ratio, positive end expiratory pressure (PEEP) and gas flow. The provision of high humidity at an adequate temperature is also vital (Tarnow-Mordi et al 1986). Initial settings commonly used are respiratory rate 30–40 min, Fio_2 0.6, peak inspiratory pressure 20 cmH_2O or less and PEEP 4–6 cmH_2O, I:E ratio 1:1, gas flow 5–10 l/min. Many babies respond to these settings which are adjusted according to the subsequent blood gases.

The spontaneous breathing rate of small babies in known to be more rapid at lower gestations. This has led to recent interest in the role of rapid rate ventilation between 60 and 140 breaths/min particularly for extremely low birth weight babies of less than 1500 g birth weight (Field et al 1984, Greenough et al 1986). These rates have resulted in improved oxygenation in a number of cases and are also associated with a reduced incidence of pneumothorax (Greenough et al 1984a). Active expiration against the ventilator is reduced (Greenough et al 1986) and this too is associated with a lower risk of air leak. Rapid rate ventilation is now finding an increasing place in the management of the very preterm infant with RDS.

High frequency ventilation utilising a jet ventilator or an oscillator pump circuit has also been evaluated (Franz et al 1983). This has been successful for short periods but has also been associated with a high complication rate including necrotising tracheobronchitis and small airway obstruction.

As the infant improves, ventilation is gradually weaned and changed to intermittent mandatory ventilation (IMV) which occurs when most of the breathing is spontaneous and the ventilator rate is less than 20 breaths/min. Continuous positive airway pressure (CPAP) is also helpful at this stage in stabilising the lungs and preventing atelectasis. Theophylline is a useful agent during the weaning phase as it stimulates the infant's intrinsic respiratory drive (Greenough et al 1985). Recently a relatively simple modification to a standard neonatal ventilator has allowed effective patient triggering even in very small babies (Mehta et al 1986) and this too may facilitate weaning.

Complications of ventilation

Pneumothorax

Complications of ventilation are not uncommon and include pneumothorax (Fig. 3.4) which may be seen in 15–40% of ventilated infants (Yu 1986c). It is also associated with other air leaks secondary to alveolar rupture with air tracking into the pulmonary lymphatics and interstitial spaces. Other associated complications include pneumomediastinum, surgical emphysema and more significantly generalised interstitial emphysema. If the air leak is

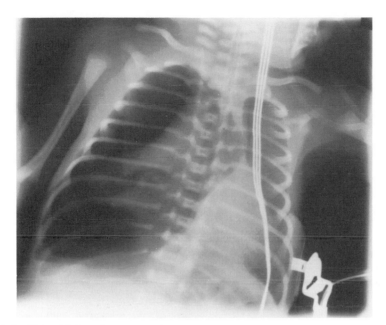

Fig. 3.4 Right sided tension pneumothorax.

under tension, there is acute collapse of lung with a rise in carbon dioxide level which is directly associated with an increased incidence of intraventricular haemorrhage (Lipscomb et al 1981). The use of selective paralysis in those who are actively expiring against the ventilator has been shown to reduce the incidence of pneumothorax and associated intraventricular haemorrhage (Greenough et al 1984a). Treatment consists of confirmation by cold light fibreoptic transillumination confirmed by X-ray if the infant's condition permits. In an emergency, the chest should be needled using a butterfly needle with its distal end under water. Should the pneumothorax be confirmed, then air should be aspirated directly and a suitably sized chest drain inserted to allow re-expansion of the lung.

Pulmonary Interstitial Emphysema (PIE)

Pulmonary interstitial emphysema is another form of air leak seen in ventilated babies; incidence figures of 19% for infants under 35 weeks gestation (Greenough et al 1984b) and 32% of infants under 1500 g (Hart et al 1983) have been described. The condition starts as an air leak into the interstitium secondary to ventilation and often spreads to develop into a pneumothorax or a pneumomediastinum. All of these conditions can result in an increase in intrapulmonary shunt with worsening of hypoxaemia. In some cases, there is gross overinflation of one or both lungs which leads to increasing difficulty in maintaining ventilation.

The chest X-ray (Fig. 3.5) typically shows hyperinflation with coarse reticular or rounded radiolucencies extending outwards from the hilum (Yu

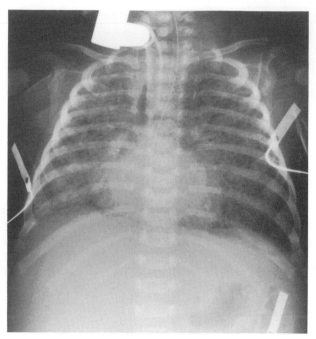

Fig. 3.5   Pulmonary interstitial emphysema.

1986c). Pneumothorax may occur in as many as 50% of cases and PIE is commonly a precursor of this condition. Hart et al (1983) found an increased incidence in babies weighing less than 1500 g and that there was a significant correlation with babies who had required active resuscitation, mechanical ventilation, or who had hyaline membrane disease. Mortality was greater in ventilated infants who developed PIE as a complication but this was not confirmed in the series described by Greenough et al (1984b).

Management consists chiefly of attempting to reduce the peak airway pressure and the end expiratory pressure, usually achieved by ventilating at a fast rate of greater than 110 per minute. This high rate of ventilation is also associated with a reduction in the incidence of pneumothorax. If this treatment fails then other procedures which have been successful include high frequency ventilation at rates of 48–72 cycles per second (Franz et al 1983), selective intubation of the contralateral lung, bronchial occlusion of the affected lung (Lewis et al 1988) or multiple needle puncture (Levine et al 1981). Surgical excision of the affected lobes has also been successful but this should be avoided if at all possible since complete recovery is usual after the acute phase of respiratory distress has passed.

Other complications of ventilation include subglottic stenosis from prolonged endotracheal intubation, secondary infection of the lungs and bronchopulmonary dysplasia (BPD) (Northway et al 1967). The long term outlook for those who have HMD is extremely good in the majority of cases, some 95% of whom may expect to survive with good intellectual and lung function (Dinwiddie et al 1974, Greenough & Roberton 1985). The mortality rate does however remain significantly greater among infants weighing less than 1 kg at birth (Yu et al 1982). The ultimate prognosis for lung function is excellent providing that there are no other major complicating factors such as chronic lung infection or BPD.

TRANSIENT TACHYPNOEA OF THE NEWBORN

This condition produces respiratory symptoms identical to those of classical hyaline membrane disease but these are much more short lived (Yu 1986d). They include the usual signs of tachypnoea, indrawing and cyanosis, but these disappear over the first 24 hours or so of life. These infants probably have retained lung fluid and this is seen on the typical X-ray (Fig. 3.6) which shows hyperinflation, prominent vascular markings, evidence of oedema with fluid in the fissures and costophrenic angles and occasionally intercostal bulging of the pleura. The condition is more common among those who are born by Caesarean section, possibly because they have a lower functional residual capacity after birth as less fluid is squeezed from the lungs during the birth process itself (Milner et al 1978). Treatment includes basic supportive measures and adequate inspired oxygen. Ventilation is unusual.

PATENT DUCTUS ARTERIOSUS (PDA)

Patent ductus arteriosus is very uncommon among normal term infants but it is extremely common in pre-term infants with HMD, occurring in as many as 40% of those under 1 kg and 20% of those with a birth weight between 1 and 1.5 kg (Ellison et al 1983). Its incidence is also increased in those who have a high fluid intake in the first few days of life (Bell et al 1980). The classical signs of patent ductus arteriosus appear 3–4 days after birth as the resistance through the pulmonary vascular bed continues to fall. The signs include tachycardia, bounding peripheral pulses, a systolic murmur in the mid-clavicular area which gradually becomes continuous and a palpable systolic thrill over the precordium. Over the next few days the shunt becomes increasingly left to right and this leads to pulmonary oedema and decreased lung compliance which is associated with an increase in ventilatory requirements. Excess fluid retention also leads to hepatomegaly. Chest X-ray shows cardiomegaly and plethoric lung fields in addition to the background pulmonary shadowing from the HMD. Echocardiography is used to confirm the diagnosis and to exclude any other underlying cardiac lesion.

Management consists of restriction of fluid intake to 60–70% of daily requirements, diuretic therapy and increased end expiratory pressure on the ventilator to reduce pulmonary oedema. If these measures fail to produce a significant response within 24–48 hours, then three doses of indomethacin, a prostaglandin synthetase inhibitor, are given in a dose of 0.2 mg/kg at intervals of 12–24 hours. This has resulted in a satisfactory response in a large number of infants entered into a multicentre trial (Gersony et al 1983). Even though in a significant proportion the duct reopens, in many cases the initial response is sufficient to allow the infant to be weaned from ventilation. Indomethacin is not without side effects. It is capable of displacing bilirubin from albumin so should not be used in those with significant jaundice. It can interfere with platelet function making thrombocytopenia a contraindication to its use. It causes a reduction in renal blood flow and can precipitate or exacerbate renal failure. If these medical approaches to ductal closure are unsuccessful, then surgical ligation should be undertaken. This can be performed on the neonatal unit itself without the need for transfer to an operating theatre.

PERSISTENT PULMONARY HYPERTENSION (PERSISTENT FETAL CIRCULATION)

Persistent fetal circulation (PFC) occurs when the normal reduction in pulmonary vascular resistance fails to occur after birth. The normal stimuli for this process include the relative increase in Pao_2 which occurs after air breathing begins and the changes in circulatory pressures which take place with clamping of the cord. In some infants these changes fail to occur and there is persistent pulmonary hypertension exacerbated by associated hypercapnia and acidosis which themselves also stimulate pulmonary arteriolar vasoconstriction (Cook et al 1963). The condition may complicate underlying HMD. It is also seen in meconium aspiration syndrome (Fox et al 1977) and in those with group B streptococcal pneumonia and septicaemia (Table 3.6). It is difficult to distinguish from underlying cyanotic congenital heart disease, particularly transposition of the great vessels and pulmonary atresia. These conditions can readily be excluded by echocardiography.

Treatment consists of ventilatory support in an attempt to increase the pH to more than 7.48 and hyperventilation to reduce the $Paco_2$ to 3.5 to 4 kPa (25–30 mmHg) may assist in this process (Drummond et al 1981). Provided the $Paco_2$ is not elevated administration of sodium bicarbonate is sometimes indicated to increase pH. If hyperventilation fails to produce an adequate response infusion of tolazoline in a dose of 1–2 mg/kg sometimes

Table 3.6 Clinical associations with persistent fetal circulation

Antenatal hypoxia	Hypothermia
Placental insufficiency	Hyperviscosity syndrome
Birth asphyxia	Hydrops fetalis
Meconium aspiration syndrome	Septicaemia
Hyaline membrane disease	Group B streptococci
Diaphragmatic hernia	Hypoglycaemia
Congenital pneumonia	Metabolic acidosis
Pulmonary hypoplasia	

produces an improvement in Pao_2. If there is a beneficial response this should be followed by a continuous infusion at the same dose/kg per hour. Systemic hypotension is common with this agent and the baby may need simultaneous support with colloid in the form of blood or plasma or an inotropic agent such as dopamine.

MECONIUM ASPIRATION SYNDROME (MAS)

The passage of meconium before birth is seen in 8 to 15% of deliveries. In a study of 1000 consecutive births Gregory et al (1974) demonstrated the wide variability of X-ray changes and clinical severity of disease. The overall incidence of symptomatic meconium aspiration was 1.6% of all deliveries. The disease is most commonly seen in term or postmature infants and is much less common in preterm infants (Ting & Brady 1975). The condition is potentially preventable by adequate antenatal care including the avoidance of intrauterine hypoxia and the early delivery of those who show evidence of fetal distress. The major risk for the baby is the aspiration of meconium into the lower respiratory tract before or after birth. Intrauterine asphyxia and fetal gasping in the presence of meconium in the upper airway results in inhalation into the trachea or more peripherally into lungs, and this can cause a wide variety of disease. Large plugs obstruct the trachea and major bronchi causing acute asphyxia. Smaller plugs are aspirated into the peripheral airways where they cause partial obstruction and a chemical pneumonitis resulting in air trapping, or the risk of air leak. Air leak, including pneumothorax and pneumomediastinum is very common, occurring in as many as 40–50% of significantly affected infants. The chest X-ray (Fig. 3.7) shows generalised overinflation and areas of patchy consolidation. Persistent pulmonary hypertension may be an accompanying problem and compounds the hypoxia which is present in those with the worst disease (Fox et al 1977).

Treatment is supportive, including correction of acid–base imbalance, antibiotics because of possible secondary bacterial infection and ventilation when indicated clinically and by deteriorating blood gases. Those who fail to respond to ventilation with persistent hypoxia have a very poor prognosis (Vidyasgar et al 1975). Paralysis during ventilation may be helpful (Runkle & Bancalari 1984) and tolazoline should be given to those who have evidence of significant pulmonary hypertension. MAS continues to carry a small but significant mortality and some survivors have chronic lung disease such as bronchopulmonary dysplasia or bronchial hyper-reactivity secondary to airway damage caused by the high pressures required to ventilate them. The long term outcome for those with mild aspiration is usually excellent, however asthmatic symptoms and increased bronchial reactivity does appear to be more common at age 6–11 years among those who have had moderate to severe meconium aspiration in the neonatal period (Macfarlane & Heaf 1988).

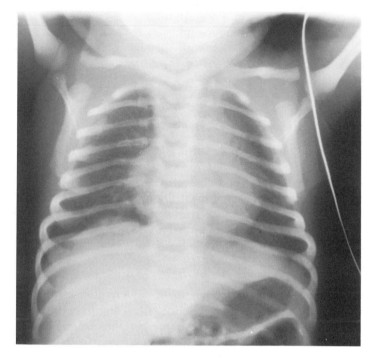

Fig. 3.6   Transient tachypnoea of the newborn.

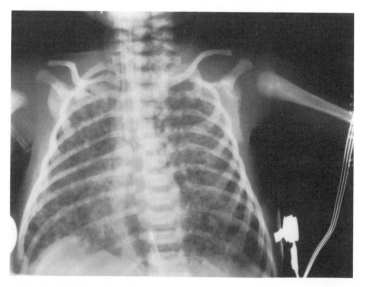

Fig. 3.7   Meconium aspiration syndrome.

INFECTIONS

Group B streptococcal pneumonia

Pneumonia in the neonatal period is extremely common especially among babies who have other respiratory problems and who require ventilation. The organisms can be bacterial, viral or fungal, and may be acquired before, during or after birth. The most serious bacterial pneumonia at present is due to group B beta haemolytic streptococcus. As many as 15% of mothers in the UK carry this organism in the birth canal but less than 1% of infants delivered vaginally by these patients become symptomatic (Pyati et al 1981). The mortality among affected infants however may be as high as 50%. Predisposing factors include prolonged rupture of the membranes, preterm delivery, birth asphyxia and fetal distress. Presenting features resemble HMD with tachypnoea, indrawing, respiratory distress and cyanosis. Chest X-ray (Fig. 3.8) shows a ground glass appearance with bilateral generalised opacity indistinguishable from HMD. In these cases the condition is rapidly fatal unless early and appropriate antibiotics are given. Most babies are also septicaemic and many show other complicating features such as disseminated intravascular coagulation and persistent fetal circulation. Treatment consists of circulatory support, correction of acid–base balance, ventilation and antibiotics, usually penicillin and gentamicin, or a third generation cephalosporin such as ceftazidime.

A number of other bacteria may cause neonatal pneumonia: *Staphylococcus epidermidis* is the commonest cause of septicaemia in the neonate at present

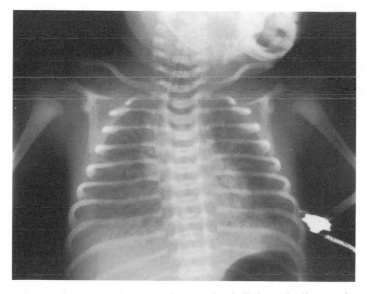

Fig. 3.8   Group B Streptococcal pneumonia; note the similarity to hyaline membrane disease.

and *Staphylococcus aureus*, although much less common is still a cause of pneumonia in some infants. *Listeria monocytogenes* is occasionally seen and the Gram-negative organisms particularly *E.coli*, *Klebsiella* and *Pseudomonas aeruginosa* can also be pathogenic especially in infants who have chronic lung disease requiring prolonged ventilation.

Chlamydia and fungi

Chlamydia trachomatis causes pneumonia in the newborn and should be considered in those who have a history of neonatal conjunctivitis. The typical chest X-ray appearance is shown in Fig. 3.9. This organism should also be looked for in those who have persistent symptoms or those who fail to respond to antibiotic treatment for the common bacterial pathogens (Frommell et al 1979). Fungi, including *Candida albicans*, are also found more often among those who have chronic lung disease, who may be undernourished and who have had repeated courses of antibiotics. Extended treatment with appropriate parenteral antifungal agents is required.

Viral pneumonia

Viral pneumonia, particularly due to organisms such as Cytomegalovirus is also being increasingly recognised in the neonatal period. It has been shown

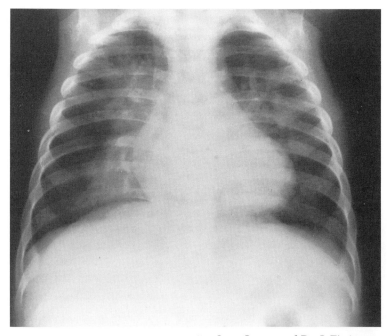

Fig. 3.9   Chlamydia pneumonia: typical perihilar flare. Courtesy of Dr G Fischer.

that as many as 0.3–1% of neonates have passively acquired cytomegalovirus in the upper airway at the time of birth (Peckham et al 1983). These infants occasionally develop persistent pneumonitis which leads to recurrent episodes of wheezing and clinically evident respiratory infection. The organism is readily cultured in the urine in such cases. Rubella rarely causes interstitial pneumonitis in the first few months of life (Boner et al 1983). Herpes simplex types I and II can cause generalised infection including pneumonia which is usually fatal. In view of the high mortality and associated morbidity from encephalitis among survivors specific treatment with acyclovir is indicated.

RECURRENT APNOEA

This is very common among pre-term babies and should not be regarded as a distinct disease entity but rather a clinical event with varied aetiology. It is particularly prevalent in the infant who is less than 1 kg at birth and who has not previously developed HMD. Significant apnoea may be defined as episodes of cessation of breathing lasting longer than 20 seconds or less than 20 seconds if accompanied by bradycardia of significance (American Academy of Pediatrics 1978). Apnoea may occur due to failure of respiratory drive because of immaturity of the respiratory centres. Apnoeic attacks can also be a symptom of any serious underlying disease including infection such as pneumonia, meningitis, septicaemia or urinary tract infection, metabolic acidosis, hypoglycaemia, or a form of seizure. It also occurs secondary to intracranial haemorrhage, respiratory depression from sedative drugs or exhaustion in relation to respiratory or cardiac failure. Upper airway obstruction such as choanal atresia, micrognathia or cleft palate can also contribute to these episodes. Before treatment is started the infant should be fully investigated for other underlying disorders which should be corrected whenever possible.

Some infants who are weaned from ventilation and recently extubated show progressive atelectasis of the lungs leading to hypoxia. In this situation supplementary oxygen with CPAP by nasal prong is often sufficient to prevent further recurrence. CPAP maintains the efficiency of the respiratory muscles by splinting the chest wall during REM sleep when the muscle tone of the intercostals and diaphragm is reduced.

When no underlying pathology is found, apart from immaturity of the respiratory system, parenteral or oral theophylline is an effective form of treatment (Jones 1982). Serum theophylline levels should be carefully monitored as there is considerable individual variation in the rate at which the drug is metabolised, especially in the very pre-term infant. It is also important to ensure that the baby is not hypothermic, anaemic, chronically hypoxic or acidotic as correction of these abnormalities will reduce the incidence of apnoeic attacks. Those who have severe episodes require ventilation until such time as their respiratory system has matured and they are able to maintain an adequate breathing pattern spontaneously.

PULMONARY HAEMORRHAGE

This condition used to be common and was probably due to haemorrhagic pulmonary oedema secondary to inappropriate fluid management. Currently, disseminated intravascular coagulation and generalised bleeding disorders are the more usual antecedent. It occurs most frequently in the second to fourth days of life and is predisposed to by birth asphyxia, underlying infection, rhesus disease, meconium aspiration syndrome or acute left heart failure. The fluid which is produced consists of haemorrhagic oedema (Cole et al 1973). Treatment consists of correction of clotting abnormalities with the use of fresh frozen plasma and Vitamin K, replacement of haemoglobin with packed cells and mechanical ventilation with appropriately raised end expiratory pressure to overcome pulmonary oedema. Despite intensive treatment the mortality for this condition remains high.

BRONCHOPULMONARY DYSPLASIA (CHRONIC LUNG DISEASE)

Bronchopulmonary dysplasia (BPD) is one of a number of chronic lung conditions affecting the increasing numbers of neonates who survive after intensive respiratory support utilizing high concentrations of oxygen and mechanical ventilation. Classical BPD with hyperinflated lungs was originally described by Northway et al (1967) but in recent years an increasing number of infants are being seen who, after mechanical ventilation during the first week of life, remain oxygen dependent at 28 days and have persistent areas of opacity on the chest X-ray without hyperinflation. Bancalari (1985) has described this entity as 'chronic lung disease' rather than BPD. Thus nowadays two types of long term lung disease are recognised although there is a considerable overlap between them.

The incidence of BPD varies between 6% and 25%, the median value being 15–17% of ventilated infants weighing less than 2.5 kg at birth. It is also more common in those with a birthweight of less than 1 kg (Yu et al 1983a). The incidence of the other forms of chronic lung disease is not yet clear but the types of illness which are seen are shown in Table 3.7. Most patients cope remarkably well with these problems but a minority develop more severe disease and may be persistently symptomatic for weeks, months

Table 3.7 Causes of chronic lung disease other than BPD

Acute or chronic infection (bacterial, viral or fungal)

Retained lung secretions (impaired mucociliary clearance)

Hypersecretory state

Patent ductus arteriosus

Recurrent aspiration

Wilson-Mikity syndrome

Metabolic bone disease of prematurity

or even years. Although their numbers are small they involve a great deal of time and resources not only for their physical needs but particularly for the emotional and family stress which their care involves. They represent one of the major outstanding problems of perinatal and infant care.

Northway et al (1967) described the typical progression of lung changes from hyaline membrane disease through a period of pulmonary plethora to a bubbly cystic appearance, finally emerging into the classical pattern of overinflated lower lobes with patchy and often linear streaky opacities throughout the upper zones. As the condition progresses one pattern merges into the next although as more infants under 1 kg survive, the final stage is becoming less common as these infants more usually demonstrate generalised haziness throughout both lung fields.

Bancalari et al (1979) gave a useful definition of BPD as follows:

1. Intermittent positive pressure ventilation (IPPV) during the first week of life lasting for at least 3 days.
2. Chronic respiratory distress characterised by tachypnoea, retractions and rales persisting for over 28 days.
3. Oxygen therapy for more than 28 days to maintain Pao_2 greater than 7 kPa (50 mmHg).
4. X-ray changes showing strands of increased density alternating with patterns of increased lucency.

However, in the most severe cases these X-ray changes worsen over a period of time before improvement begins and also vary in severity according to the presence of intercurrent infection or pulmonary oedema secondary to cardiac failure. The aetiology of BPD and of chronic lung disease in preterm infants is multifactorial and the major factors are shown in Table 3.8.

The most important precipitating factors are the presence of hyaline membrane disease, requiring for its treatment the administration of oxygen, and artificial ventilation (Coalson 1986). Many of the other factors shown compound the lung injury because of the underlying immaturity of this organ. The two most important aetiological factors are barotrauma from ventilation and local tissue damage from high oxygen concentration. The

Table 3.8   Aetiology of BPD and chronic lung disease

Pulmonary immaturity	Recurrent infection
Birth asphyxia	Artificial ventilation
Oxygen therapy	Poor mucociliary clearance
High fluid intake	Patent ductus arteriosus
Surfactant deficiency (hyaline membrane disease)	Metabolic bone disease
High fluid intake	Vitamin deficiency (A, D or E)
Pulmonary air leak (interstitial emphysema)	Persistent fetal circulation

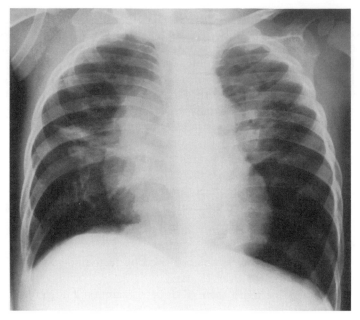

a

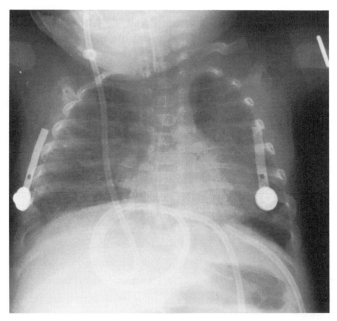

b

Fig. 3.10 (a) Bronchopulmonary dysplasia. Small, low volume upper lobes and overinflated lower lobes. (b) Chronic lung disease. Generalised hazy shadowing throughout both lung fields affecting upper and lower zones.

role of protection against oxygen toxicity by enzymes such as superoxide dysmutase is not clear and requires further study (O'Brodovich & Mellins 1985a). It is known that high concentrations of oxygen produce an acute inflammatory response in the lung which must contribute to the chronic changes which are seen in these infants. The use of an antioxidant such as vitamin E in pharmacological doses has not been shown to be beneficial in the prevention of BPD (Bancalari 1985b). The role of metabolic bone disease of prematurity is important. The poor mineralisation of the chest wall makes it soft and floppy and compromises the mechanics of breathing at a time when the lungs are stiff and fibrotic. The characteristic chest X-ray appearances of BPD and chronic lung disease are shown in Fig. 3.10.

Treatment

Treatment of chronic lung disease and especially BPD is complex and requires attention to all aspects of the baby's general condition as well as the need for respiratory support (Table 3.9). The ultimate cure for this disease is the natural growth and maturation of normal lung tissue which occurs with increasing age and weight gain. The achievement of this goal can sometimes be extremely difficult in those who remain persistently hypoxic or who need a very restricted fluid intake because of the severity of their disease and associated cor pulmonale (Yu et al 1983b).

Oxygen therapy is required by definition, it is useful to maintain the Pao_2 greater than 8 kPa (60 mmHg), 90% saturation, and to provide extra oxygen during periods of stress. These infants have marked pulmonary arterial muscle hyperplasia and quickly develop acute pulmonary hypertension due to vasoconstriction during procedures or when distressed. When ventilation is no longer required, oxygen is given by a catheter placed either just inside the nose or across the upper lip (Dinwiddie 1981, Campbell et al 1983). Low flow oxygen therapy may be needed for several months in those with the worst disease but it is quite practical to manage this at home. Fluid restriction is frequently required in very small infants with severe BPD, as there is an element of interstitial pulmonary oedema present; this is exacerbated in those with patent ductus arteriosus who have a left to right shunt. Early closure of the duct is therefore important. Diuretics are also useful

Table 3.9   Treatment of BPD and chronic lung disease

Oxygen	Antibiotics for infections
Ventilation	Adequate vitamins (A, D and E)
Fluid restriction	Diuretics
Close PDA	Adequate nutrition
Theophylline	Bronchodilators
Steroids	Ipratropium, β agonists

and a number of infants exhibit diuretic dependency becoming more hypoxic if these agents are withdrawn. Severe fluid restriction however, limits nutritional input which is vital for their recovery. Theophylline can be helpful in weaning from ventilation, by stimulating diaphragm function and central respiratory drive, and also has a mild diuretic effect and may cause bronchodilation (Rooklin et al 1979). These infants often develop acute wheezy episodes due to airway obstruction and nebulised bronchodilator agents such as ipratropium bromide or a beta sympathomimetic (Kao et al 1984) may be indicated.

Infection plays a major role in the pre-term infant with BPD or other chronic lung disease; they are particularly susceptible to this because of the disturbance of mucociliary clearance due to chronic intubation and ventilation, introduction of pathogenic hospital organisms, interstitial pulmonary oedema, relative immaturity of the immune system and lack of transfer of maternal antibodies. Organisms such as CMV can be introduced via blood transfusion (Yeager et al 1981) and human immune deficiency virus (HIV) has also been introduced via this route and led to the later development of opportunistic lung infection. The agents responsible for infection include the common hospital pathogens such as *Staphylococcus*, *Streptococcus*, *E. coli*, *Klebsiella* and *Pseudomonas*. Fungal infection with organisms such as *Candida albicans* is also being seen more frequently. Acute viral infection with respiratory syncitial virus (RSV) is another major hazard for these children and many succumb with increasing respiratory failure during such acute episodes. These patients are therefore candidates for treatment with Ribavirin which has to be given by a special nebuliser (Barry et al 1986). Other viruses such as CMV may also be present in the respiratory tract at birth (Peckham et al 1983) and this can lead to chronic lung disease with interstitial pneumonitis (Yu 1986e) or with recurrent wheezing in infancy. *Chlamydia trachomatis* has also caused chronic lung disease in very pre-term infants.

Because of these recurrent infections frequent courses of antibiotics and sometimes antifungal or antiviral agents are needed — many of these agents have potential toxic side-effects and measurement of blood levels, especially when using ototoxic agents such as the aminoglycosides, is vital. Whenever possible immunisation against pertussis should be performed and should start some 3 months post birth at any gestation.

Recurrent reflux and aspiration may be a more common complication than has previously been recognised. The very preterm infant has poorly developed sucking and swallowing reflexes and may have an impaired cough, particularly after extubation following a period of airway support. These conditions predispose to the aspiration of upper respiratory secretions and milk into the lower respiratory tract. The gastro-oesophageal sphincter is less developed in this age group and this, in conjuction with large diaphragmatic movements caused by increased work of breathing, must also increase the risk of regurgitation and aspiration. Some units employ nasal jejunal feeding in order to avoid this problem. It is probably useful to keep the baby propped up at an angle of 30° and to use thickened feeds or introduce solids at a relatively early age in infancy for those who have chronic lung problems. Theophylline also relaxes the gastro-oesophageal sphincter and so should be withdrawn in those who have obvious reflux clinically.

Prevention of vitamin deficiency is also important. Adequate intake of Vitamin A (Zachman 1986), Vitamin D (Lancet 1987) and Vitamin E is essential in the effort to minimise lung damage. These vitamins should be replaced at physiological levels as it has not been shown that giving pharmacological doses is of any long term benefit. Steroids have also been shown to be effective in BPD — Mammel et al (1983) showed a response in six infants with a mean birth weight of 1049 g. All were weaned from ventilation but three later died from intercurrent infection. Steroid therapy may have to be given over an extended period with all the associated complications that this can produce. The role of steroids in BPD is currently under investigation by a multicentre trial.

The outcome for those with severe BPD has improved over the last few years but there is still a very significant mortality during the first year of life from cor pulmonale during acute intercurrent respiratory infections. Most infants show gradual improvement over a period of time as their lungs develop. They have more frequent episodes of upper and lower respiratory tract infection, particularly during the first 2 years. Many develop bronchial hyper-reactivity which is probably secondary to airway damage caused by ventilation. A number of these children go on to have persistent lung function abnormalities for several years (Bancalari 1985).

Smyth et al (1981) found airway obstruction, hyperinflation and increased bronchial lability in nine BPD survivors age 7–9 years. Gerhardt et al (1983) found increased airway resistance up to the age of 2 years. Lindroth & Mortensson (1986) found persistent hyperinflation and pulmonary fibrosis on chest X-ray at 4–6 years of age in 13 of 14 post BPD patients. Bader et al (1987) reported persistent respiratory symptoms in eight of 10 BPD survivors with a mean age of 10.4 years. They also found significant reduction in FVC and FEV_1 and an increased residual volume. Five of the 10 showed exercise-induced bronchospasm. These studies all indicate that there is a significant risk of lifelong lung damage from BPD. Further studies of lung function will be required in adult life to answer this important question.

WILSON MIKITY SYNDROME

This condition was first described by Wilson & Mikity in 1960 and is typically seen in very low birthweight infants under 1500 g. The baby usually has mild respiratory distress initially and does not require ventilation. Subsequently chronic respiratory difficulty develops towards the end of the first or second week of life. Chest X-ray shows a bubbly appearance with streaky shadows alternating with more obviously cystic areas. Some infants show multiple rib fractures as well. The aetiology is not known but it probably represents the effects of a number of stress factors on the immature lung.

Treatment is supportive with oxygen therapy and occasionally ventilation, especially during intercurrent respiratory infection. A few develop cor pulmonale. Most patients show gradual resolution of the symptoms and signs over a period of several months. The long term outlook for those who survive this period is excellent.

REFERENCES

American Academy of Pediatrics 1978 Task force on prolonged apnea. Pediatrics 61: 651–652

Avery M E, Mead J 1959 Surface properties in relation to atelectesis and hyaline membrane disease. American Journal of Diseases of Children 97: 517–523

Bader D, Ramos A D, Lew C D, Platzkker A C G, Stabile M W, Keens T G 1987 Childhood sequelae of infant lung disease: exercise and pulmonary function abnormalities after bronchopulmonary dysplasia. Journal of Pediatrics 110: 693–699

Ballard P L 1984 Combined hormonal treatment and lung maturation. Seminars in Perinatology 8: 283–292

Bancalari E, Abdenour G E, Feller R, Gannon J 1979 Bronchopulmonary dysplasia: clinical presentation. Journal of Pediatrics 95: 819–823

Bancalari E 1985 Bronchopulmonary Dysplasia. In: Milner A D, Martin R J (eds) Neonatal and pediatric respiratory medicine. Butterworths, London, pp 54–80

Barry W, Cockburn F, Cornall R, Price J F, Sutherland G, Vardag A 1986 Ribavirin aerosol for acute bronchiolitis. Archives of Disease in Childhood 61: 593–597

Bell E, Warburton D, Stonestreet B S, Oh W 1980 Effect of fluid administration on the development of symptomatic PDA and congestive heart failure in premature infants. New England Journal of Medicine 302: 598–604

Bell E F 1986 Prevention of bronchopulmonary dysplasia: vitamin E and other antioxidants. In: Farrell P M, Taussig L M (eds) Bronchopulmonary dysplasia and related chronic respiratory disorders. Report of ninetieth Ross Conference on pediatric research. Ross Laboratories, Columbus, Ohio, pp 77–85

Boner A, Wilmott R W, Dinwiddie R, Jeffries J G, Matthew D J, Marshall W C et al 1983 Desquamative interstitial pneumonia and antigen antibody complexes in two infants with congenital rubella. Pediatrics 72: 835–839

Campbell A N, Zarfin Y, Groenveld M, Bryan M H 1983 Low flow oxygen therapy in infants. Archives of Disease in Childhood 58: 795–798

Cashore W J, Stern L 1984 Neonatal problems of the preterm infant. Clinics in Obstetrics and Gynaecology 11: 391–414

Coalson J J 1986 Animal models for bronchopulmonary dysplasia research, particularly primate studies. In: Farrell P M, Taussig L M (eds) Bronchopulmonary dysplasia and related chronic respiratory disorders. Report of ninetieth Ross Conference on pediatric research. Ross Laboratories, Columbus, Ohio, p 7

Cole V A, Normand I C S, Reynolds E O R, Rivers R P A 1973 Pathogenesis of haemorrhagic pulmonary oedema and massive pulmonary haemorrhage in the newborn. Pediatrics 51: 175–187

Collaborative Group on Antenatal Steroid Therapy 1981 Effect of antenatal dexamethasone administration on the prevention of respiratory distress syndrome. American Journal of Obstetrics and Gynaecology 141: 276–286

Cook C D, Drinker P A, Jacobson H N, Levison H, Strang L B 1963 Control of pulmonary blood flow in the foetal and newly born lamb. Journal of Physiology 169: 10–29

Dawes G S, Mott J C, Widdicombe J G, Wyatt D G 1953 Changes in the lungs of the newborn lamb. Journal of Physiology 121: 141–162

Dawes G S, Rudolph A M, Heymann M A 1966 Response of the pulmonary vasculature to hypoxia and H^+ ion concentration changes. Journal of Clinical Investigation 45: 399–411

Dawes G S 1968 Foetal and neonatal physiology: a comparative study of changes at birth. Year Book Medical Publishers, Chicago, pp 141–159

Dinwiddie R 1981 Long term oxygen therapy via nasal catheter. Journal of Maternal and Child Health 6: 426

Dinwiddie R, Mellor D H, Donaldson S H C, Tunstall M E, Russell G 1974 Quality of survival after artificial ventilation of the newborn. Archives of Disease in Childhood 49: 703–710

Drew J 1982 Immediate intubation at birth of the very low birthweight infant: effect on survival. American Journal of Diseases of Children 136: 207–210

Drummond W H, Gregory G A, Heymann N A, Phibbs R A 1981 The independent effects of hyperventilation, tolazoline and dopamine infusions on infants with persistent pulmonary hypertension. Journal of Pediatrics 98: 603–611

Ellison R C, Peckham G J, Lang P, Talver N S, Lever T S, Lin L et al 1983 Evaluation of the preterm infant for patent ductus arteriosus. Pediatrics 71: 364–372

Field D J, Milner A D, Hopkin I E 1984 High and conventional rates of positive pressure ventilation. Archives of Disease in Childhood 59: 1151–1154

Field D, Milner A D, Hopkin I E 1986 Efficiency of manual resuscitators at birth. Archives of Disease in Childhood 61: 300–302

Fox W W, Gewitz M H, Dinwiddie R, Drummond W H, Peckham G J 1977 Pulmonary hypertension in the perinatal aspiration syndromes. Pediatrics 59: 205–209

Franz I D, Westhammer J, Stark A R 1983 High frequency ventilation in premature infants, adequate gas exchange at lower tracheal pressure. Pediatrics 71: 483–488

Frommell G J, Rothenberry R, Wang S, McIntosh K 1979 Chlamydial infection of mothers and their infants. Journal of Pediatrics 95: 28–32

Fujiwara T, Maeta H, Morita T, Watabe Y, Chida S, Abe T 1980 Artificial surfactant therapy in hyaline membrane disease. Lancet 1: 55–59

Gerhardt T, Tapia J L, Goldman S L, Hehre D, Feller R, Bancalari E 1983 Serial lung function measurements in infants with chronic lung disease (CLD). Pediatric Research 17: 376A

Gersony W M, Peckham G J, Ellison R S, Miettiner O S, Nadas A S 1983 Effects of indomethacin in premature infants with patent ductus arteriosus. Results of a national collaborative study. Journal of Pediatrics 102: 895–906

Gluck L, Kulovich M V 1973 L/S ratios in amniotic fluid in normal and abnormal pregnancies. American Journal of Obstetrics and Gynaecology 115: 539–552

Greenberg M I, Roberts J R, Baskin S I 1981 Use of endotracheally administered epinephrine on a pediatric patient. American Journal of Diseases of Children 135: 767–768

Greenough A, Roberton N R C 1985 Morbidity and survival of neonates ventilated for the respiratory distress syndrome. British Medical Journal 290: 597–600

Greenough A, Dixon A K, Roberton N R C 1984a Pulmonary interstitial emphysema. Archives of Disease in Childhood 59: 1046–1051

Greenough A, Morley C J, Wood S, Davies J A 1984b Pancuronium prevents pneumothoraces in ventilated premature babies who actively expire against positive pressure inflation. Lancet 1: 1–3

Greenough A, Elias-Jones A C, Pool J, Morley C J, Davis J A 1985 The therapeutic actions of theophylline in preterm ventilated infants. Early Human Development 12: 15–22

Greenough A, Morley C J, Pool J 1986 Fighting the ventilator — are fast rates an effective alternative to paralysis? Early Human Development 13: 189–194

Gregory G A, Gooding C A, Phibbs R H, Tooley W H 1974 Meconium aspiration in infants, a prospective study. Journal of Pediatrics 85: 848–852

Haddad G G, Mellins R B 1977 The role of airway receptors in the control of respiration in infants: a review. Journal of Pediatrics 19: 281–266

Harrison V C, Heese H de V, Klein M 1968 The significance of grunting in hyaline membrane disease.Pediatrics 41: 549–559

Hart S M, McNair M, Gamsu H, Price J F 1983 Pulmonary interstitial emphysema in very low birthweight infants. Archives of Disease in Childhood 58: 612–615

Hey E N, Katz G 1970 The optimum thermal environment for naked babies. Archives of Disease in Childhood 45: 328–332

Hoskyns E W, Milner A D, Hopkin I E 1987 A simple method of face mask resuscitation at birth. Archives of Disease in Childhood 62: 376–378

Howie P W, Patel N B 1984 Obstetric management of preterm labour. Clinics in Obstetrics and Gynaecology 11: 373–390

Ingemarsson I, Westgren M, Svenningsen N W 1978 Long term follow up of preterm infants in breech presentation delivered by Caesarean section. Lancet ii: 172–175

Jones R A K 1982 Apnoea of prematurity. 1. A controlled trial of theophylline and face
   mask continuous positive airway pressure. Archives of Disease in Childhood 57: 761–764
Kao L C, Warburton D, Platyker A C G, Keens T C 1984 Effect of isoproterenol
   inhalation on airway resistance in chronic bronchopulmonary dysplasia. Pediatrics
   7: 509–514
Karlberg P, Cherry R B, Escardo F E, Koch G 1962 Respiratory studies in newborn
   infants II Pulmonary ventilation and mechanics of breathing in the first few minutes of
   life, including the onset of respiration. Acta Paediatrica Stockholm 51: 121–136
Kelnar L J H, Harvey D (eds) 1987 Respiratory problems. In: The sick newborn baby.
   Ballière–Tindall, London, p 113
Kennedy E P, Weiss S B 1956 The function of cytidine coenzymes in the biosynthesis of
   phospholipids. Journal of Biological Chemistry 222: 193–214
Lamont R F, Dunlop P D M, Crowley P, Elder M G 1983 Spontaneous preterm labour
   and delivery under 34 weeks gestation. British Medical Journal 286: 454–457
Lancet 1987 Editorial. Metabolic bone disease of prematurity. 1: 200
Lindroth M, Mortensson W 1986 Long-term follow up of ventilator treated low
   birthweight infants. I. Chest X-ray, pulmonary mechanics, clinical lung disease and
   growth. Acta Paediatrica Scandinavica 75: 819–825
Levine D, Trump D S, Waterkotte G 1981 Unilateral pulmonary intestitial emphysema. A
   surgical approach to treatment. Pediatrics 68: 510–514
Lewis S, Pelausa E, Ojah C, Paes B 1988 Pulmonary interstitial emphysema: selective
   bronchial occlusion with a Swan-Ganz catheter. Archives of Disease in Childhood
   63: 313–315
Lipscomb A P, Thorburn R J, Reynolds E O R et al 1981 Pneumothorax and cerebral
   haemorrhage in preterm infants. Lancet 1: 414–416
Lou H C, Lassen N A, Frus-Hansen B 1979 Impaired autoregulation of cerebral blood
   flow in the distressed newborn infant. Journal of Pediatrics 94: 118–121
MacFarlance P I, Heaf D P 1988 Pulmonary function in children after neonatal meconium
   aspiration syndrome. Archives of Disease in Childhood 63: 368–372
Mammel M C, Green T P, Johnson D E, Thompson T R 1983 Controlled trial of
   dexamethasone therapy in infants with bronchopulmonary dysplasia. Lancet 1: 1356–1358
Mehta A, Callan K, Wright B M, Stacey T E 1986 Patient triggered ventilation in the
   newborn. Lancet II: 17–19
Milner A D, Saunders R A, Hopkin I E 1978 Effect of delivery by Caesarean section on
   lung mechanics and lung volume in the human neonate. Archives of Disease in
   Childhood 53: 545–548
Milner A D, Vyas H 1982 Lung expansion at birth. Journal of Pediatrics 101: 879–886
Morley C J 1984 Surfactant treatment for respiratory distress syndrome — a review.
   Journal of the Royal Society of Medicine 77: 788–792
Northway W H, Rosan R C, Porter D Y 1967 Pulmonary disease following respirator
   therapy of hyaline membrane disease. Bronchopulmonary dysplasia. New England
   Medical Journal 276: 357–368
O'Brodovich H M, Mellins R B 1985 Bronchopulmonary dysplasia. Unresolved acute
   neonatal lung injury. American Review of Respiratory Disease 132: 694–709
O'Souya S W, Black P, Cadman J, Richards B 1983 Umbilical venous pH: a useful aid in
   the diagnosis of asphyxia at birth. Archives of Disease in Childhood 58: 15–19
Pagtakhan R D, Faridy E E, Chernick V 1971 Interaction between arterial Po_2 and Pco_2
   in the limitation of respiration of foetal sheep. Journal of Applied Physiology
   30: 382–387
Pattle R E 1955 Properties, nature and function of the alveolar lining layer. Nature
   175: 1125–1126
Peckham C S, Chin K S, Coleman J C, Henderson K, Hurley R, Preece P M 1983
   Cytomegalovirus infection in pregnancy: preliminary findings from a prospective study.
   Lancet 1: 1352–1355
Platt L D, Manning F A 1980 Fetal breathing movements: an update. Clinics in
   Perinatology 7: 423–433
Primhak R A, Herber S M, Whincup G, Milner R D G 1984 Which deliveries require
   paediatricians in attendance. British Medical Journal 289: 16–18
Pyati S P, Pildes R S, Ramamurthy R S, Jacobson 1981 Decreasing mortality in neonates
   with early onset group B streptococcal infection: reality or artefact. Journal of Pediatrics
   98: 625–627

Rigatto H, Davi M, Frantz I D et al 1989 Division of Lung Diseases. National Heart, Lung and Blood Institute, National Institute of Health, Bethesda. New England Journal of Medicine (320) 2: 83–93

Roberton N R C 1982 Advances in respiratory distress syndrome. British Medical Journal 284: 917–918

Roberton N R C (ed) 1986 Disorders of the respiratory tract. In: A manual of neonatal intensive care. Edward Arnold, London, pp 72–142

Rooklin A R, Moomjian A S, Shutack J G, Schwartz J G, Fox W W 1979 Theophylline therapy in bronchopulmonary dysplasia. Journal of Pediatrics 95: 882–885

Rudolph A M, Heymann M A 1974 Fetal and neonatal circulation and respiration. American Review of Physiology 36: 187–207

Rudolph A M 1977 Fetal and neonatal pulmonary circulation. American Review of Respiratory Diseases 115: 11–18

Runkle B, Bancalari E 1984 Acute cardiopulmonary effects of pancuronium bromide in mechanically ventilated newborn infants. Journal of Pediatrics 104: 614–617

Schönberger W, Grimm W, Emmrich P, Gempp J 1981 Reduction of mortality rate in premature infants by substitution of thyroid hormones. European Journal of Pediatrics 135: 245–253

Smyth J A, Tabachnik E, Duncan W J, Reilly B J, Levison H 1981 Pulmonary function and bronchial hyperreactivity in long-term survivors of bronchopulmonary dysplasia. Pediatrics 68: 336–340

Stanley F J, Alberman E D 1978 Infants of very low birthweight: I Perinatal factors affecting survival. Developmental Medicine and Child Neurology 20: 300–312

Strang L B (ed) 1977a Oxygen transport in the blood. In: Neonatal respiration — physiological and clinical studies. Blackwell Scientific, Oxford, pp 138–160

Strang L B (ed) 1977b Morphology of lung development. In: Neonatal respiration — physiological and clinical studies. Blackwell Scientific, Oxford, pp 1–19

Sykes G S, Molloy P M, Johnson P et al 1982 Do Apgar scores indicate asphyxia? Lancet i: 494–496

Tarnow-Mordi W O, Sutton P, Wilkinson A R 1986 Inadequate humidification of respiratory gases during mechanical ventilation of the newborn. Archives of Disease in Childhood 61: 698–700

Ten Centre Study Group 1987 Ten centre trial of artificial surfactant (artificial lung expanding compound) in very premature babies. British Medical Journal 294: 991–996

Thompson A J, Searle M, Russell G 1977 Quality of survival after severe birth asphyxia. Archives of Disease in Childhood 52: 620–626

Ting P, Brady J 1975 Tracheal suction in meconium aspiration. American Journal of Obstetrics and Gynecology 122: 767–771

Vidyasgar D, Yeh T F, Harris V, Pildes R S 1975 Assisted ventilation in infants with meconium aspiration syndrome. Pediatrics 56: 208–213

Vyas H, Milner A D, Hopkin I E, Boon A W 1981 Physiological responses to prolonged and slow rise inflation in the resuscitation of the asphyxiated newborn infant. Journal of Pediatrics 99: 635–639

Walters D V, Olver R E 1978 The role of catecholamines in lung liquid absorption at birth. Pediatric Research 12: 239–242

Whitelaw A 1989 Intervention after birth asphyxia. Archives of Disease in Childhood 64: 66–68

Wilson M E, Mikity Y G 1960 A new form of respiratory disease seen in premature infants. American Journal of Diseases of Childhood 99: 489–499

Yeager A S, Grumet F C, Hafleigh E B, Arvin A M, Bradley J S, Prober C G 1981 Prevention of transfusion acquired cytomegalovirus infections in newborn infants. Journal of Pediatrics 98: 281–287

Yu V Y H, Zhao S M, Bajuk B 1982 Results of intensive care for 375 very low birth weight infants. Australian Paediatric Journal 18: 188–192

Yu V Y H, Orgill A A, Lim S V, Bajuk B, Astbury J 1983a Bronchopulmonary dysplasia in very low birthweight infants. Australian Paediatric Journal 19: 233–236

Yu V Y H, Orgill A A, Lim S V, Bajuk B, Astbury J 1983b Growth and development of very low birthweight infants recovering from bronchopulmonary dysplasia. Archives of Disease in Childhood 58: 791–794

Yu V Y H (ed) 1986a Perinatal respiratory physiology. In: Respiratory disorders in the newborn. Churchill Livingstone, Edinburgh, pp 8–17

Yu V Y H (ed) 1986b Perinatal asphyxia. In: Respiratory disorders in the newborn. Churchill Livingstone, Edinburgh, pp 18–28

Yu V Y H (ed) 1986c Pulmonary air leak. In: Respiratory disorders in the newborn. Churchill Livingstone, Edinburgh, pp 86–99

Yu V Y H (ed) 1986d Transient tachypnoea of the newborn. In: Respiratory disorders in the newborn. Churchill Livingstone, Edinburgh pp 74–76

Yu V Y H (ed) 1986e Pneumonia. In: Respiratory disorders in the newborn. Churchill Livingstone, Edinburgh, pp 54–72

Zachman R D 1986 Vitamin A. In: Farrell P M, Taussig L M (eds) Bronchopulmonary dysplasia and related chronic respiratory disorders. Report of ninetieth Ross Conference on pediatric research. Ross Laboratories, Columbus, Ohio, pp 86–89

RECOMMENDED READING

Harvey D, Cooke R W I, Levitt G A (eds) 1989 The baby under 1000 g. Wright, London

Roberton N R C (ed) 1986 A manual of neonatal intensive care — 2nd Edition. Edward Arnold, London

Yu V Y H (ed) 1986 Respiratory disorders in the newborn. Churchill Livingstone, Edinburgh

4. Developmental anomalies of the respiratory tract

Developmental anomalies of the respiratory tract occur at any level throughout the system and include abnormalities of the nose, palate and upper airway, larynx, tracheobronchial tree, abnormalities of the lungs themselves and the rib cage. They are best sub-divided anatomically by region in order to understand causation and treatment. The major anomalies which are seen are shown in Table 4.1.

UPPER RESPIRATORY TRACT

Pierre Robin Syndrome and choanal atresia frequently require intervention and airway support and are therefore considered in detail in chapter 5 under ear, nose and throat problems. Cleft lip and palate (Table 4.2) occur in 1 per 600 births. They result from failure of fusion of various embryological

Table 4.1 Congenital abnormalities of the respiratory tract

Upper respiratory tract	Extrinsic lesions
Pierre Robin syndrome	Duplication cyst
Goldenhar syndrome	Vascular ring
Treacher-Collins syndrome	Intrapulmonary lesions
Chonal atresia	Congenital lobar emphysema
Cleft lip and palate	Congenital lung cysts
Larynx	Cystic adenomatoid malformation
Laryngomalacia	Lobar sequestration
Stenosis	Pulmonary agenesis
Atresia	Pulmonary aplasia
Cleft	Pulmonary hypoplasia
Web	Diaphragmatic hernia or eventration
Vocal cord paralysis	Rib cage anomalies
Local obstructive lesions	Neuromuscular disease
Hemangioma	Pulmonary A–V fistula
Laryngeal cysts	
Papilloma	
Tracheobronchial lesions	
Stenosis	
Atresia	
Tracheomalacia	
Bronchial stenosis	
Tracheo-oesophageal fistula and	
oesophageal atresia	
Tracheal pouch	

Table 4.2 Distribution and sex ratio of cleft lip and palate (Fogh-Andersen 1968)

	% of all cases	sex ratio
Cleft lip alone	25%	60% male
Cleft palate alone	25%	59% female
Cleft lip and palate	50%	70% male

In 75% of cases the cleft was unilateral.

structures and are best regarded separately. Cleft lips are further subdivided into those which are anterior to the incisor foramen behind the incisor teeth in the hard palate and those which are posterior to this level and involve the palate itself. There is a genetic component to these conditions in which the anterior clefts are inherited separately to isolated clefts of the hard and soft palate (Dickson 1985). The recurrence rate in siblings is approximately 5% for cleft lip lesions with or without cleft palate and 3% for isolated cleft palate; this increases to about 10% if there are two affected children in the family (Fraser 1958). The incidence of other congenital malformations including chromosome defects is also increased in children with cleft lip or palate.

Children with combined lesions have a high incidence of upper respiratory tract infection due to swallowing problems with repeated regurgitation of milk into the nasal passages causing oedema and obstruction of the Eustachian tubes (Paradise et al 1969). These children also have a high incidence of aspiration into the lungs secondary to swallowing inco-ordination and breathing difficulties during feeding. The feeding problems can present major difficulties and may need to be dealt with in various ways, such as tube feeding, use of a cleft palate teat or a cup and spoon. Some babies are able to breast feed quite well despite their abnormality. The mode of feeding varies from one infant to another.

Cleft lip repair is usually carried out at the age of 3 months, although an increasing number of surgeons now perform this immediately after birth. The most important factor is the long term result, especially in relation to appearance and function. Where there is any evidence of obstruction to the airway, particularly in conditions such as Pierre Robin Syndrome, palatal repair should be delayed until significant growth has occurred to avoid a recurrence of airway obstruction when the posterior pharyngeal space is again physically reduced in size and when there may be postoperative oedema. Early aggressive repair of the palate in Pierre Robin syndrome has resulted in death on a number of occasions. The normal age for repair of the cleft palate is around 15 months. It is important that speech is allowed to develop normally and this may be inhibited by hearing problems secondary to the recurrent middle ear infections to which these children are prone. Careful evaluation of the correct time for surgery is, therefore, important. The best care of these children is provided by a team approach involving plastic surgeons, orthodontists, audiologists and speech therapists.

LARYNX

Laryngomalacia

This is by far the commonest cause of persistent stridor in infancy. Its incidence outstrips all other causes put together and accounts for 60–70% of the cases seen (Holinger 1980). The infant classically presents with inspiratory stridor, frequently from birth. The noise varies with respiration and increases when a higher negative intrathoracic pressure is created, such as during crying or with mild airway obstruction secondary to upper respiratory tract infection. Some children show indrawing of respiratory muscles and mild respiratory distress but this diminishes with age as the laryngeal tissue becomes firmer and the chest wall compliance improves. If the symptoms are typical and the child is thriving and feeding normally, further intervention is not required. When there is any doubt as to the diagnosis, further investigation, including lateral neck X-ray, chest X-ray, high KV filter picture, barium swallow to exclude extrinsic tracheal and oesophageal compression, and laryngoscopy are indicated. The vast majority of children with laryngomalacia will outgrow this problem in the first 2–3 years of life (Cinnamond 1987). They very seldom require any other treatment.

Laryngeal abnormalities

A variety of laryngeal abnormalities may be seen. Laryngeal stenosis may be congenital or acquired secondary to prolonged endotracheal intubation (Cinnamond 1987) which may also cause vocal cord damage. Children with congenital stenosis may present with inspiratory stridor (Table 4.3) and evidence of airway obstruction but often not until several weeks or months of age when they have developed an intercurrent respiratory infection. Airway support is often needed immediately and careful assessment by an expert laryngoscopist is required. Major obstructive lesions will require urgent tracheostomy.

Laryngeal webs occur at any level in relation to the larynx — above, within, or below it. The most common types are glottic or subglottic. Symptoms will depend on the degree of airway narrowing and will often produce hoarseness of the voice and airway obstruction. Congenital vocal cord palsy is considered in Chapter 5 under ENT problems.

Table 4.3 Causes of stridor

Laryngomalacia	Acute allergic oedema of the larynx
Acute epiglottitis	Laryngeal cleft
Laryngotracheitis, viral or bacterial	Vascular ring
Subglottic stenosis, congenital or acquired	Hemangioma
Foreign body inhalation	Laryngeal cyst
Subglottic hemangioma	Mediastinal tumour
Vocal cord palsy, central or peripheral	Papillomatosis
Laryngeal web	Diphtheria

Cleft larynx occurs where there is a posterior cleft of the laryngeal cartilage allowing communication between the upper trachea and the oesophagus (Petterson 1955). These children present with persistent cough and recurrent episodes of aspiration pneumonitis. Symptoms occur particularly during feeding and also while asleep with spasmodic outbursts of coughing due to spillover of saliva into the upper trachea. Identification is by direct laryngoscopy. Minor lesions are best treated medically with thickening of the feeds or tube feeding initially. Larger clefts require surgical intervention, although this can be a major procedure in the young child (Kauten et al 1984).

A number of rare lesions may affect a larynx, including multiple papillomatosis (Strong 1987). These children can develop severe problems including acute airway obstruction and death. Many require tracheostomy and repeated laser treatment to control the papillomata. Occasionally, isolated lesions are seen and these have a much better prognosis. Haemangioma of the larynx is also a rare occurrence but inspection of the child may reveal haemangiomas elsewhere (Garfinkel & Handler 1980). Laryngeal cysts occur in association with glossal abnormalities, but may also arise de novo from abnormalities of development of the larynx. These usually have a good prognosis (Suhonen et al 1984).

TRACHEA

Tracheal atresia is an extremely rare lesion and usually not compatible with life. It is commonly associated with major oesophageal abnormality due to their common embryonic origin. Subglottic stenosis may be congenital or acquired. These children present with biphasic stridor and respiratory difficulty which may not necessarily be seen at birth and only come to light in the course of an intercurrent respiratory tract infection. Some children present with wheeze due to retention of secretions and secondary small airway obstruction below the level of the narrowing. The most common cause of this problem nowadays is a complication of prolonged endotracheal intubation in the neonatal period. Some children will require tracheostomy to relieve the obstruction; reconstructive surgery for the trachea in these cases is described in Chapter 5. Tracheal stenosis is also an occasional associated finding in cases with oesphageal atresia and tracheo-oesophageal fistula. Direct tracheal surgery in severe cases of congenital tracheal stenosis is very difficult and carries an extremely high mortality, particularly in the younger age groups.

Tracheomalacia

This is due to softening of the tracheal wall usually due to a cartilage abnormality but frequently found in association with an extrinsic compressive lesion such as a vascular ring. It is a common association at the site of a tracheo-oesophageal fistula. The lesion results in dynamic airway changes during respiration and these may be visualised on screening of the chest, particularly from the lateral view. During expiration, when there is a positive expiratory pressure in the lungs, the tracheal wall may collapse and this leads to airway obstruction (Gordon et al 1987). In a few cases, this may be so severe as to produce major apnoea and require positive pressure from the upper airway to relieve it. More commonly, it results in retention of secretions within the bronchial tree leading to recurrent infection, persistent cough and sputum production and small airway obstruction with the onset of wheeze. Investigation will include full imaging of the trachea with postero-anterior and lateral chest X-ray, filter picture of the large airways, chest screening and barium swallow to exclude extrinsic compressive lesions. Most children will require endoscopy to assess the level and extent of the tracheomalacia.

Treatment consists of correction of any underlying abnormalities such as a tracheo-oesophageal fistula or division of a vascular ring with re-routing of any anomalous blood vessel lying between the trachea and oesophagus. An aortopexy in which the aorta is stitched forward onto the back of the sternum so stabilising the trachea is sometimes helpful (Filler et al 1976). Some children with congenital tracheomalacia require tracheostomy to support the trachea in the weakened area and also to allow easy application of positive pressure for resuscitation from above should the trachea collapse completely on expiration. A small number of rare congenital abnormalities are seen in the trachea or major bronchi. These include tracheal pouch and peripheral bronchial stenosis. These children usually have an associated parenchymal lung abnormality as well and may present either with stridor or with wheezing. A large airway abnormality beyond the trachea is extremely difficult to correct surgically and frequently only symptomatic treatment is available.

EXTRINSIC LESIONS

Lesions outside the trachea and major bronchi can produce tracheomalacia or respiratory obstruction because of extrinsic pressure. These include a bronchogenic cyst or a vascular ring. A bronchogenic cyst may lie anywhere along the trachea or the main bronchi but most commonly occurs in the area of the carina. It does not usually communicate with the tracheo-bronchial tree but can cause compression of the large major bronchi resulting in an increased angle below the carina. The usual imaging procedures should be performed initially, but thoracic CT scan may be the most accurate way of delineating the size and position of such a lesion nowadays (Gordon et al 1987). It requires surgical removal in order to relieve the tracheomalacia and to allow normal growth of the airways to continue.

Cystic hygroma may occasionally produce tracheal compression if it is in the upper mediastinum or if there is sudden spontaneous haemorrhage into the lesion itself. This will also require surgical removal or decompression if total removal is not possible.

Vascular ring

Abnormal development of the large blood vessels involving the aorta, ductus arteriosus and pulmonary artery can result in a variety of vascular ring abnormalities. These are shown in Table 4.4. Not all of these lesions produce strictly ring-like abnormalities; they do produce tracheal compression and often associated tracheomalacia (Fig. 4.1) (Roesler et al 1983). They are occasionally familial (Westaby et al 1984). The innominate artery may rarely produce anterolateral tracheal wall compression by a late take off (Strife et al 1981).

Treatment for most cases is surgical with rerouting of the aberrant blood vessel and ligation and division of the ductus or ligamentum arteriosum if necessary to relieve the pressure on the trachea. Aortopexy may be necessary if the tracheal wall is weak (Filler et al 1976) to pull it away from the tracheal wall and thus relieve the compression. Most children make good progress after such procedures and show gradual resolution of the tracheomalacia over the ensuing months or years.

Table 4.4   Types of vascular ring

Double aortic arch

Right sided aortic arch with patent ductus arteriosus or ligamentum arteriosum

Aberrant right subclavian with patent ductus arteriosus or ligamentum arteriosum

Aberrant left pulmonary artery

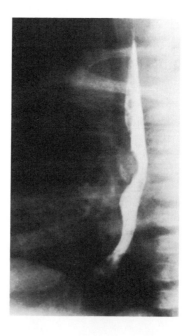

Fig. 4.1   Aberrant left pulmonary artery lying between oesophagus and trachea, causing mid-oesophageal indentation and tracheomalacia.

A few have more generalised tracheobronchomalacia and this is much more difficult to treat especially in infancy. During expiration there may be dynamic compression of the airways as intrathoracic pressure rises — this is particularly likely to occur during crying. Some of these infants have life threatening obstructive apnoeic episodes when there is massive air trapping causing overinflation of the lungs which compress the trachea. These patients may require active resuscitation by squeezing of the chest to push the air out. In severe cases a tracheostomy can stabilise the trachea sufficiently to allow more normal breathing or to facilitate manual ventilation during apnoeic episodes. The long term prognosis is reasonably good if they survive infancy.

ABNORMALITIES OF THE LUNG

Congenital lung cysts

Cysts of the lung may be seen on chest X-ray (Fig. 4.2) under a number of circumstances — they are either congenital or associated with acute infection. They may be seen as an incidental finding on a routine chest X-ray or can develop in the course of an infection especially with staphylococci or klebsiella — these are more common in children with an associated immune deficiency such as the hyper IgE syndrome. The cyst can be single or there may be several lesions of varying size. Congenital lung cysts frequently become infected or may indeed develop during the course of an infection itself. It is important to treat the infection vigorously and to follow the patient carefully to ensure resolution. This usually occurs in the case of staphyloccocal pneumatocele, but if this does not occur then the possibility of a congenital lung cyst with secondary infection must be considered. These lesions require surgical removal since they are liable to develop recurrent infection and this may spread to other areas of the lung causing further damage. Careful investigation should precede surgery as some cysts are present in sequestered lobes of the lung to which there will be a systemic blood supply making surgery more difficult. Ventilation/perfusion scan, digital vascular imaging or pulmonary angiography helps to delineate these problems. The results of surgery are usually excellent.

Cystic adenomatoid malformation

This abnormality may be diagnosed by ultrasound antenatally but more often presents in the neonatal period with persistent shadowing on the chest X-ray (Fig. 4.3) indicating poor aeration of an area of lung; it can affect any lobe. Multiple cysts may be seen within the lesion and these can give the appearance of localised emphysema. The area either does not ventilate at all or ventilates poorly on lung scan and is also poorly perfused. The cysts may produce compression of adjacent areas of lung or large airways leading to acute respiratory distress (Yu 1986). Histologically three different types are

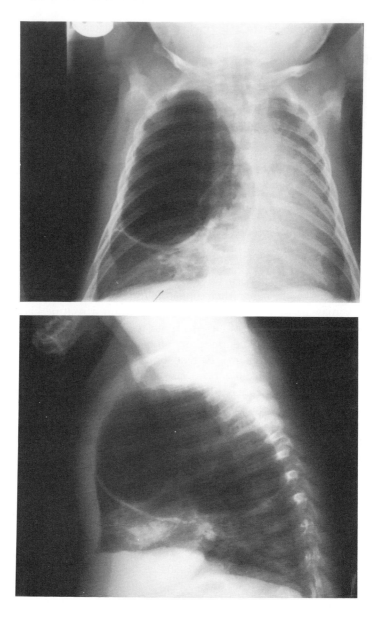

Fig. 4.2   Congenital lung cysts — right upper and left lower zones.

recognised (Stocker et al 1977). Type 1 lesions consist of single or multiple large cysts which are lined with ciliated pseudostratified epithelium. Smooth muscle elastic tissue and mucous secreting cells may be present along with normal alveolar tissue between the cysts. The larger cysts may cause mediastinal shift but the prognosis after surgery is usually good. Type 2 lesions consist of multiple small cysts less than 1 cm in diameter. These

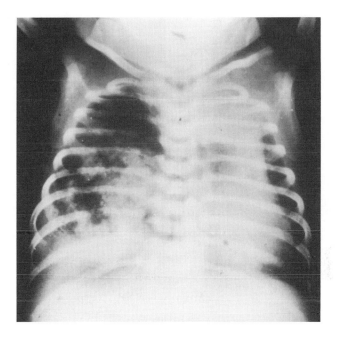

Fig. 4.3 Cystic adenomatoid malformation of the right lower lobe.

resemble dilated terminal bronchioles lined by ciliated cuboidal or columnar epithelium. Smooth muscle cells are sometimes present but mucous glands and cartilage are not seen. Type 3 lesions form a firm solid airless mass consisting of cystic bronchioles lined by ciliated cuboidal epithelium. This type carries a poor prognosis. A few cases have been described where this abnormality has been found incidentally on chest X-ray. It is important not to confuse the chest X-ray appearance with that of a diaphragmatic hernia, especially on the left side. Particular attention should be paid to the position of the gastric bubble. If there is any doubt a barium meal will differentiate the two conditions.

Any acute infection should be treated first and the patient's condition stabilised prior to surgical removal of the affected lobe which is required in all cases. The prognosis after removal of the cysts is extremely good and the rest of the lung compensates well for the area which has been removed (Frenckner & Freyschuss 1982).

Congenital lobar emphysema

This condition results in overinflation of a lobe of the lung to varying degrees (Fig 4.4). The younger the patient, the greater the overinflation present and the more likely it is to produce significant pressure on adjacent lobes. It is thought to be due to intrinsic deficiency of bronchial cartilage and possibly elastic tissue. Some cases are secondary to an extrinsic lesion,

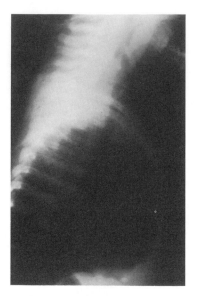 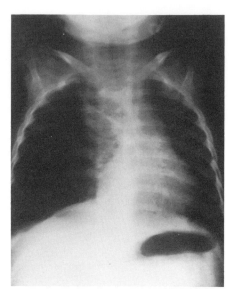

Fig. 4.4 Congenital lobar emphysema, right upper and middle lobes.

such as an aberrant or enlarged blood vessel pressing on the lobar bronchus.

A significant proportion of affected infants present in the first few weeks of life with tachypnoea, wheezing and increasing respiratory difficulty. On examination there is obvious respiratory distress with increased percussion note over the affected side and reduced air entry. The airway obstruction may also result in wheezing. A few patients present later, sometimes when an incidental chest X-ray is taken during a respiratory tract infection; in these cases, the overinflation is much less.

The lobes most affected occur in the following order of frequency: left upper (47%), right middle (28%), right upper (20%) and rarely right lower or left lower (De Luca & Wesselhoeft 1978). Sometimes the lesion is mistaken for a pneumothorax and a needle or drain is inserted which may result in a bronchopleural fistula. Fourteen per cent of patients have an associated congenital heart lesion (Yu 1986). Diagnosis is made by full radiographic examination, including chest screening and ventilation/perfusion lung scan.

Treatment consists of lobectomy for those who have significant compressive symptoms and absent ventilation and perfusion on lung scan, particularly in the youngest age groups. Those with less symptomatic lesions discovered after the first few months of life may be treated conservatively and most will show gradual improvement with age. The long term lung function after surgery is good (McBride et al 1980). Rarely, another lobe may over-distend and further surgery could be indicated if the patient has sufficient residual lung function to cope with a further lobar resection, although this is very unusual.

Lobar sequestration

This is an area of non-functioning lung tissue caused by abnormal embryonic development and which has an aberrant airway connection to the tracheobronchial tree and a blood supply which is systemic in origin. There are two major groups: the extralobar or accessory type and the intralobar type. The extralobar or accessory type has its own separate pleura and a systemic arterial blood supply usually from the aorta. It may have a communication with the tracheobronchial tree or occasionally with the gut. Intralobar sequestration lies within the visceral pleura and is intimately associated with normal lung tissue. It has been suggested that it derives from an extra tracheobronchial bud in early embryonic development.

The lesions are not primarily cystic in nature and if they do have a tracheobronchial communication may ventilate quite well (Gordon et al 1987). Those which do cause symptoms commonly present with secondary infection of the affected lobe and the appearance of multiple cyst formation on chest X-ray. They are seen in the left lower lobe more commonly than the right lower lobe in the ratio of 2:1. Treatment consists of antibiotics for the acute infection followed by further investigation when the infection has cleared. Typically, there are persistent cystic changes on chest X-ray and the ventilation/perfusion scan shows poor ventilation and no perfusion because of the systemic blood supply. Direct vascular imaging is then undertaken and if the lesion is confirmed then lobar resection is indicated since further infections will occur if it is left untreated.

Pulmonary agenesis

Bilateral pulmonary agenesis is extremely rare and incompatible with life. Unilateral pulmonary agenesis, although uncommon, may be asymptomatic. There is a significant association with other congenital malformations, particularly cardiovascular and rib cage anomalies. Some children present with lower respiratory tract infection or with a mild degree of scoliosis, chest wall asymmetry and diminished air entry on the affected side with mediastinal shift. The chest X-ray (Fig. 4.5) shows an opaque hemithorax with the heart shifted to the affected side. There is no specific treatment and the prognosis for the isolated lesion is good since the other lung is normal.

Pulmonary hypoplasia

Bilateral pulmonary hypoplasia is seen in approximately 1 per 1000 births (Knox & Barson 1986). It may happen spontaneously but is often associated with oligohydramnios during prenatal life secondary to fetal urological abnormalities. Severe bilateral pulmonary hypoplasia is classically found in Potter's Syndrome where it is associated with renal agenesis. Another important factor which contributes to pulmonary hypoplasia is prolonged

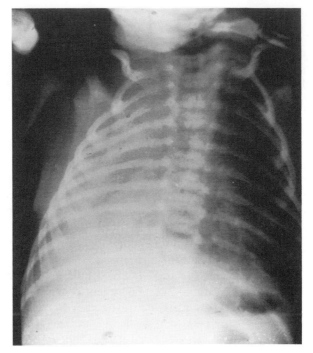

Fig. 4.5   Right pulmonary agenesis.

rupture of the membranes (Nimrod et al 1984). The outcome for babies born with bilateral hypoplasia is very variable and depends on the underlying lesion; it is worse for those who have associated renal abnormalities (Moessinger et al 1987).

Unilateral pulmonary hypoplasia can be asymptomatic and may occur spontaneously without other associated abnormalities. Either lung may be affected and some children present with recurrent respiratory tract infection. Chest X-ray (Fig. 4.6) shows mediastinal and tracheal deviation to the affected side, the hemithorax is smaller and the ribs appear 'crowded' together. The lung tissue appears more radiodense on the affected side and this pathology must be distinguished by radiological investigation from chronic collapse-consolidation. The long term outlook is usually very good. Bilateral lung hypoplasia is also seen in association with other lesions especially cardiac defects.

Dysplastic right lung (Scimitar syndrome)

The Scimitar syndrome is a dysmorphic condition of the right lung which includes pulmonary hypoplasia (Partridge et al 1988). The hypoplasia is associated with anomalous venous drainage usually to the right atrium or inferior vena cava and there are often systemic arterial collateral vessels of varying size as well. Patients may present with recurrent respiratory infec-

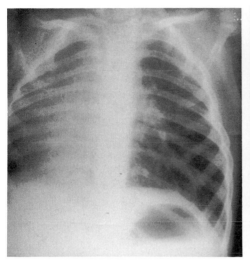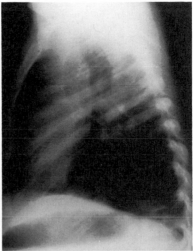

Fig. 4.6 Pulmonary hypoplasia of right lung; note compensatory overinflation of left lung.

tion or the abnormality may be detected on an incidental chest X-ray. This shows a small right lung with mediastinal shift to the right and an indistinct right heart border. The 'Scimitar' sign is caused by an abnormal vertical right upper lobe pulmonary vein running into the right atrium. Surgical correction of the vascular anomalies is recommended although the right lung usually functions well.

Diaphragmatic hernia

This occurs principally on the left side in the ratio of 4:1 compared to the right. The incidence varies from 1 in 2200–3500 births (Yu 1986). It usually occurs on the left as a posterolateral lesion through the foramen of Bochdalek. Unless the hernia has occurred very late during pregnancy, which is unusual, there is an accompanying hypoplasia of the lung on the affected side. This lung in particular suffers from a reduction in alveolar number as a consequence. The contralateral lung is also smaller than expected and has a reduced number of alveoli because of compression due to mediastinal shift during intrauterine life.

Chest X-ray (Fig. 4.7) shows bowel in the chest with lung compression on both sides. As the bowel distends with air the lung compression worsens and this is associated with increasingly severe respiratory distress. The differential diagnosis includes cystic adenomatoid malformation. The presence of a normally placed gastric bubble below the diaphragm should help to distinguish the two lesions. The passage of a nasogastric tube will deflate the bowel in diaphragmatic hernia and in other conditions will point out the correct position of the stomach. If there is any doubt then a barium swallow should be done. Treatment is surgical — the abdominal viscera are replaced

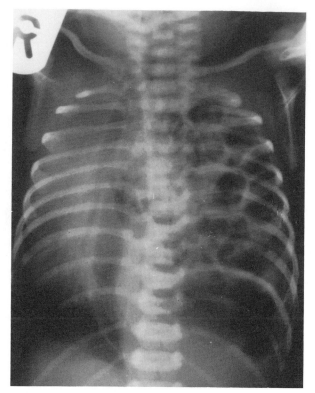

Fig. 4.7 Left-sided diaphragmatic hernia.

and the defect in the diaphragm is closed. The condition still carries a high mortality rate of about 60%. Persistent fetal circulation is not an uncommon complication and may require treatment with pulmonary vasodilators (Sumner & Frank 1981). The long term outcome depends on the underlying degree of pulmonary hypoplasia but the degree of lung growth may be quite satisfactory (Thurlbeck et al 1979). Approximately 5% of children with a diaphragmatic hernia present later after the neonatal period; some are even discovered as an incidental finding on chest X-ray.

Eventration of the diaphragm is due to a very thin layer of tissue representing the diaphragm muscle itself. This is usually non-functional and results in a 'high diaphragm' seen on the affected side of the chest X-ray. If it is of significant size it will require surgical plication.

Chylothorax

Chylothorax occurs for a number of reasons. In some cases it is congenital and is present at birth. At this stage the fluid is yellow and straw coloured as the infant has not yet had any fat in the diet. Congenital chylothorax usually resolves spontaneously after pleural tapping and sufficient drainage of the chest to allow expansion of the underlying lung. This form of neonatal chylothorax is more common in males than females and occurs slightly more often on the right side than the left. The baby should be started on a medium chain triglyceride milk to decrease the flow of chyle.

Chylothorax occurs later in association with underlying infection, malformation of the lymphatics, tumours and post-thoracic surgery. The treatment is similar and includes drainage to allow the underlying lung to re-expand and stick to the pleural surface. Prolonged drainage should be avoided as it leads to major protein loss and lymphocyte depletion (Yu 1986). If drainage fails then thoracotomy is required to cauterise the affected areas which are oozing chyle. In severe cases pleurectomy is usually effective. Chemical pleurodesis may also be used but is painful.

Rib cage anomalies

These are usually evident in the neonatal period and are often lethal if they result in severe reduction of rib cage size and hypoplasia of the underlying lung. Conditions in which this occurs include asphyxiating thoracic dystrophy (Jeune's syndrome), achondroplasia, thanatotrophic and camptomelic dwarfism. It is also seen in Ellis van Creveld syndrome (chondroectodermal dysplasia). Other conditions associated with severe respiratory difficulty include hypophosphatasia and osteogenesis imperfecta.

Asphyxiating thoracic dystrophy or Jeune's syndrome (Jeune 1955) is an autosomal recessive disorder characterised by a small thoracic cage with abnormal rib development which results in pulmonary hypoplasia. Associated anomalies include short limbs, hypoplastic iliac wings and renal dysplasia. The chest X-ray (Fig. 4.8) typically demonstrates a small thoracic cage with short ribs and irregularly widened costochondral junctions. Pelvic films confirm the ileal hypoplasia.

The degree of thoracic cage abnormality is variable and some children have relatively mild disease while others succumb to severe respiratory failure at an early age. The associated renal abnormality, which is usually manifested as chronic nephritis, can also lead to early death (Smith 1982).

Children with any type of severe rib cage anomaly who survive the neonatal period may have frequent episodes of cor pulmonale due to pulmonary hypertension which occurs during intercurrent infections thus stressing the infant's limited respiratory reserve. A number of cases have however survived with intensive respiratory support and some following successful surgery to enlarge the chest cavity. These patients may have further respiratory failure at puberty if the lungs fail to keep up with systemic growth.

Neuromuscular disease

A number of infants are born with congenital neuromuscular disease which presents at birth or in the first few days or weeks of life. The commonest

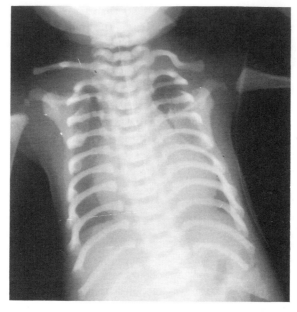

a

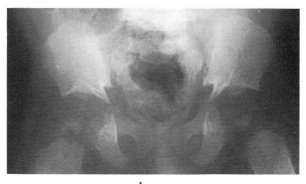

b

Fig. 4.8   a,b Jeune's asphyxiating thoracic dystrophy. Small short ribs, irregular widened costochondral junctions, small thoracic cage. Hypoplasia of ileal wings. Courtesy of Dr C M Hall.

condition causing this problem is spinal muscular atrophy (Werdnig-Hoffman disease). Severe birth asphyxia may also produce similar signs.

Werdnig-Hoffman disease is an autosomal recessive disorder. The onset of muscle weakness can occur during fetal life and be noticed as reduced intrauterine movements. Most other infants present at birth or in the first few months. The typical features which are seen in any infant with early muscle weakness include poor respiratory effort, a soft floppy rib cage, feeding and swallowing difficulty leading to recurrent aspiration (Volpe 1987). Fasciculation of the tongue is also present. The chest X-ray in these

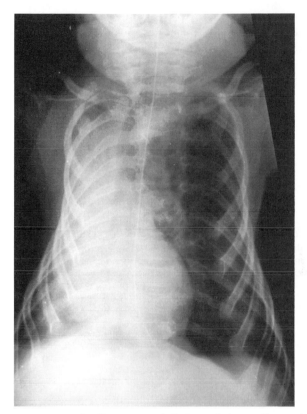

Fig. 4.9 Severe neuromuscular disease; note bell shape of chest wall secondary to muscle weakness.

children (Fig. 4.9) typically shows a 'bell-shaped' chest due to intercostal muscle weakness failing to overcome the intrinsic retractile forces of the lungs. There is no specific treatment and more than 50% of infants with Werdnig-Hoffman disease die in the first year of life.

Other conditions which present in this way include neonatal myotonic dystrophy, type II glycogen storage disease (Pompe's disease) and congenital myasthenia gravis. Myasthenia gravis in this age group is usually secondary to maternal disease although truly congenital and familial cases have been reported (Seybold & Lindstrom 1981). Treatment of neonatal myasthenia is with the judicious use of oral pyridostigmine following a diagnostic test with tensilon (edrophonium). Infants with myasthenia secondary to maternal disease usually recover by 4–6 weeks of age.

Arteriovenous fistula

Pulmonary arteriovenous fistula is a rare abnormality which is usually congenital in children. As many as 60% are associated with hereditary haemorrhagic telangiectasia (Rendu-Osler-Weber disease) which is inherited as an autosomal dominant. Many patients are asymptomatic but the classical presentation is with effort dyspnoea, cyanosis and clubbing. Chest X-ray typically shows a circumscribed noncalcified lesion most commonly in a lower lobe which is single in two-thirds of cases (Prager et al 1983). Further investigation requires digital subtraction or direct pulmonary angiography. Treatment is by intravascular embolisation or by localised surgical removal if possible.

REFERENCES

Cinnamond M J 1987 Congenital disorders of the larynx, trachea and bronchi. In: Evans J N G (ed) Scott-Brown's otolaryngology. Butterworths, London, pp 412–416
De Luca F G, Wesselhoeft C W 1978 Surgically treatable causes of neonatal respiratory distress. Clinics in Perinatology 5: 377–394
Dickson J A S 1985 Surgical Disorders. In: Harvey D, Kovar I (eds) Child health. A textbook for the DCH. Churchill Livingstone, Edinburgh, pp 264–282
Filler R M, Rossello P J, Lebnowitz R L 1976 Life threatening anoxic spells caused by tracheal compression after repair of esophageal atresia: correction by surgery. Journal of Pediatric Surgery 11: 739–748
Fogh-Anderson P 1968 Lips, palate, face and ear. In: Love M (ed) Bailey and Love's short practice of surgery, 14th edn. H K Lewis, London, p 452
Frenckner B, Freyschuss U 1982 Pulmonary function after lobectomy for congenital lobar emphysema and congenital cystic adenomatoid malformation. A follow up study. Scandinavian Journal of Thoracic and Cardiovascular Surgery 16: 293–298
Fraser F C 1958 Genetic counselling in some common paediatric diseases. Pediatric Clinics of North America 5: 475–491
Garfinkel T J, Handler S D 1980 Hemangioma of the head and neck. Journal of Otolaryngology 9: 435–450
Gordon I, Matthew D, Dinwiddie R 1987 Respiratory system. In: Gordon I (ed) Diagnostic imaging in paediatrics. Chapman and Hall, London, pp 27–57
Hollinger L D 1980 Etiology of stridor in the neonate, infant and child. Annals of Otology, Rhinology and Laryngology 89: 397–400
Jeune M, Beraud C, Carron R 1955 Dystrophie thoracique asphyxiante de caractere familial. Archives Francais Pediatrie 12: 886
Kauten J R, Konrad H R, Wichterman K A 1984 Laryngotracheoesophageal cleft in the newborn. International Journal of Pediatric Otolaryngology 8: 61–71
Knox W F, Barson A J 1986 Pulmonary hypoplasia in a regional perinatal unit. Early Human Development 14: 33–42
McBride J T, Wohl M E, Strieder D J et al 1980 Lung growth and airway function after lobectomy in infancy for congenital lobar emphysema. Journal of Clinical Investigation 66: 962–970
Moessinger A C, Fox H E, Higgin A, Rey H R, Al Haideri M 1987 Fetal breathing movements are not a reliable indicator of continued lung development in pregnancies complicated by oligohydramnios. Lancet ii: 1297–1300
Nimrod C, Varela-Gittings G, Machin G, Campbell D, Wesenberg R 1984 The effect of very prolonged membrane rupture on fetal development. American Journal of Obstetrics and Gynecology 148: 540–543
Paradise J L, Bluestone C D, Felder H 1969 The universality of otitis media in 50 infants with cleft palate. Pediatrics 44: 35–42
Partridge J B, Osborne J M, Slaughter R E 1988 Scimitar etcetera. The dysmorphic ring lung. Clinical Radiology 39: 11–19
Petterson G 1955 Inhibited separation of the larynx and upper part of the trachea from the esophagus in the newborn: report of a case sucessfully operated on. Acta Chirurgica Scandinavica 110: 250–254
Prager R L, Laws K H, Bender H W 1983 Arteriovenous fistula of the lung. The Annals of Thoracic Surgery 36: 231–239

Roesler N, De Leval M, Chrispin A, Stark J 1983 Surgical management of vascular ring. Annals of Surgery 197: 139–146

Seybold M E, Lindstrom J M 1981 Myasthenia gravis in infancy. Neurology 31: 476–480

Smith D W (ed) 1982 Recognisable patterns of human malformation. Major problems in clinical pediatrics VII, Saunders, Philadelphia, pp 244–245

Stocker J T, Madewell J E, Drake R M 1977 Congenital cystic adenomatiod malformation of the lung. Human Pathology 8: 155–171

Strife J L, Baumel A S, Scott Dunbar J 1981 Tracheal compression by the innominate artery in infancy and childhood. Radiology 139: 73–75

Strong 1987 Recurrent respiratory papillomatosis. In: J N G Evans (ed) Scott-Brown's otolaryngology. Butterworths, London, pp 466–470

Suhonen H, Kero P O, Puhakka H, Vilkki P 1984 Saccular cyst of the larynx in infants. International Journal of Pediatric Otorhinolaryngology 8: 73–78

Sumner E, Frank J D 1981 Tolazoline in the treatment of congenital diaphragmatic hernias. Archives of Disease in Childhood 56: 350–353

Thurlbeck W M, Kida K, Langston C et al 1979 Postnatal lung growth after repair of diaphragmatic hernia. Thorax 34: 338–343

Volpe J J (ed) 1987 Neuromuscular disorders: levels above the lower motor neuron to the neuromuscular junction. In: Neurology of the newborn. Saunders, Philadelphia, pp 477–507

Westaby S, Dinwiddie R, Chrispin A R, Stark J 1984 Pulmonary artery sling in identical twins. Thoracic and Cardiovascular Surgery 32: 182–183

Yu V Y H (ed) 1986 Congenital respiratory anomalies. In: Respiratory disorders of the newborn. Churchill Livingstone, Edinburgh, pp 133–150

5. Ear, nose and throat problems

J. N. G. Evans   R. J. Black

PIERRE ROBIN SYNDROME

The well recognised combination of micrognathia, glossoptosis and cleft palate is known as the Pierre Robin syndrome. It is preferable to consider this disorder as a nonspecific anomalad which may occur as an isolated defect or as part of a broader pattern of malformations (Gorlin et al 1976). The most common conditions associated with the Robin anomalad are Stickler syndrome (Herrman et al 1975), Camptomelic syndrome (Storer & Grossman 1974) and persistent left superior vena cava syndrome (Gorlin et al 1970). A range of other cardiovascular, skeletal and ocular abnormalities have also been described (Smith & Stowe 1961, Gewitz et al 1978).

Pathogenesis

The primary defect is probably arrested development of the mandible resulting in hypoplasia (Latham 1966). This prevents normal descent of the tongue between the palatal shelves, which therefore cannot come together and fuse. It occurs in approximately 1:30 000 live births (Schuknecht 1974).

Clinical features

At birth the facies is striking with a small symmetrically receded mandible producing an 'Andy Gump' appearance. The micrognathia provides very little support for the tongue musculature and this allows it to fall downwards and backwards (glossoptosis). In this position, it produces airway obstruction on inhalation particularly in the supine position or when relaxed during sleep. The palatal defect may vary from a cleft uvula to that which involves two-thirds of the hard palate. A cleft lip is not a part of this anomalad. Associated feeding problems occur as a result of both the cleft palate and inadequate control of the tongue. The difficulty in nursing, cyanotic episodes and choking fits may suggest tracheoesophageal fistula or choanal atresia. Because of the distinct appearance, however, diagnosis should not be difficult.

Management

Respiratory obstruction

A number of techniques have been used to overcome the respiratory obstruction such as glossopexy or nursing prone with the aid of a special frame or with the head suspended in a stockinette taped to the scalp. The most successful way of relieving the obstruction is with the use of a nasopharyngeal airway (Fig. 5.1). This results in the abolition of cyanotic episodes, relief of heart failure, improved blood gases and better weight gain when compared with those nursed in a prone position (Heaf et al 1982). Careful placement of the nasopharyngeal airway is necessary with lateral neck radiography (Fig. 5.2) to check the position. The ideal site is for the tip to be just above the level of the epiglottis. There is a positive correlation between the length of the nasopharyngeal tube and crown/heel length (Fig. 5.3) but this is only useful in providing initial guidelines. Optimal position must still be confirmed by clinical assessment.

High caloric intake is provided and supplemented by nasogastric feeds for those unable to cope with oral feeds. Both this and the decreased metabolic demands on breathing from accurate positioning of the

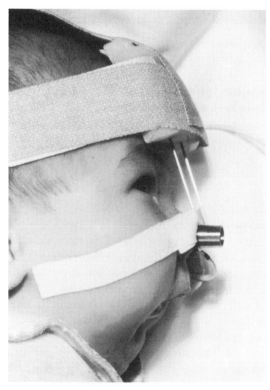

Fig. 5.1   Long term nasopharyngeal airway to overcome the respiratory obstruction in Pierre Robin syndrome.

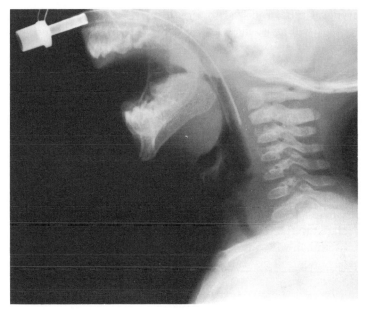

Fig. 5.2   Lateral neck X-ray to show correct position of nasopharyngeal tube in Pierre Robin syndrome behind the tongue but above the epiglottis.

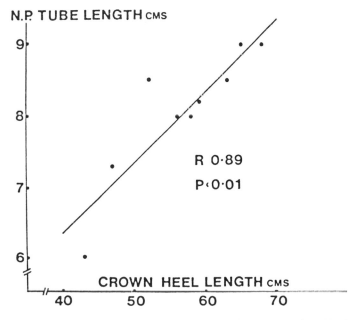

Fig. 5.3   Nasopharyngeal tube length for use in Pierre Robin syndrome (from Heaf et al 1982, reproduced by kind permission from *Journal of Pediatrics*).

nasopharyngeal tube, will lead to a rapid increase in body weight (Heaf et al 1982). This will assist in the natural resolution which occurs with mandibular growth.

Cleft palate

The optimal timing of palate surgery is a subject of considerable debate. Early establishment of velopharyngeal competency may benefit speech development although there is evidence that palatal surgery may inhibit facial growth (Schuller & Krause 1979). In any case, the rate of growth of the mandible will determine the timing of closure of the cleft palate (Campbell & Watson 1980). For those with palatal defects, long term dental care is mandatory with orthodontic and prosthodontic treatment being directly related to the timing of surgery and the results obtained. It requires personnel familiar with the related abnormalities and able to provide long term management. This can be divided into three phases (Schuller & Krause 1979):

1. Expansion of the maxillary segments.
2. Treatment of the mixed abnormalities of deciduous dentition.
3. Full band appliances for proper occlusion of permanent dentition.

The efficacy of speech therapy in improving articulation has been demonstrated by Van Demark (1974) but this is not the only role of the speech therapist. Diagnostic functions utilizing speech assessment, manometric pressure measurement and palatal screening are important and allow conclusions to be drawn regarding the effectiveness of velopharyngeal closure.

Otologic problems

Chronic secretory otitis media is common in the cleft palate patient. Even following palatal repair there is still altered function of the tensor palati muscle (which opens the Eustachian tube) because its tendon is usually slipped off the hamulus to facilitate palatal closure (Schuller & Krause 1979). The hearing loss produced will significantly affect auditory processing skills and language unless treated (Lewis 1976) by aspiration of the fluid and insertion of ventilating tubes (Pappas 1974). The authors recommend that adenoids not be removed as velopharyngeal competence may be disturbed.

Once the general condition has been stabilized with the nasopharyngeal airway and the baby is feeding satisfactorily, there is no reason why they cannot be successfully managed at home. Adequate local nursing and medical supervision must be ensured, however. Because of the multisystem involvement and long term management required, a team approach is emphasised. This will also assist in giving considerable support to the parents.

CHOANAL ATRESIA

The term choanal atresia implies occlusion of the nasal airway. There are a number of causes of nasal obstruction when considering the differential diagnosis. Less common ones to be borne in mind in the neonate include encephaloceles, gliomas and dermoids. However, generally the term is taken to mean congenital posterior choanal atresia.

Embryology

There are three commonly accepted theories as to the cause. First, persisting bucconasal membrane; second, persisting buccopharyngeal membrane; and third, adhesions. A detailed explanation of the embryological development of the nose is given by Cinnamond (1987). It appears that a persisting bucconasal membrane is the most likely explanation since the atretic segments are situated anterior to the foramen of Lushka (representing the site of the embryonic Rathke's pouch); are invariably bony (the buccopharyngeal membrane does not have a core of mesoderm); and are remarkably symmetrical (unlikely if due to adhesions).

Types and incidence

Choanal atresia may be unilateral or bilateral, complete or incomplete, bony or membranous. Approximately 60% are unilateral (Pracy 1978a) and a significant preponderance of these occur on the right side. Complete bony obstruction occurs in 90% of cases and the male to female ratio is 3:2 (Kaplan 1985). Forty-eight per cent of cases have other congenital abnormalities of which 80% are major defects of other systems such as cardiac defects, craniosynostosis or renal dysplasia. Choanal atresia is especially associated with the so called CHARGE syndrome (Pagon et al 1981) in which there is: 'C' colobomata of the eyes, 'H' heart disease, 'A' atresia of the choanae, 'R' retarded growth and development, 'G' genital hypoplasia in males and 'E' ear deformities (Kaplan 1985).

Clinical features

By instinct, a newborn baby breathes through the nose; mouth breathing is a technique acquired slowly. Thus the main potential danger in bilateral choanal atresia is death from asphyxia but it is important to be aware that the same possibility can occur in unilateral atresia if the patent side of the nose becomes obstructed for other reasons. The history is fairly typical. Immediately post-partum, the baby cries and during this period there is no evidence of respiratory distress. When the baby settles down the classic cycle of events is seen: there is obvious respiratory obstruction with suprasternal and intercostal recession and cyanosis. All these symptoms are relieved dramatically when the baby cries. Feeding difficulties are experienced because of the inability to suck and breathe at the same time.

The symptoms of unilateral choanal atresia are less well defined. Although degrees of respiratory obstruction and feeding difficulties are likely to occur in the neonatal period, the presenting symptom is frequently a mucoid nasal discharge some months later. Snoring is not a symptom of unilateral or bilateral atresia.

Diagnosis and management

In the delivery room, the diagnosis is frequently suspected on the typical clinical features plus not being able to pass a suction catheter through the nose to remove mucus from the upper respiratory tract. The latter is a routine procedure immediately following birth.

Establishing oral respiration is of immediate importance. This is best achieved by inserting a Guedel airway size 00 into the mouth and fixing it with adhesive tape. This stabilises the situation and allows formal examination and assessment of the baby. Another attempt should be made to pass a catheter through the nose. If there is any doubt about the diagnosis contrast X-rays should be performed. Computerised tomography (CT) is also useful in demonstrating abnormality of the lateral wall of the nasal cavity and the bony fusion if present (Wetmore & Mahboubi 1986). In view of the high incidence of other congenital abnormalities, general paediatric assessment is vital and any necessary investigations should be commenced.

Arrangements should then be made for immediate surgical correction. There is no place, in our opinion, for medical management unless, due to prematurity or other congenital abnormalities, the overall prognosis is poor. We feel the risks of pneumonia from inadequate pulmonary ventilation and inhalation of food are a common sequel to medical management. This may prejudice survival particularly if there are other congenital problems.

The baby is fed as necessary by an orogastric tube. Surgical correction is not an emergency procedure and can be performed on a routine operating list (usually within one or two days). Blood should be available but transfusion is rarely necessary.

Operative treatment

In the past, a tracheostomy was performed to safeguard the airway (Pracy 1978a) but most authorities now agree this is not necessary. The two most common approaches for repair of the choanal atresia are endonasal and transpalatal (Maniglia & Goodwin 1981) but transeptal and transantral approaches have been described for the older patient. The subject has been well reviewed by Pirsig (1986) and Cinnamond (1987).

The current policy of the senior author (JNGE) is to perform endonasal repair. The technique is as follows: a Boyle Davis tonsillectomy gag is inserted to give access to the post nasal space, the atretic segment is perforated endonasally using a curved urethral sound, the perforation is enlarged using an electric drill and diamond burr, portex tubing is inserted as a splint to prevent re-stenosis (Fig. 5.4).

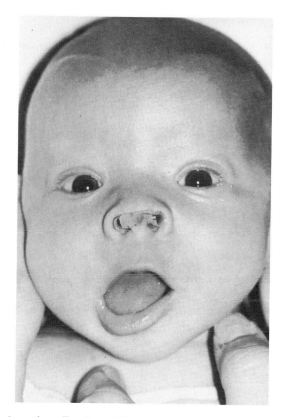

Fig. 5.4 Choanal atresia: splints in position.

Postoperatively the baby should be nursed in an incubator with high humidity. Normal feeding may be commenced within 12 hours. There still may be difficulties with feeding, however, because of mucoid nasal discharge partially blocking the tubes. The parents need to be instructed in how to keep the tubes clear and they are supplied with portable suckers for this purpose. The tubes are removed in the outpatient department in 6 weeks. Routine bouginage by the parents is not advocated since they find it unpleasant to do and therefore frequently perform it inadequately.

The parents are naturally concerned about the prognosis but reassurance can be given that the local condition itself is not of a serious nature. This encouragement should be given, however, with the information that more than one operation may be required (e.g. dilatation, formal revision by endonasal or transpalatal route).

The risk of hereditary transmission is approximately 6% (Evans & Machlachlan 1971) but it is very difficult to know how accurate this is from the small numbers reported. If the parents are particularly concerned, genetic counselling would be desirable and a case could be made for future confinements taking place in hospital.

TONSIL AND ADENOID PROBLEMS

The literature on the tonsil and adenoid problem is extensive with divergent opinions and experience being expressed (Jazbi 1980, Hibbert 1987). The authors here present the indications for surgery currently in practice at The Hospitals for Sick Children, London (Table 5.1) and briefly discuss the basis for each situation.

Biopsy to define possible malignancy

Tonsillectomy, or even unilateral tonsillectomy, in order to obtain tissue for histological proof of a suspected malignancy is a procedure that would undoubtedly be accepted by all medical practitioners.

Obstructive sleep apnoea

Cor pulmonale due to chronic upper airway obstruction was first described in children by Menashe et al (1965). There are two major factors in the genesis of the obstruction (Bailey & Croft 1987). Loss of tone in postural muscles is a normal part of the neurological changes during sleep, being pronounced during the rapid eye movement (REM) phase. The flaccid tongue and pharyngeal wall do not cause obstruction in normal children, but when combined with partial obstruction of the upper airway, obstructive sleep apnoea occurs. The site of obstruction is variable but in the child is most commonly related to tonsil and adenoid hypertrophy (Kravath et al 1977). A well defined sequence of events occurs: the hypoventilation leads to hypoxia and hypercapnia until the patient is rescued by central arousal mechanisms. The blood gases then return to normal and the child drifts back to sleep.

By definition, obstructive sleep apnoea is diagnosed when at least 30 apnoeic episodes of 10 seconds or longer occur in a 7 hour period (Guillemi-

Table 5.1   Indications for tonsillectomy and adenoidectomy

Tonsillectomy and adenoidectomy
    Obstructive sleep apnoea

Tonsillectomy
    Definite indication
        Biopsy, to confirm possible maligancy
        Obstructive sleep apnoea
        Peritonsillar abscess
    Relative indication
        Recurrent tonsillitis
        ± poor weight gain

Adenoidectomy
    Nasal obstruction from adenoid hypertrophy
    Secretory otitis media

nault et al 1976). This recurrent nocturnal hypoxia and hypercapnia produces the following major symptoms (Sullivan 1980):

1. Excessive daytime sleepiness from reduced synthesis of neurotransmitters although sleep fragmentation is a likely contribution;
2. Pulmonary hypoventilation and right ventricular hypertrophy from the induced increase in pulmonary vascular resistance;
3. Bradycardia and arrythmias via a vagally mediated reflex resulting from hypoxia without lung expansion.

The diagnosis may be difficult with poor performance at school due to excessive daytime sleepiness being the major presenting problem. The physical examination is often unremarkable. The diagnosis can be confirmed, however, by observation and continuous percutaneous Po_2 and Pco_2 or oxygen saturation measurement while the child is asleep (Rowe et al 1980). In advanced cases, the pulmonary arterial structural changes persist (Levy et al 1967). Hence greater awareness of this syndrome is essential so it may be recognised and treated early. There is increasing evidence that this condition may be completely cured by adenotonsillectomy (Eliaschar et al 1980, Mauer et al 1983). Adenoidectomy alone, however, does not consistently cure all symptoms (Massumi 1969).

Peritonsillar abscess (Quinsy)

A peritonsillar abscess has significant complications (Lee et al 1973):

1. Inflammatory swelling combined with medial and downward displacement of the tonsil causing upper airway obstruction;
2. Spontaneous rupture with aspiration;
3. Dissection into the parapharyngeal space with base of skull involvement;
4. Involvement of the retropharyngeal space and mediastinum.

Because of this and the fact that recurrent abscesses frequently occur (Kornblut & Kornblut 1980), tonsillectomy is advised. Initial drainage of the abscess followed by an interval tonsillectomy is the commonly accepted practice although primary tonsillectomy in the acute phase is advocated by Beeden & Evans (1970).

Recurrent tonsillitis

The authors feel that tonsillectomy is indicated in children when chronic persistent or recurrent acute tonsillitis results in loss of significant amounts of time from school and requires considerable expenditure of time and money in providing medical care. Careful selection criteria are necessary with the most important being accurate diagnosis and documentation of the episodes of tonsillitis. The history from the parent or child is unreliable

(Paradise et al 1978) and this has resulted in unsatisfactory surgical results in the past. There are many arguments against performing a tonsillectomy but the authors wish to draw the reader's attention to the following facts:

1. The overwhelming majority of instances of tonsillitis are not bacterial in origin (Kisch 1976). It is thought to be a recurrent bacterial-viral illness with the virus being primarily Epstein-Barr Virus (EBV) and adenovirus being a poor second (Sprinkle et al 1980). Once EBV is acquired in the B-cells of the tonsils or adenoids, the genome remains permanently. Medical treatment in the form of antibiotics may not solve the problem permanently.

2. Children who suffer from recurrent tonsillitis have been shown to have an abnormal bacterial-viral microflora (Sprinkle et al 1980). This is converted to normal following adenotonsillectomy.

3. While there is no satisfactory prospective controlled trial reported to date which supports the role of tonsillectomy (Jazbi 1980), there is also no evidence that tonsil disease can be modified by medical treatment (Editorial 1977).

4. The tonsils and adenoids are an integral part of the gut-associated lymphoid tissue but represent a very small percentage of the total. Removal has repeatedly failed to compromise the immunological competence in animals and humans (Sprinkle & Veltri 1979). By rigidly applying the proper indications for tonsillectomy, the authors feel the child's quality of life can be improved and the abnormal or impaired function of the throat returned to normal.

Nasal obstruction from adenoid hypertrophy

Hypertrophied adenoids can obstruct the posterior choanae; interfering with nasal airflow and causing stasis of secretions, this may predispose to chronic sinusitis. Adenoid enlargement is best confirmed by lateral radiograph which also gives an assessment of the size of the airway (Hibbert 1987). If there is significant nasal obstruction, mouth breathing, snoring and persistent low grade nasal congestion without major allergic precipitants then adenoidectomy is indicated. Using these criteria adequate nasal breathing can then be re-established.

Secretory otitis media

Secretory otitis media develops when eustachian tube dysfunction disturbs the complex mucociliary transport system of the middle ear cleft (Potsic 1980). Clinical conditions that predispose to this are:

1. Anatomical deformities such as cleft palate and craniofacial anomalies;
2. Inflammatory conditions of the upper respiratory tract;

3. Systemic disorders such as hypoparathyroidism and mucopolysac-
charidosis;
4. Nasopharyngeal obstruction as seen with tumours and adenoid hypertrophy.

Treatment must take into account the middle ear effusion (MEE) and
any underlying predisposition must be searched for. The general approach
to both aspects must be aggressive because of the potential serious effects
on language and speech development (Lewis 1976), the associated risk of
infection producing sensorineural hearing loss and the possibility of retraction and cholesteatoma developing. The MEE is treated by myringotomy
and insertion of grommets (Editorial 1981). The adenoids should be
removed when they cause or contribute to the eustachian tube dysfunction.
They need not physically obstruct the eustachian tube as their influence on
nasal airflow and frequency of swallowing will affect the volumetric and air
pressure changes occurring routinely in the upper respiratory tract (Smyth
1980).

TRACHEOSTOMY

The first successful tracheostomy in a child was recorded in 1766 (Rogers
1987). Until the early part of this century, tracheostomy was the only procedure available for the relief of upper airway obstruction and for repeated
aspiration of the lower respiratory tract. With the development of paediatric
anaesthesia and increased understanding of the respiratory problems of
small infants, long term nasotracheal intubation is possible (Pracy 1978b).
This enables the surgeon to avoid a tracheostomy and its associated complications in many cases. Also with the development of endolaryngeal
microsurgery, many cysts and tumours can be removed endoscopically.
Hence, a tracheostomy is required in only a small percentage of infants
and neonates with respiratory problems.

Indications for tracheostomy

A tracheostomy is indicated in those infants and children in whom:

1. Acute upper airway obstruction which cannot be bypassed by an
   endotracheal tube (e.g. facial trauma, supraglottitis, epiglottitis);
2. Chronic upper airway obstruction exists (e.g. laryngeal webs, subglottic
   stenosis, subglottic haemangioma, vocal cord palsy);
3. Respiratory failure requires intermittent positive pressure ventilation
   for a considerable period.

As well as relieving the obstruction, the tracheostomy will facilitate
aspiration of tracheobronchial secretions and reduce the anatomical dead
space, thus decreasing ventilatory resistance.

INVESTIGATION OF UPPER AIRWAY OBSTRUCTION

History and examination

It is imperative that a correct diagnosis of the cause of respiratory distress be made before considering a tracheostomy. The only exception is a severe airway problem that demands immediate intervention. The clinician should be mindful of the wide variety of other conditions which can cause respiratory distress even without airway obstruction (Cotton & Richardson 1981), for example intracranial haemorrhage or large abdominal mass. A careful history and full examination are vital.

Stridor is the cardinal sign of laryngeal problems. It is of particular value to determine the time of onset, whether it is intermittent or continuous, positional or associated with dysphagia. Variation in the quality and pitch of the stridor depends on the degree and level of obstruction. Auscultation of the neck also assists in estimating the level of obstruction.

Appropriate X-rays of the upper airway include a lateral view of the neck, AP and lateral view of the chest and high kV filter view (Gordon et al 1987). Xerograms are occasionally useful (Benjamin 1979) but the radiation dose is high. A barium swallow is routinely performed to exclude vascular lesions causing extrinsic tracheal compression. Thoracic CT scan will be necessary for certain selected cases.

Endoscopic assessment

At the completion of the above, the surgeon generally has a reasonable idea of the site and nature of the lesion. However, endoscopy must be performed to determine the exact diagnosis. The use of the ancillary investigations should not replace the need for this as the incidence of erroneous diagnoses based on their results is high (Cohen et al 1980). These tests serve only to indicate whether additional therapy might be necessary at the time.

Tracheostomy should be carried out under general anaesthetic in an operating theatre with full aseptic technique. A selection of tracheostomy tubes must be readily available and the connections must be checked in every case. The authors routinely use the Great Ormond Street pattern plastic tracheostomy tube (Searle) (Fig. 5.5). The actual surgical technique is well described by Rogers (1987). At the completion, the tube must be securely fixed in position with tapes and stay sutures.

Postoperative care

The tracheostomised infant should be nursed initially in an environment of high humidity since nasal respiration has been bypassed. The need for this will decline. Frequent aspiration of the tracheobronchial tree is necessary and must be performed with full aseptic precautions. Normal saline (0.5 ml) is instilled prior to this to loosen secretions. Feeding may be difficult in the

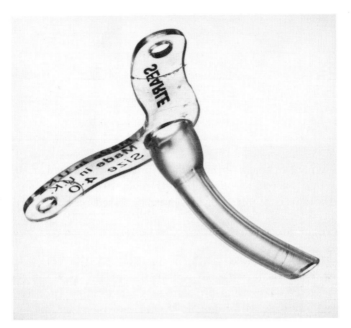

Fig. 5.5 Great Ormond Street pattern plastic tracheostomy tube (Searle).

early postoperative period and supplementation via a nasogastric tube may be necessary. The wound should be dressed, the tapes changed daily, and the tube changed every week (or sooner if secretions are a problem). The first tube change should be performed by the surgeon.

When the primary pathology which necessitated the tracheostomy is limited to the upper airway, the child makes rapid progress. If a long term tracheostomy appears likely, the child does not have to stay in hospital; the parents can be taught the skills of home tracheostomy care and provided with the necessary equipment. A specially prepared booklet (Singh & Innes 1981) gives details of the operation itself, suction, care and changing of tubes, and everyday hints. The child is not discharged until the parents are confident and arrangements have been made with the General Practitioner, Health Visitor and local hospital.

Complications

In a review by Rodgers et al (1979), of 108 children with a tracheostomy, the overall mortality rate from all causes was 44% with 6.5% being due to complications of the tracheostomy itself. Table 5.2 enumerates the most common possibilities but most of these should be avoidable by proper technique at the time of operation and scrupulous postoperative care.

Bacterial colonisation of the tracheobronchial tree almost always occurs (Aass 1975) and is possibly more common in children (Espinoza et al 1974).

Table 5.2   Complications of tracheostomy

Operative	Postoperative	
	Early	Late
Haemorrhage	Infection	Tracheomalacia
Air embolus	Obstruction of tubes	Stenosis
Damage to nearby structures	Accidental decannulation	Fistula
Apnoea	Pneumomediastinum/pneumothorax	
	Tracheal erosion and haemorrhage	

The development of tracheobronchitis or pneumonia, however, appears unrelated to this bacterial colonisation (Brook 1979). Therefore, whether antibiotic therapy is required or not must be based on clinical criteria.

Decannulation

Once the primary pathology which necessitated the tracheostomy has resolved or been dealt with, decannulation is the next objective. The simplest method for assessing the readiness for decannulation is to occlude the tracheostomy tube with a finger. If the child tolerates this for a minute without distress, then decannulation should be possible. Even with an apparently adequate airway, difficulties may be encountered and are often related to the duration of the tracheostomy. Part of the problem is psychological (Pracy et al 1981) because the child is used to breathing through a tracheostomy and cannot adjust to normal. This so called 'decannulation panic', however, is insufficient to explain the problem. Definite mechanical problems do exist and are likely to occur in children rather than adults as air passages are both absolutely and relatively smaller. Re-establishment of the normal pathway of breathing results in an increase in dead space and consequent increased resistance to airflow. Here, decannulation on a controlled and gradual basis is advocated using an Alder Hey Hospital fenestrated silver tracheostomy tube (Fig. 5.6) (Downs Surgical Ltd). This can be serially blocked and has the advantage of permitting evaluation of the ability to ventilate effectively and can be easily reversed if difficulties occur. When the tube can be blocked for 24 hours, it may be removed and the fistula covered with a sterile dressing.

VOCAL CORD PALSY

Aetiology

Abduction paralysis of the vocal cord may be unilateral or bilateral corresponding approximately to a peripheral or central aetiology. It is important to consider the differential diagnosis (Table 5.3) and search for the cause. Congenital paralysis is the most likely but its aetiology will remain uncertain in many cases (Holinger et al 1976a, Emery & Fearon 1984). Bilateral paralysis is commonly associated with central nervous system problems. Intracerebral bleeding during birth, meningocele,

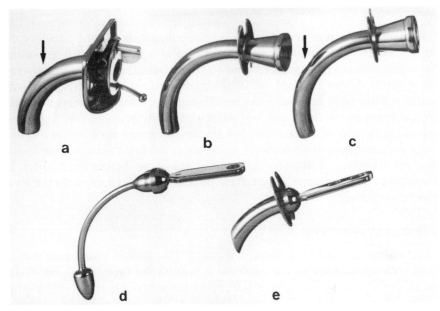

Fig. 5.6 Alder Hey Hospital silver tracheostomy tube (20 FG): (a) outer tube with an adjustable flange to alter position of the fenestration (arrowed); (b) inner tube without fenestration (sleeping tube); (c) inner tube with speaking valve and fenestration (arrowed); (d) introducer; (e) blocker.

encephalocele, Arnold-Chiari malformation, hydrocephalus, cerebral agenesis, and dysgenesis of the nucleus ambiguus are the most common (Cotton & Richardson 1981).

Unilateral paralysis is the most commonly encountered (Fearon & Ellis 1971). The one normally functioning vocal cord often provides adequate laryngeal respiratory function with a weak cry and occasional stridor when agitated being the main symptoms. The stridor is louder when the infant is awake and may be positional. Bilateral paralysis is associated with more serious respiratory obstruction and marked inspiratory stridor. The cry, however, may be relatively normal. Intermittent aspiration and cyanosis during feeding can occur due to inco-ordination of the cricopharyngeus muscle and loss of sensation in the area if the superior laryngeal nerve function is abnormal.

Table 5.3 Differential diagnosis of vocal cord palsy

Congenital	Acquired
Unilateral	CNS
Associated with abnormalities of	Trauma (including iatrogenic)
cardiovascular/respiratory systems and	Inflammation
upper gastrointestinal tract	Neoplastic
Birth trauma	Vascular
Bilateral	Idiopathic
Central nervous system	

Management

Endoscopic evaluation provides the definitive diagnosis of cord paralysis although electromyography has been suggested as a means of differentiating between this and cricoarytenoid joint fixation (Guindi et al 1981). Management of the airway is based on symptomatic criteria with a tracheostomy being performed if necessary. As mentioned previously, a diligent search for the aetiology should be pursued with appropriate neurological, radiological and laboratory investigations. If a tracheostomy has been necessary, the child is endoscoped at six-monthly intervals in the hope there will be spontaneous recovery. A number of years must lapse before cord palsy is assumed to be permanent. Thereafter, three alternatives exist as to the long term management:

Valved tracheostomy tube

This allows the child to inspire through the tracheostomy but expire through a fenestration on the converse surface of the tube, thus permitting air to traverse the larynx. Thereafter phonation is possible (Biller & Lawson 1980). There is still the disadvantage, however, that the need for a tracheostomy is not eliminated.

Lateralization of the vocal cord

Whether this is performed endoscopically or as an extralaryngeal arytenoidectomy (Biller & Lawson 1980), the result is to provide an adequate airway and thus permit decannulation. The major disadvantage with this procedure is that the voice may be significantly weakened.

Laryngeal reinervation

A technique for selective reinervation of the posterior cricoarytenoid muscle has been described (Tucker 1980). This utilises a neuromuscular pedicle derived from branches of the ansa cervicalis nerve to the strap muscles. This has the theoretical advantage of improving the airway without adversely affecting phonation. However, the lack of proper documentation of postoperative results (Biller & Lawson 1980) seriously questions the validity of this procedure. Also, it would certainly have no role to play when there is a central aetiology for the palsy.

A delicate balance always exists between airway and quality of voice. The decision as to the most appropriate treatment is based on the particular needs of the patient, associated presence or absence of cricoarytenoid joint fixation, and the judgement of a surgeon experienced in this area.

SUBGLOTTIC STENOSIS

The incidence of acquired subglottic stenosis in infants and children appears to be increasing (Cotton 1978) and may be explained by the use of long term endotracheal intubation as a means of respiratory support. However, it is also reasonable to assume that the initial mortality may have been higher prior to the development of long term endotracheal intubation and increased understanding of respiratory problems in small infants. The incidence of congenital subglottic stenosis may also be higher than is generally assumed because of symptoms mistakenly attributed to other entities. For example, a subglottic stenosis with marginal obstruction may present a serious problem only when there is a superimposed laryngotracheobronchitis.

Embryology of congenital subglottic stenosis

The larynx begins developing at the fourth week of fetal life. In the seven week embryo there is marked epithelial proliferation obliterating the lumen with recanalisation occurring at nine weeks. Failure to recanalise completely may result in atresia, webs or stenosis. The subglottic region of the larynx is formed by the conus elasticus and the rigid circumferential cricoid cartilage. The underlying pathology of congenital subglottic stenosis, therefore, is an abnormality of the cricoid cartilage. The normal cartilagenous diameter in the newborn full term infant is 5.5 mm with an effective intramucosal diameter of 4.5 mm (Fearon & Cotton 1972). Symptoms begin to occur when this diameter is reduced to 4 mm.

Stridor is the cardinal symptom and must be fully investigated. The need for, and timing of, a tracheostomy is based on clinical criteria; it is usual policy to manage all patients conservatively in the first instance. This is because the infant larynx is not only absolutely smaller but also relatively smaller than an adult larynx (Tucker & Tucker 1979). As the child grows, therefore, the airway may improve and the symptoms resolve. Children who have not required a tracheostomy are reviewed regularly in the outpatient department and the parents are advised to contact the hospital if symptoms worsen. In those children with a tracheostomy, endoscopy is performed at three monthly intervals to assess laryngeal growth. If there has not been significant improvement in 12 months, surgical intervention is considered. Although dilatation of the stenosis is advocated by Holinger et al (1976b) the results are disappointing (Cinnamond 1987). Open surgical correction of the stenosis at a relatively early stage appears justified as it may circumvent some of the morbidity and mortality associated with a long term tracheostomy (Rodgers et al 1979). Also, experimental (Calcaterra et al 1974) and clinical (Cotton & Evans 1981) evidence indicate that surgery on the growing larynx does not interfere with the normal growth potential.

Operative reconstruction

Cotton (1978) describes splitting the cricoid cartilage anteriorly and inserting a costal cartilage rib graft to widen the airway. Difficulties in accurate maintenance of the graft in the correct position are sometimes encountered.

Grahne (1971) describes splitting the cricoid posteriorly although there is a risk of damage to the arytenoid cartilages thus affecting the voice.

The current practice at The Hospitals for Sick Children, London is to perform a laryngo-tracheoplasty (Figs 5.7 and 5.8) (Evans & Todd 1974, Evans 1987). Briefly, the surgical technique involves a castellated incision of the larynx and upper trachea to enter the subglottis. A rolled silastic stent is placed in the glottis, subglottis and upper trachea to guide the mucosa in its healing process and the segments of cartilage are sewn together in a distracted position. The stent is removed endoscopically at 6 weeks. Decannulation should then be possible soon after.

All conservative efforts to establish an airway must be considered prior to surgical intervention. Following this, external laryngotracheal reconstruction has the advantage of early extubation and a relatively shorter hospital stay with reduction in the number of anaesthetics.

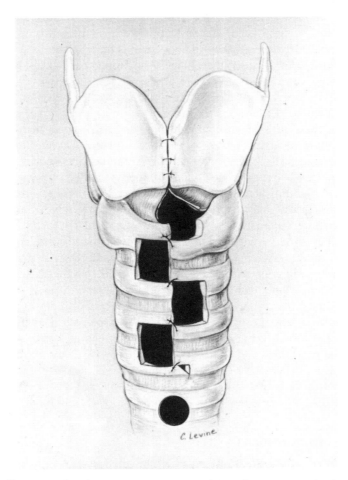

Fig. 5.7 Laryngotracheoplasty: castellated incision with cartilage sewn together in a distracted position to increase the airway lumen.

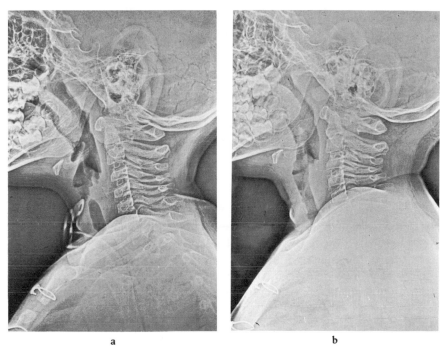

a   b

Fig. 5.8 Xerograms showing (a) complete respiratory obstruction due to subglottic stenosis, and (b) the same child after relief of the obstruction by laryngotracheoplasty (reproduced by kind permission from Hatch D J, Sumner E 1981 Neonatal Anaesthesia, Edward Arnold, London).

CLEFT LARYNX

A laryngotracheoesophageal cleft occurs because of failure of rostral development of the tracheoesophageal septum (Cotton & Richardson 1981). This normally occurs at 35 days gestation and results in failure of dorsal fusion of the cricoid cartilage 10 days later. It is a very rare condition. A posterior cleft limited to the larynx is an anomaly compatible with life and any symptoms may subside with medical management. Its occurrence, therefore, is difficult to determine accurately. The more extensive laryngo-tracheoesophageal cleft is incompatible with life unless surgically repaired.

The chief presenting symptom is aspiration with the length of the defect determining the severity (Cinnamond 1987b). A large cleft will result in aspiration of all secretions with choking and cyanosis. X-ray evidence of aspiration pneumonitis occurs early. Those with a small cleft may well be able to cope with endogenous secretions but oral feedings, being only liquids in the neonate, will produce similar problems. Stridor is not a feature and, if present, is usually expiratory, resulting from tracheobronchial obstruction from aspirated secretions. In 30% of cases reported (Cotton & Richardson 1981), there had been a history of maternal hydramnios. Other congenital malformations have been associated with this anomaly and a separate tracheoesophageal fistula co-exists in 20% of cases.

This unusual anomaly and its extent can only be diagnosed reliably by direct visualisation. Endoscopy, however, still has its difficulties and often the only way is for the surgeon to be aware of the possibility and to look specifically and carefully for a posterior cleft. The differential diagnosis of aspiration problems in the neonate is complex and involves many areas (other anatomical defects, central nervous system lesions, neuromuscular disorders) and is beyond the scope of this chapter. Full physical examination with plain and contrast radiological assessment is necessary before endoscopy. This will yield the highest success rate in making a definitive diagnosis.

Management

The neonate with a small cleft who can cope with his own secretions may well be managed medically with thickened feeds. In the majority, however, gastric decompression and alimentation is required either via a nasogastric tube or gastrostomy. A tracheostomy is usually required, not so much for maintenance of an airway but to cope with the frequent aspiration. The problem with a large defect is that the tracheostomy tube may slip over the superior edge into the oesophagus. Once the general condition has been stabilised, surgical repair can be undertaken. A lateral pharyngotomy is advocated and offers the best visualisation. Closure is only taken up to the level of the true vocal cords in order to prevent posterior glottic stenosis and oesophageal stricture.

Even following successful repair, aspiration may still be a problem. This is presumably due to the disordered anatomy and muscular inco-ordination in combination with the fact that the baby has never been fed orally. Patient nursing and parental care are required and the situation will improve with time. Tracheostomy decannulation is not contemplated until normal swallowing is established along with adequate protective reflexes of the airway.

REFERENCES

Aass A S 1975 Complications to tracheostomy and long term intubation: a follow-up study. Acta Anaesthesia Scandinavica 19: 127–133
Bailey C M, Croft C B 1987 Stertor, sleep apnoea and velopharyngeal insufficiency. In: Evans J N G (ed) Scott-Brown's otolaryngology, 5 edn. vol 6. Paediatric Otolaryngology. Butterworths, London, pp 350–367
Beeden A G, Evans J N G 1970 Quinsy tonsillectomy — a further report. Journal of Laryngology and Otology 84: 443–448
Benjamin B 1979 Xeroradiography of the upper airway in paediatrics. Australian Radiology (Sydney) 23: 214–224
Biller H F, Lawson W 1980 Arytenoidectomy, arytenoidopexy and the valve tube. In: Snow J B (ed) Controversy in otolaryngology. Saunders, Philadelphia, pp 37–42
Brook I 1979 Bacterial colonisation, tracheobronchitis and pneumonia following tracheostomy and long term intubation of paediatric patients. Chest 76: 420–424
Calcaterra T C, Mclure R, Ward P H 1974 Effect of laryngofissure on the developing canine larynx. Annals of Otology, Rhinology and Laryngology 83: 810–813
Campbell J L, Watson A C H 1980 Management of the neonate. In: Edward M, Watson

A C H (eds) Advances in the management of cleft palate. Churchill Livingstone, Edinburgh, pp 123–133

Cinnamond M J 1987a Congenital anomalies of the nose. In: Evans J N G (ed) Scott Brown's otolaryngology, 5th edn, vol 6. Paediatric Otolaryngology. Butterworths, London, pp 218–225

Cinnamond M J 1987b Congenitial disorders of the larynx, trachea and bronchi. In: Evans J N G (ed) Scott Brown's otolaryngology, 5th edn, vol 6. Paediatric Otolaryngology. Butterworths, London, pp 412–419

Cohen S R, Geller K A, Seltzer S, Thompson J W 1980 Papilloma of the larynx and tracheobronchial tree in children: a retrospective study. Annals of Otology, Rhinology and Laryngology 89: 497–503

Cotton R 1978 Management of subglottic stenosis in infancy and childhood. Annals of Otology, Rhinology and Laryngology 87: 649–657

Cotton R, Evans J N G 1981 Laryngeal reconstruction in children: five year follow-up. Annals of Otology, Rhinology and Laryngology 90: 516–520

Cotton R, Richardson M A 1981 Congenital laryngeal anomalies. Otolaryngologic Clinics of North America 14: 203–218

Editorial 1977 Clinical Otolaryngology 2: 79–84

Editorial 1981 Otitis media and grommets. British Medical Journal 282: 501–502

Eliaschar J, Lavie P, Halperin E, Gordon C, Alroy G 1980 Sleep apnoeic episodes as indication for adenotonsillectomy. Archives of Otolaryngology 106: 492–496

Emery P J, Fearon B 1984 Vocal cord palsy in pediatric practice: a review of 71 cases. International Journal of Pediatric Otorhinolaryngology 8: 147–154

Espinoza H, Palmer C L, Kisch A L, Ulrich J, Eberle B, Reed W P 1974 Clinical and immunological response to bacteria isolated from tracheal secretions following tracheostomy. Journal of Thoracic and Cardiovascular Surgery 68: 432–439

Evans J N G, Maclachlan R F 1971 Choanal atresia. Journal of Laryngology and Otology 85: 903–929

Evans J N G, Todd G B 1974 Laryngotracheoplasty. Journal of Laryngology and Otology 88: 589–597

Evans J N G (ed) 1987 Stenosis of the larynx. In: Evans J N G (ed) Scott Brown's otolaryngology, 5th edn, vol 6. Paediatric Otolaryngology. Butterworths, London, pp 495–502

Fearon B, Cotton R 1972 Subglottic stenosis in infants and children: the clinical problem and experimental surgical correction. Canadian Journal of Otolaryngology 1: 281–289

Fearon B, Ellis D 1971 The management of long term airway problems in infants and children. Annals of Otology, Rhinology and Laryngology 80: 669–667

Gewitz M, Dinwiddie R, Yuille T, Hill E, Carter C O 1978 Cleft palate and accessory metacarpal of index finger syndrome: possible familial occurrence. Journal of Medical Genetics 15: 162–164

Gordon I, Matthew D J, Dinwiddie R 1987 Respiratory system. In: Gordon I (ed) Diagnostic imaging in paediatrics. Chapman and Hall, London, pp 27–57

Gorlin R J, Cervenka J, Anderson R C, Savk J J, Bevis W D 1970 Robin's syndrome: a probably x-linked subvariety exhibiting persistence of left superior vena cava and atrial septal defect. American Journal of Diseases in Children 119: 176–179

Gorlin R J, Pinborg J J, Cohen M M 1976 Syndromes of the head and neck, 2nd edn. McEwens-Hill Book Co, New York, pp 132–136

Grahne B 1971 Operative treatment of severe chronic traumatic laryngeal stenosis in infants up to three years old. Acta Otolaryngologica 72: 134–137

Guilleminault C, Tilkian A, Dement W C 1976 The sleep apnoea syndromes. Annual Review of Medicine (Palo Alto) 27: 465–484

Guindi G M, Higgenbottom T W, Payne J K 1981 A new method for laryngeal electromyography. Clinical Otolaryngology 6: 271–278

Heaf D P, Helms P J, Dinwiddie R, Matthew D J 1982 Nasopharyngeal airways in Pierre Robin syndrome. Journal of Pediatrics 100: 698–703

Herrman J, France T D, Spranger J W et al 1975 The Stickler syndrome (hereditary arthro-opthalmopathy). Birth Defects 11: 76–103

Hibbert J 1987 Tonsils and adenoids. In: Evans J N G (ed) Scott Brown's otolaryngology. 5th edn, vol 6. Paediatric Otolaryngology. Butterworths, London, pp 368–383

Holinger L D Holinger P C, Holinger P H 1976a Etiology of bilateral vocal cord paralysis: a review of 389 cases. Annals of Otology, Rhinology and Laryngology 85: 428–436

Holinger P H, Kutnick S L, Schild J A, Holinger L D 1976b Subglottic stenosis in infants and children. Annals of Otology, Rhinology and Laryngology 85: 591–599

Jazbi B 1980 Tonsillectomy and adenoidectomy: a controversial problem. In: Jazbi B (ed) Paediatric otorhinolaryngology: a review of ear, nose and throat problems in children. Appleton-Century-Crofts, New York, pp 239–252

Kaplan L C 1985 Choanal atresia and its associated anomalies. Further support for the CHARGE association. International Journal of Pediatric Otolaryngology 8: 237–242

Kisch A L 1976 Principles of antimicrobial therapy of head and neck infections. Otolaryngologic Clinics of North America 9: 751–769

Kornblut A, Kornblut A D 1980 Tonsillectomy and adenoidectomy. In: Paparella M M, Shumrick D A (eds) Otolaryngology. vol III. Head and Neck. Saunders, Philadelphia, pp 2283–2301

Kravath R E, Pollack C P, Borowiecki B 1977 Hypoventilation during sleep in children who have lymphoid airway obstruction treated by nasopharyngeal tube and T and A. Pediatrics 59: 865–871

Latham R A 1966 The pathogenesis of cleft palate associated with the Pierre Robin syndrome. British Journal of Plastic Surgery 19: 205–214

Lee K J, Traxler J H, Smith H W et al 1973 Tonsillectomy treatment of peritonsillar abscess. Transactions of the American Academy of Ophthalmology and Otolaryngology 77: ORL 417–423

Levy A, Tabakin B, Hanson J, Narkewicz R 1967 Hypertrophic adenoids causing pulmonary hypertension and severe congestive heart failure. New England Journal of Medicine 277: 506–510

Lewis N 1976 Otitis media and linguistic incompetence. Archives of Otolaryngology 102: 387–390

Maniglia A J, Goodwin W J 1981 Congenital choanal atresia. Otolaryngological Clinics of North America 14: 167–173

Massumi R 1969 Tonsillar hypertrophy, airway obstruction, alveolar hypoventilation and cor pulmonale in twin brothers. Diseases of the Chest 55: 110–114

Mauer K W, Staats B A, Olsen K D 1983 Upper airway obstruction and disordered nocturnal breathing in children. Mayo Clinic Proceedings 58: 349–353

Menashe D, Farrehi C, Miller M 1965 Hypoventilation and cor pulmonale due to chronic upper airway obstruction. Journal of Pediatrics 67: 198–203

Pagon R A, Graham J M, Zonana J, Yong S L 1981 Coloboma, congenital heart disease and choanal atresia with multiple anomalies: CHARGE association. Journal of Pediatrics 99: 223–227

Pappas J J 1974 Middle ear ventilation tubes. Laryngoscope, St Louis 84: 1098–1117

Paradise J L, Bluestone C D, Bachman R Z et al 1978 History of recurrent sore throats as an indication for tonsillectomy. New England Journal of Medicine 298: 409–413

Pirsig W 1986 Surgery of choanal atresia in infants and children: historical notes and updated review. International Journal of Pediatric Otorhinolaryngology 11: 153–170

Potsic W P 1980 The role of adenoidectomy in secretory otitis media. In: Snow J B (ed) Controversy in Otolaryngology. Saunders, Philadelphia, pp 154–159

Pracy R 1978a Posterior choanal atresia. In: Rickman P P, Lister J, Irving I M (eds) Neonatal surgery, 2nd edn. Butterworths, London, pp 143–147

Pracy R 1978b Tracheostomy. In: Rickham P P, Lister J, Irving I M (eds) Neonatal surgery. 2nd edn. Butterworths, London, pp 149–151

Pracy R, Siegler J, Stell P M, Rogers J 1981 Ear, nose and throat surgery and nursing. Hodder and Stoughton, London, p 187

Rodgers B M, Rooks J J, Talbert J L 1979 Pediatric tracheostomy: long term evaluation. Journal of Pediatric Surgery 14: 258–263

Rogers J H 1987 Tracheostomy and decannulation. In: Evans J N G (ed) Scott Brown's Otolaryngology, 5th edn, vol 6, Paediatric Otolaryngology. Butterworths, London, pp 471–486

Rowe L D, Hansen T N, Nieson D, Tooley W 1980 Continuous measurement of skin surface oxygen and carbon dioxide tensions in obstructive sleep apnoea. Laryngoscope. (St Louis) 90: 1797–1803

Schukneckt H F 1974 Pathology of the ear. Howard University Press, Cambridge, Massachusetts, p 179

Schuller D E, Krause C J 1979 Cleft lip and palate. In: Maran A G D, Stell P M (eds) Clinical otolaryngology. Blackwell Scientific, Oxford, pp 514–521

Singh A, Innes A J 1981 Tracheostomy: a guide for parents. Department of Medical
   Illustration. The Hospitals for Sick Children, London
Smith J L, Stowe F R 1961 The Pierre Robin syndrome (glossoptosis, micrognathia, cleft
   palate): a review of 39 cases with emphasis on associated ocular lesions. Pediatrics
   27: 128–133
Smyth G D L 1980 Chronic ear disease. Churchill Livingstone, Edinburgh, pp 9–13
Sprinkle P M, Veltri R W 1979 Tonsils and adenoids: tonsils. In: Maran A G D, Stell P M
   (eds) Clinical otolaryngology. Blackwell Scientific, Oxford, pp 475–484
Sprinkle P M, Veltri R W, Wainwright W H, McLung J E 1980 Epstein-Barr virus and
   adenotonsillitis. In: Jazbi B (ed) Pediatric otolaryngology: a review of ear, nose and
   throat problems in children. Appleton-Century-Crofts, New York, pp 231–238
Storer J, Grossman H 1974 The Camptomelic syndrome. Radiology 111: 673–681
Sullivan C E 1980 Disorders of breathing in sleep. Modern Medicine of Australia
   (March): 7–17
Tucker H M 1980 Neuromuscular pedicle reinervation for paralysis of the vocal cord. In:
   Snow J B (ed) Controversy in otolaryngology. Saunders, Philadelphia, pp 43–55
Tucker J A, Tucker G F 1979 A clinical perspective on the development and anatomical
   aspects of the infant larynx and trachea. In: Healy G B, McGill T J I (eds)
   Laryngo-tracheal problems in the pediatric patient. Charles C Thomas, Springfield,
   Illinois, pp 3–8
Van Demark D R 1974 Assessment of articulation for children with cleft palate. Cleft
   Palate Journal 11: 200–208
Wetmore R F, Mahboubi S 1986 Computed tomography in the evaluation of choanal
   atresia. International Journal of Pediatric Otorhinolaryngology 11: 265–274

RECOMMENDED READING

Evans J N G (ed) 1987 Scott-Brown's otolaryngology, 5th edition, volume 6. Paediatric
   Otolaryngology. Butterworths, London

6. Respiratory tract infection

Respiratory tract infection is the commonest cause of illness in the childhood population accounting for an estimated 15 million deaths per year under the age of 5 worldwide (Lancet 1985). They cause up to 30% of General Practice consultations in the UK amounting to some 560 per GP per annum (Styles 1985). A number of different organisms affect the respiratory system in various ways depending on the site of infection and on the age and natural resistance of the child. Epidemiological factors have also been shown to increase the predisposition of children to more frequent or severe respiratory infections. These include age, particularly infancy and the preschool years, lower socioeconomic status and overcrowding which increases severity but not frequency of infection, poor nutrition, male sex, parental smoking, seasonal and geographical variation (Colley 1976). Also the presence of intrinsic factors such as congenital malformations, especially of heart or lungs, or damage to respiratory tract by previous disease, for example bronchopulmonary dysplasia. The overall manifestation of the disease may be seen on the basis of a balance between a number of factors shown in Table 6.1.

It has been estimated that up to 90% of respiratory tract infections in childhood have a viral aetiology, the most important pathogen in this respect is respiratory syncytial virus (RSV). Viruses which are known to affect the respiratory tract in children are shown in Table 6.2.

Table 6.1 Factors in respiratory tract infection

Infectious agent	Host
Type of organism	Age
Dose	Low birth weight
Virulence	Male sex
Level of maximum impact on respiratory	Obesity
tract	Immunity — active or passive
	Allergy
	Socioeconomic
	Home — overcrowding
	School
	Smoking — active or passive
	Previous lung damage

Table 6.2 Non-bacterial causes of respiratory illness

Respiratory syncytial virus	Mycoplasma pneumonia
Rhinovirus	Rubella
Para-influenza virus	Chlamydia trachomatis
Influenza A and B	Cytomegalovirus
Adenovirus	Varicella
Epstein-Barr virus	Herpes simplex
Coxsackie A and B	Measles
Echo	Human immunodeficiency virus

RSV is by far the most common virus causing major respiratory tract infection in children. The incidence is quoted at 110 per 1000 children per year (Godfrey 1984) and the hospital admission rate in the UK is 12 to 25 per 1000 infants per year (Clarke et al 1978). The major illness which it causes is bronchiolitis which is highly prevalent in infancy and occurs in epidemics from late autumn to early spring. It is also the commonest cause of pneumonia under the age of one year (Lancet 1988). Parainfluenza viruses, particularly type 1, cause large airway disease including laryngo-tracheobronchitis or croup; type 3 more often produces a bronchiolitic type of infection in the small airways. Influenza viruses are common at all times in an endemic form, particularly types A and B. However there may be occasional worldwide pandemics due to new strains which cause a much higher incidence of disease.

Adenovirus is potentially a much more serious cause of lower respiratory tract infection since it can produce severe lung damage in the form of obliterative bronchiolitis (Simpson & Mok 1985). This is more prevalent in those patients who are immunosuppressed or who have had a recent episode of measles (Sly et al 1984). Rhinoviruses mainly cause common cold symptoms and less commonly lower respiratory tract infection. Coxsackie A and B usually confine themselves to the upper respiratory tract and outbreaks are common in young children attending nursery or play school where there is higher incidence of nosocomial spread of infection.

Measles can produce an acute tracheobronchitis in those who are immunocompetent during the course of classical measles infection. It can also produce a much more serious and usually fatal interstitial 'giant cell' pneumonitis in the immunosuppressed, especially the lymphopenic (Enders et al 1959); this is most frequently seen in patients with malignant disease on chemotherapy. This is one reason why measles immunisation should be given to every child whenever possible.

TYPES OF RESPIRATORY ILLNESS

It is useful in the understanding of the pathophysiology and treatment of respiratory tract infections in children to divide the illnesses seen into two major groups, namely those affecting either the upper or the lower respiratory tract and within these to subdivide the areas affected anatomically. The upper respiratory tract is divided into ears, nose, throat, tonsils, pharyngeal area and sinuses. The lower respiratory tract is divided into larynx, trachea, bronchi, bronchioles, alveoli and pleura.

Nasopharyngitis (acute coryza or the common cold)

The nose and throat are the most frequent areas to be infected by the common viral upper respiratory tract infections. It is important to remember that in the young child the Eustachian tube is short and the infant spends a great deal of time in the horizontal position so spread of infection to the middle ear is common. The vast majority of infections are viral and present with a febrile illness in association with rhinorrhea, sneezing, poor feeding, and coughing but relatively little in the way of systemic upset. A small number of cases are due to bacteria, particularly pneumococcus and group A streptococci, although these will often cause a more purulent nasal discharge. Treatment is symptomatic, encouraging fluid intake and reducing fever with paracetamol. Antibiotics are not indicated unless there is persistence of symptoms, obvious toxicity or marked purulent nasal discharge. If there is evidence of associated otitis media, however, antibiotics should be given because of potential complications secondary to bacterial infection. In the larger child, ephedrine nose drops can be effective if there is marked nasal oedema and obstruction but there is little evidence that they are of value in the young child. Oral 'decongestants' are of little value and can cause behavioural problems and nightmares in some children so are best avoided. Infection confined more specifically to the pharyngeal area is less common as this is usually involved in the inflammatory process of acute tonsillitis. Most purely pharyngeal infections are again viral but other organisms, including the beta-haemolytic streptococcus, can cause this problem.

Acute tonsillitis

Acute tonsillitis is another common infection in young children and, although the majority are viral, a significant number are due to the bacterial pathogens such as the group A beta-haemolytic streptococcus. In these cases there may be an exudative tonsillitis with white pustules present on the tonsils as part of the acute inflammatory response; it is not possible to differentiate viral from bacterial tonsillitis by inspection alone. Most children will also have cervical adenopathy as part of the illness but this too is not a differentiating feature. It is for this reason that virtually all children with obvious acute tonsillitis should be treated with oral penicillin which is effective against group A streptococcus. This policy, together with improved nutritional and public health measures, has resulted in the virtual eradication of rheumatic fever in this country. Acute glomerulonephritis, another post-streptococcal complication, is also seen less frequently. The treatment of children with recurrent tonsillitis causing systemic upset and disturbance of the general growth pattern is described in Chapter 5.

Adenoiditis

Inflammation of the adenoids is extremely common with all upper respiratory infections including the common cold and also with many bacterial infections. The major problems in relation to the adenoids occur when the nasal passages are small, as in infancy, and when the adenoids show chronic, persistent enlargement which does not reduce sufficiently to relieve nasal obstruction between infections. In the infant and young child this may affect feeding and growth and, in a few cases, produces major upper airway obstruction resulting in sleep apnoea. In the worst cases, this can lead on to recurrent hypoxia, right ventricular hypertrophy, pulmonary hypertension and cardiac failure. These children require adenoidectomy even at quite a young age (from 1–3 years) to relieve the airway obstruction (Hibbert 1987). The role of adenoidectomy in the child with recurrent infection in association with tonsillitis is discussed in Chapter 5.

Acute otitis media

This is an extremely common illness of the pre-school child (Pukander et al 1982). Many cases are viral in origin but the commonest bacterial pathogen is *Streptococcus pneumoniae* accounting for 25 to 50% of infections, followed by *Haemophilus influenzae*, group B streptococci and a number of other less common bacteria and viruses such as influenza, parainfluenza and RSV (Drug and Therapeutics Bulletin 1984). The child presents with acute symptoms including fever, irritability and rubbing of the ears. The infant may head bang and, if old enough, he may complain of severe pain in one or both ears. Inspection of the tympanic membrane demonstrates loss of light reflex and the normal anatomical markings. It is acutely inflamed and may be bulging; in severe cases spontaneous acute perforation occurs. If vesicles are seen on the tympanic membrane, this may be a sign of mycoplasma infection. Treatment of the acute infection involves symptomatic measures to relieve the pain and reduce the fever which would normally include the administration of paracetamol. Antibiotics are commonly used, the most frequent being penicillin, amoxycillin, erythromycin or trimethoprim. Many cases resolve spontaneously and a number of clinical trials have failed to show significant benefit from the use of antibiotics acutely. It is likely, however, that their administration has reduced the incidence of more serious complications including mastoiditis (Hibbert 1987) and meningitis and possibly the onset of chronic or suppurative otitis media. Treatment is usually given for 5 days but may be longer if inspection of the tympanic membrane does not reveal a satisfactory response. The use of decongestants and antihistamines, while widely practiced, has not been shown to be of significant benefit (Olsen et al 1978). The treatment of chronic otitis media is considered in Chapter 5.

Sinusitis

The maxillary antra and ethmoid air cells are sufficiently large at birth to develop infection even during the first few months of life. The maxillary sinuses gradually increase in size and are usually visible on X-ray between 2 and 4 years. At this stage, the sphenoidal sinuses are also developing and they too may become infected. The frontal sinuses, although present, are rarely involved in acute infection until school age. The presenting features of sinusitis include fever, headache, pain and localised tenderness, particularly on percussion over the face. There are usually associated signs of a more generalised upper respiratory tract infection and a mucopurulent nasal discharge. Pathogenic organisms causing this problem include pneumococci, group A streptococci, *Haemophilus influenzae* and occasionally staphylococci. Treatment consists of symptomatic measures to reduce pain and fever and the administration of antibiotics including amoxycillin, erythromycin or trimethoprim. The presence of chronic sinusitis should make one consider another underlying diagnosis. These include allergic disorders, cystic fibrosis, immune deficiency or rare conditions such as ciliary dyskinesia or Kartagener's syndrome (especially if there is dextrocardia and evidence of recurrent lower respiratory tract infection). The treatment of chronic sinusitis is dealt with in Chapter 5.

Larynx

Acute laryngotracheobronchitis or croup is a common condition of young children, most frequently seen between the ages of 6 months and 4 years. The most common aetiological organisms include the parainfluenza and influenza viruses, RSV and rhinovirus. Bacterial infection also occurs due to *Staphylococcus aureus* and, less commonly, to *Streptococcus pneumoniae*. The aetiology of this condition is different to that of acute epiglottitis which is due to *Haemophilus influenzae* type B. In the young child there is acute swelling and oedema of the airway which may result in significant laryngeal obstruction and, in severe cases, in respiratory failure. The classic presentation is with the gradual onset of a brassy cough with inspiratory stridor, fever and evidence of upper respiratory infection. If more significant airway obstruction develops, then there will be inspiratory indrawing and obvious difficulty with breathing and the child will become restless and irritable, especially if hypoxia is present. Fortunately, only a few children go on to have major airway obstruction or require respiratory support but some require elective intubation to relieve airway obstruction during the acute phase of the illness. Treatment consists of symptomatic measures including humidity, paracetamol to reduce fever and the administration of adequate fluids. Oxygen may be required for those who are restless or hypoxic, although blood gases should only be performed when clinically indicated as it is better not to disturb the patient in order to avoid exacerbating the oedema and airway obstruction already present. Nebulised adrenaline may temporarily relieve acute respiratory obstruction but this should only be used in hospital. Antibiotics are not usually required unless the child is particularly toxic or there is suggestive evidence of bacterial aetiology such as purulent sputum production which may occur if there are staphylococci present.

Other causes of acute croup should also be considered, chiefly epiglottitis, but one should also think of foreign body inhalation, an acute allergic reaction or retropharyngeal abscess. Diphtheria should not be forgotten if the child has not been immunised. Lateral neck X-ray may help to delineate some of these problems but should not be undertaken until acute epiglottitis has been ruled out by other means. A small number of children have recurrent episodes of croup. These may be viral or allergic in origin and an underlying abnormality of the airway such as subglottic stenosis can predispose to this. These children may require elective laryngobronchoscopy to exclude other pathology.

Acute epiglottitis

This is an extremely dangerous condition, usually seen in the age range 6 months to 6 years with a peak incidence in the second to fourth year of life. The vast majority of cases are caused by *Haemophilus influenzae* type B, although beta-haemolytic streptococcus, pneumococcus and *Staphylococcus aureus* are occasionally seen (Freeland 1987). Haemophilus with outer membrane subtype 1 appears to be the most common pathogen (Takala et al 1987). Systemic infection with the organism is quite common and it is often cultured from the blood at the same time. Rapid bacterial antigen screening of blood now frequently leads to identification of the causative organism within an hour or two of admission to hospital. The onset is usually acute, the patient presenting with fever, toxicity and sore throat progressing to respiratory obstruction over a few hours. Inspiratory stridor appears with indrawing of the respiratory muscles and evidence of increasing airway obstruction. This results in hypoxia and hypercarbia, producing restlessness and cyanosis. The child often holds the neck in an extended position to ease the passage of air through the obstructed airway. Acute and potentially fatal airway obstruction may occur at any time.

If epiglottitis is suspected, no attempt should be made to visualise the throat and no instruments should be put in the mouth because of the risk of acute airway obstruction.

The diagnosis is suspected by history and external examination. The child should be taken directly to hospital where visualisation of the epiglottis should be undertaken in the operating theatre only by experienced personnel who can intubate immediately or, if this fails, perform a tracheostomy to relieve the airway obstruction. Typically, a large swollen oedematous cherry red epiglottis is seen. A lateral neck X-ray is not recommended as a diagnostic procedure because the additional handling and extension of the neck to obtain proper views may precipitate acute obstruction. If acute epiglottitis is excluded by careful and proper inspection under the appropriate circumstances, a lateral neck X-ray may then be performed to exclude other pathology lower in the trachea. Treatment should be supportive, initially consisting of added oxygen and the provision of adequate humidity. The patient should be handled as little as possible, especially prior to airway inspection, and procedures such as venepuncture, blood gases and the siting of intravenous infusion should preferably be left until after inspection of the airway. In an acute emergency, the passage of a large bore needle into the trachea, below the cricoid cartilage, may be lifesaving. Intravenous antibiotics should be given after a blood culture has been taken. Chloramphenicol or a third generation cephalosporin is used since an increasing number of *Haemophilus influenzae* are resistant to ampicillin. After inspection of the airway, intravenous fluids are given to maintain hydration until oral fluids can be taken once again.

Airway support is vital and is required in 60–70% of cases admitted to hospital. The preferred route is nasotracheal intubation (Mitchell & Thomas 1980) and this is performed at the time of inspection of the airway under light anaesthesia. If intubation proves impossible then a tracheostomy may be necessary although this is rare in present day practice. The condition carries a small but significant mortality of 0.9% (Cautrell et al 1978). Death usually occurs secondary to acute obstruction when attempts are made to inspect the airway without full supportive staff and resuscitative measures being available. Further morbidity occurs secondary to severe hypoxic cerebral insult, either secondary to airway obstruction or following difficulties with intubation or blockage of the endotracheal tube. The airway can usually be removed after 3–4 days and the patient takes oral fluids 24 hours after tube removal. The use of steroids, such as dexamethasone, to reduce oedema is not proven but they are commonly administered for 24 hours prior to extubation when the endotracheal tube is fitting tightly and does not have a leak round it. The prognosis for children who recover from acute epiglottitis is excellent and recurrence of this condition is uncommon, unlike other forms of croup.

Pertussis

This is an acute lower respiratory tract infection usually caused by the organism *Bordetella pertussis*. The disease principally affects infants and young children but may be seen in adults. It occurs in epidemics at intervals of 3–4 years. The incidence (Fig. 6.1) has greatly increased in recent years due to reduced uptake of the vaccine. During 1986, 66 000 cases were notified to the Communicable Disease Surveillance Centre in the UK (Communicable Disease Report 1987). The uptake of vaccine has now improved to around 65% of infants in this country.

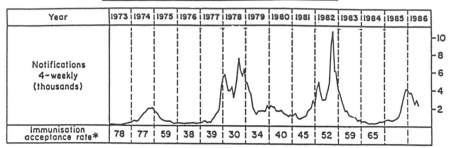

WHOOPING COUGH : ENGLAND AND WALES 1973–86

Fig. 6.1   Whooping cough notifications, England and Wales 1973–1986 (reproduced by kind permission from PHLS Communicable Disease Surveillance Centre, Colindale, London).

The clinical features take the form of an initial coryzal type of illness which lasts 7–10 days and begins one to two weeks after contact with the organism. The coryzal phase is followed by the onset of the classical 'whooping' cough. This comes in short bursts one after the other without an inspiratory pause, and causes acute facial congestion followed by cyanosis during severe spasms. The eyes may bulge and stream with tears and subconjunctival haemorrhage can occur. At the end of the coughing spasm, there is a typical 'whoop' as air is drawn into the lungs and at this point a small amount of thick tenacious mucus is coughed up. The spasms may result in vomiting and apnoeic spells in infants and young children. Other complications include epistaxis and convulsions if there is significant hypoxia during the coughing spell; this is more common in infants. Paroxysms of cough are often precipitated by mild activity such as exercise, excitement or laughter. They can induce severe bronchospasm in wheezy children especially those with asthma. The spasmodic phase typically lasts for 6–8 weeks but often longer. It has been described as 'the 100 day cough'. It gradually lessens in severity during this period but may return again if another respiratory tract infection occurs during the ensuing months. Pneumonia is not uncommon as a primary consequence of the disease itself or as the result of secondary bacterial infection with organisms such as pneumococci, staphylococci or *Haemophilus influenzae*. This complication may be seen in as many as 20% of cases (Dinwiddie 1981).

Typical X-ray changes (Fig. 6.2) include increase in perihilar bronchial wall thickening and, in the more severe cases, patches of overinflation and other areas of collapse or consolidation. Mediastinal and subcutaneous emphysema are occasionally seen although pneumothorax is uncommon. The risk of long term lung damage is, however, surprisingly small in children who have had pertussis who are otherwise normal (Johnson et al 1983). Those who have pertussis complicated by apnoeic episodes or a fit may have a worse intellectual outcome (RCGP 1987).

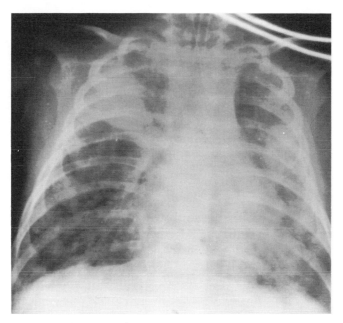

Fig. 6.2 Pertussis bronchopneumonia.

Treatment

General supportive measures and careful nursing are of prime importance in the care of the affected child. Particular attention should be paid to adequate nutritional and fluid intake, especially during the paroxysmal phase. Antibiotics do not influence the course of the primary illness, although they may shorten the period of excretion of the organism and thus its infectivity to others (Bass et al 1969). Erythromycin is the treatment of choice although the organism may be sensitive to other antibiotics such as ampicillin and co-trimoxazole. Oral salbutamol may have a role in the reduction of paroxysms and should be given three to four times daily (Simpson 1987). A small number of infants with frequent apnoeic attacks or respiratory failure will require artificial ventilation and full intensive care.

Prevention

Active immunisation with pertussis vaccine undoubtedly reduces the incidence, morbidity and mortality of the disease. The uptake of the vaccine has greatly reduced in recent years because of public fears about side effects. These appear to be very uncommon in those who are otherwise healthy. Specific contraindications should now only include a previous history of convulsions in the patient or first degree relative (excluding febrile convulsions) or significant adverse reaction to previous immunisation. It is only by increasing the resistance of the whole population that the prevalence of this disease will once again fall.

Bronchiolitis

Bronchiolitis is an acute infection at bronchiolar level caused by respiratory syncytial virus (RSV) in as many as 70% of cases (Clarke et al 1978) although other viruses including parainfluenza, influenza and adenovirus can cause similar symptoms. It occurs most commonly during the first 6 months of life but is seen throughout the first year. Seasonal epidemics occur with peak incidence from late autumn to early spring. RSV infection is also the commonest cause of pneumonia during the first year of life.

Pathology

The organism produces a marked local tissue reaction at epithelial level leading to necrosis and destruction of cilia and epithelial cells. The acute inflammatory response in the submucosal region leads to oedema, disruption of airway architecture and small airway obstruction (Godfrey 1984). These changes result in widespread bilateral hyperinflation. As the airway obstruction increases, blood gas changes occur due to abnormal ventilation/perfusion ratios which lead to hypoxia and hypercapnia. These changes are especially seen in infants who have other underlying lung disease such as bronchopulmonary dysplasia.

The infant presents with fever, coryzal signs and a dry cough. As the illness progresses tachypnoea and wheeze appear together with increasing respiratory difficulty and indrawing of the muscles of breathing on inspiration. Widespread inspiratory crepitations and expiratory rhonchi are heard on auscultation. Rapid diagnosis can be made by the use of viral immunofluorescent techniques which demonstrate the virus present in a large number of cases during the early phase of the illness (Kaul et al 1978).

The typical X-ray changes (Fig. 6.3) include bilateral hyperinflation with patchy areas of increased density which are due to patchy collapse or secondary pneumonic consolidation. Although the liver is often palpable below the costal margin, this is seldom due to concurrent cardiac failure unless there is some other underlying condition; it is usually secondary to hyperinflation of the lungs. A few infants present with acute apnoeic attacks and convulsions or evidence of mild encephalitis. These signs may present before the lung disease is clinically evident and probably account for a small number of sudden infant deaths.

Treatment

Treatment of this viral infection is mainly supportive. The infant is placed in an oxygen tent or head box with added humidity and sufficient oxygen is given to relieve the underlying hypoxaemia. Adequate fluid intake is important, although this should not be in excess of 75–80% of normal requirement since inappropriate antidiuretic hormone (ADH) secretion can occur during the acute phase of the illness. Infants over the age of 6 months

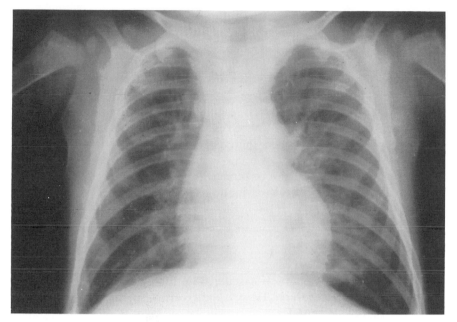

a

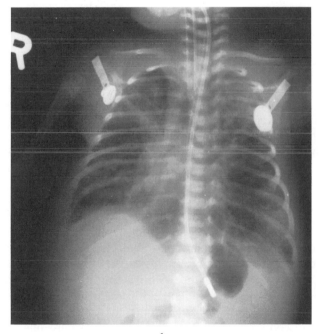

b

Fig. 6.3   (a) RSV bronchiolitis, (b) fatal RSV bronchiolitis complicating severe combined immune deficiency (SCID).

who have severe wheeze can usefully be given nebulised ipratropium bromide or salbutamol although there is little objective evidence that either produces significant bronchodilation at this age (Silverman 1984). Those who develop significant respiratory failure will need ventilation and full intensive care. The antiviral agent ribavirin may be effective in reducing the duration and severity of the illness (Barry et al 1986) but as this is an expensive form of treatment it is best reserved for those with other underlying pulmonary or heart disease or severe respiratory failure (Conrad et al 1987). Antibiotics are not given unless there is evidence of secondary bacterial infection which is more likely to occur in those who are ventilated. Infants with severe disease should also be screened to exclude other underlying conditions such as cystic fibrosis or immune deficiency either of which may present in this way.

Prognosis

The vast majority of infants with acute RSV bronchiolitis appear to make a complete clinical recovery. However there is a significant incidence of recurrent wheezing episodes which may be as high as 40–50% (Godfrey 1984) when these children are followed up. Whether this is due to underlying atopy, bronchial lability or caused by the illness is a matter of debate (Godfrey 1984, Simpson & Mok 1985).

Obliterative bronchiolitis

This is a much more severe form of bronchiolitis in which there is permanent damage to the growing lung at the bronchiolar level and beyond (Simpson & Mok 1985). The usual causative agent is adenovirus which can infect the lungs on its own or after an episode of measles (Sly et al 1984). These children have persistent symptoms of dyspnoea, cough, wheezing, and hyperinflation of the chest. The initial X-ray changes consist of peribronchial shadowing with areas of patchy collapse and consolidation which fail to clear. These are followed by evidence of reduced peripheral perfusion in the lungs indicating obliteration of small blood vessels at this level. These children often require extended treatment with a number of medications including bronchodilators and steroids, although there is no firm evidence that the latter are of value. Lung function tests show widespread overinflation and air trapping suggesting decreased lung compliance and a high airway resistance. This is only partially reversible with bronchodilator therapy. A few patients with this problem go on to develop permanent bilateral lung disease or the unilateral hyperlucent lung syndrome (McLeod's or Swyer-James syndrome), where one lung shows diminished vascularity and evidence of pruning of the peripheral bronchioles secondary to the acute infection (Cumming et al 1971). The typical X-ray changes are reviewed in Chapter 13.

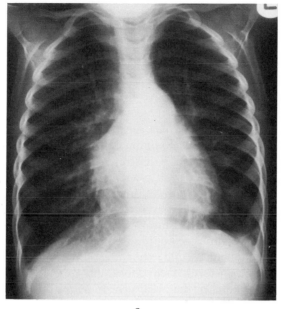

a

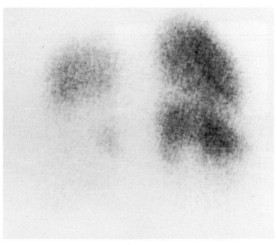

b

Fig. 6.4 (a) Obliterative bronchiolitis. Pruning of peripheral airways and small blood vessels; (b) Posterior perfusion scan in obliterative bronchiolitis — marked decrease in blood flow to left lower lobe and at periphery of other lobes.

These children should also be checked for underlying conditions such as cystic fibrosis, immune deficiency, alpha-1-antitrypsin deficiency and ciliary dyskinesia. Unfortunately the incidence of permanent lung damage after adenovirus infection may be as high as 60% (Lang et al 1969, Sly et al 1984) and most of these patients will be symptomatic throughout life.

PNEUMONIA

Pneumonia is common at all ages but particularly in infants and young children. The commonest pathogens in the younger age group are viral, usually RSV, although the other respiratory viruses can cause severe infection, especially adenovirus (Lancet 1988). In older children, viruses continue to be important but bacterial infections become increasingly common. *Streptococcus pneumoniae* is the predominent pathogen, although the incidence of *Mycoplasma pneumoniae* increases towards adolescence. Infection with other bacteria is less common but can be severe; these include *Staphylococcus aureus*, beta-haemolytic streptococci and *Haemophilus influenzae*. Gram-negative organisms such as *E. coli*, klebsiella and *Pseudomonas aeruginosa* are seen in debilitated children or those with other underlying disorders such as immune deficiency or cystic fibrosis. *Pneumocystis carinii*, adenovirus, cytomegalovirus and measles can produce very serious interstitial pneumonia in the immunocompromised at any age.

In the infant and young child, the infection is more often bronchopneumonic with signs of fever, tachypnoea, dry cough and increased work of breathing. Auscultation of the chest reveals areas of diminished air entry and crepitations over the affected lung fields. Chest X-ray confirms widespread areas of patchy bilateral consolidation. In the older child, the infection is more commonly lobar in type, air entry is diminished over the affected area and crepitations are heard. Dullness to percussion is found and bronchial breathing heard when more complete consolidation is present. In any severe pneumonia respiratory failure can occur and may ultimately lead to cor pulmonale with circulatory failure, hypoxia and acidosis.

Identification of the causative organism is made by examination of respiratory secretions which should be cultured for the common bacteria in the usual way. Rapid viral immunofluorescence has proved most helpful in identifying viral agents. In the longer term a rise in specific viral antibodies clarifies the aetiology. Rapid bacterial antigen screen on the blood is also helpful in a number of cases. Bacterial pathogens such as *Haemophilus influenzae* are not infrequently isolated from blood culture.

Viral pneumonia

The common viruses causing respiratory infection have already been mentioned (see Table 6.2). The type of illness they produce depends on the immunocompetence of the host. The particular syndromes seen in those who are abnormal are described below. Viral pneumonia in young children is difficult to distinguish clinically from that caused by bacteria. There are usually signs of generalised illness with fever, cough, tachypnoea and indrawing of respiratory muscles. Particular clues may be given by the presence of epidemics at different seasons of the year caused by viruses such as RSV or influenza. Chest X-ray may show widespread consolidation to be present.

Treatment is supportive with adequate fluid intake, humidity and appropriate oxygen if hypoxaemia is present. Although antibiotics are not specifically indicated unless bacterial infection is suspected, patients at risk of respiratory failure may be covered by a broad spectrum agent such as erythromycin or trimethoprim. More specific therapy should be given when appropriate such as with flucloxacillin for staphylococci or amoxycillin for *Haemophilus influenzae*. If the patient is debilitated, has underlying lung disease such as bronchopulmonary dysplasia or is severely ill, then broad spectrum antibiotics, including an aminoglycoside such as gentamicin should be used in combination with penicillin, flucloxacillin or ampicillin. This therapy is most frequently required in those with severe respiratory failure requiring ventilation. If RSV is proven as the cause these children should probably be given nebulised ribavirin while on the ventilator. The older child is at greater risk of suffering from *Mycoplasma pneumoniae* infection and this should be specifically looked for on culture and treated with erythromycin if necessary.

Bacterial pneumonia

Streptococcus pneumoniae is the commonest cause of bacterial pneumonia in childhood. It is particularly prevalent in the immediate pre-school and early school years. The vast majority of children with pneumococcal infection probably never reach hospital and are treated with antibiotics at home by their GP with a satisfactory response. The spectrum of pneumonia seen in hospital practice is rather different and, although pneumococci are common and can result in severe infection leading to respiratory failure, there is a much higher incidence of infection with other less common organisms in children who are not infrequently found to have an underlying susceptibility to bacterial pneumonia due to immune deficiency, cystic fibrosis or a congenital malformation of the lung itself. Diagnosis in these cases is by similar techniques to those used to evaluate the viral pneumonias, namely sputum culture, blood culture, rapid antigen screen on blood and culture of lung fluid if this is available from either pleural or empyema fluid, preferably before antibiotics have been given. X-ray will confirm the diagnosis, usually showing lobar consolidation which will vary in extent and site depending on the severity of the disease.

Staphylococcal pneumonia

Staphylococcal pneumonia is not uncommon in children who have underlying pathology as mentioned above and is a presenting feature in a number of cases of cystic fibrosis. Congenital malformations of the lung such as lung cysts or sequestered lobes of lung should also be suspected in these cases and further investigation is required after resolution of the acute infection. The organism is particularly prone to produce pneumatoceles in the lung parenchyma (Fig. 6.5) which may be air or liquid filled. These will resolve

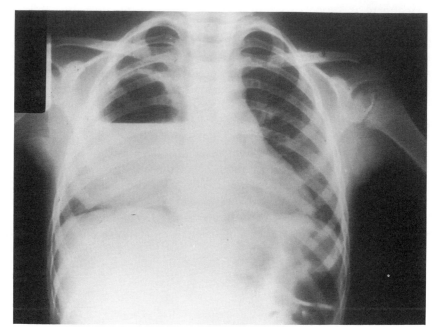

Fig. 6.5　Abscess right lung. Courtesy Dr G Fischer.

completely on X-ray over the ensuing weeks if they are due to primary staphylococcal infection. Congenital lung cysts, however, do not resolve and will require surgical removal at a later date.

Antibiotic therapy should be intensive and includes an aminoglycoside and flucloxacillin in appropriate dosage; fucidin is also commonly used. Those with significant illness should continue with oral antibiotics for 6 weeks after the initial fever has settled. In a few cases the infection spreads to other sites such as the bone or soft tissues, particularly in small or pre-term babies.

Streptococcal pneumonia

Streptococcal pneumonia is more commonly seen as a complicating factor of viral infection such as measles, influenza or varicella and it is caused by the group A beta-haemolytic streptococcus. Group B haemolytic streptococcal pneumonia is now a very important cause of acute neonatal lung infection and death in this age group. It is discussed in Chapter 3. Group A haemolytic streptococcal pneumonia has a variable onset, from the acute to the more gradual. It is sometimes associated with other complications such as pleural effusion or empyema although this is uncommon. Chest X-ray shows typical features of lobar consolidation but pneumatoceles are rare. Treatment is supportive and the organism is extremely sensitive to parenteral penicillin.

Other organisms

Pneumonia due to Gram-negative organisms such as *Haemophilus influenza*, *E. coli*, klebsiella and pseudomonas is more usually seen in children with other underlying disorders, those who have been hospitalised for some considerable period of time or who are being chronically ventilated. Fungal infection with candida or aspergillus can also occur in these children. *Pneumocystis carinii* pneumonia is seen in those with congenital or acquired immune deficiency; this specific pneumonia is discussed in Chapter 7.

Treatment

Children with pneumonia require intensive support with adequate fluid, nutrition and oxygen therapy. Underlying disease such as cystic fibrosis or immune deficiency should be sought at an early stage as this will affect treatment and prognosis. Broad spectrum antibiotics should be given initially until a specific organism is identified. This usually involves the use of an aminoglycoside such as gentamicin or tobramycin or occasionally amikacin, in combination with another agent such as a penicillin or a third generation cephalosporin. Antifungal agents such as amphotericin or 5-flucytosine are used when appropriate.

PLEURA

Inflammation of the pleura with accumulation of fluid in the pleural space — either as an effusion or pus as in empyema — although not common, is still seen in the paediatric age group. Other fluids, such as a haemorrhagic effusion or chylothorax, are seen in conditions where there is underlying malignant disease or an abnormality of the lymphatic system. Pleural inflammation, or pleurisy, is common when there is underlying pulmonary infection. Small effusions are quite frequent in this situation, although progression to empyema is much less frequent. Causative organisms include *Staphylococcus aureus*, *Streptococcus pneumoniae*, beta-haemolytic streptococcus, *E. coli*, klebsiella and pseudomonas.

Chest X-ray shows obliteration of the costophrenic angle in the erect position or the fluid may create a haziness with apical capping of the lung fields in the supine position. Lateral views show less of the normal increasing vertebral lucency as one descends the thoracic spine — this is called the 'disappearing vertebra sign'. Large effusions can obliterate the whole lung field on one side leading to complete opacity on the X-ray. Ultrasound of the chest is useful in this situation in delineating the size and extent of the pleural effusion and the structures which underlie it. Diagnosis is by the usual culture techniques from respiratory secretions plus tapping of the pleural fluid, preferably before antibiotics have been given. Rapid antigen screening should be performed on the fluid obtained which should then be cultured. Tuberculosis should never be forgotten in this clinical setting.

Treatment is by supportive measures with antibiotics, either broad spectrum until an organism has been identified, or specific chemotherapy if the organism has been isolated. Drainage of pleural fluid is important and this is initially performed using an intercostal tube, but a small open thoracotomy to break down loculated areas of pus and to place a large chest drain may be necessary for those with thick or persistent purulent effusions. The prognosis depends on the underlying pathology, but if the patient is otherwise normal it is usually excellent.

BRONCHIECTASIS

Bronchiectasis is a chronic lung condition in which there is persistent dilatation of the bronchi with chronic infection associated with persistent cough and sputum production. It is the end result of a number of different pathological processes. The major contributory factors include acute pneumonia, recurrent lower respiratory tract infection, underlying chronic disease such as cystic fibrosis and structural abnormality of the lung such as sequestered lobe or cilia dyskinesia.

In an otherwise normal child bronchiectasis can occur following a particularly severe episode of viral or bacterial pneumonia. Although the infected lobe in these cases partially recovers it is not normal and is therefore susceptible to further damage during subsequent respiratory infection. Investigation of these children including ventilation-perfusion lung scan and bronchoscopy usually demonstrates an isolated lesion only. Vigorous treatment with daily physiotherapy, physical exercise and antibiotics during further infections can lead to partial or virtually complete recovery over a number of years. Unless the affected area is collapsed and so persistently infected that it is a source of spread to other areas of the lung surgical removal is not advised. If surgery is necessary then a preoperative bronchogram should be performed in order to delineate bronchiectatic change in any of the adjacent lobes of the lung (Gordon et al 1987).

Recurrent lower respiratory tract infection leading to bronchiectasis occurs in a number of circumstances. These include the normal infections of childhood in those who are malnourished or who have a mild degree of immune deficiency and also infections in children who have any type of feeding or swallowing difficulty causing recurrent spillover into the tracheobronchial tree. Another predisposing factor is previous foreign body inhalation in which the lung may be damaged distally and thus be prone to subsequent chronic infection. Bronchiectasis in these cases is more common in the lower lobes and may be unilateral or bilateral. Investigation of the child with chronic lung disease is shown in Table 6.3. Treatment is as for bronchiectasis following a single acute infection plus alleviation of any predisposing cause if possible. Surgery is seldom indicated where there is bilateral disease. Patients with cystic fibrosis all develop some degree of bronchiectasis sooner or later and this is discussed in Chapter 10.

Table 6.3 Investigation of chronic respiratory disease

Common	Uncommon
Sputum culture, throat swab, nasal swab	Full immune function
X-ray chest, postnasal space, sinuses	Respiratory viral antibodies
Filter view of trachea	Barium swallow
Full blood count, white cell differential including eosinophil count	Chest screening
Immunoglobulins IgG, IgG, IgA, total IgE Immunoglobulin subclasses	Ventilation-perfusion lung scan
	Cilia biopsy
Skin tests	Laryngotracheobronchoscopy
Lung function tests	Oesophagoscopy
Exercise test	Digital vascular imaging
Bronchodilator response	Thoracic CT scan
Histamine challenge	Magnetic resonance imaging
Mantoux test	Pulmonary angiography
Sweat test	Bronchography
	Psychological assessment

Chronic lung infection with bronchiectasis is commonly seen in patients with disorders of the cilia (Roberton 1985). This takes various forms the most classical of which is Kartagener's syndrome in which there is an associated situs inversus and chronic sinusitis. Cilia abnormalities leading to bronchiectasis also occur without dextrocardia (Turner et al 1981, Buchdahl et al 1988). This is discussed more fully in Chapter 7. Bronchiectasis is considerably less common nowadays than it was 30–40 years ago. This is probably due to better general health and nutrition, immunisation against diseases such as pertussis, diphtheria and measles, the wider use of antibiotics during infections and better techniques of investigation and surgery for those with significant disease.

PNEUMONIA DUE TO UNUSUAL ORGANISMS

Pneumocystis carinii

Pneumocystis carinii is a widespread organism which is probably quite common even in healthy children but which is usually asymptomatic. Pifer et al (1978) found pneumocystis antibodies in the blood in more than 60% of children by the age of four. This organism is a common cause of a severe interstitial pneumonia in the susceptible host including those with primary immune deficiency, malignant disease on chemotherapy and those with HIV infection. It used to be seen in pre-term babies but this has now disappeared. The organism proliferates in the alveoli and causes a reaction within the alveolar walls leading to an interstitial pneumonitis with a secondary inflammatory response. It cannot be cultured outside the lung itself and is only seen within the alveoli using special silver staining techniques after lung biopsy (Jaffe & Maki 1981). More recently a monoclonal antibody has been produced in order to aid identification on bronchoalveolar lavage specimens (Kovacs et al 1986). The biopsy material should be screened for other opportunistic pathogens as some children may have a mixed infection. The typical histological features include cysts containing merozoites, the true 'pneumocyst', and the trophozoite, which is less common (Roberton 1985).

The disease begins with the insidious onset of chest signs including tachypnoea without respiratory indrawing and a dry cough. Initially there is a low grade fever but as the disease progresses this becomes more fluctuant. Exercise tolerance is gradually reduced to the point where minimal exercise or indeed any movement produces a considerable increase in the respiratory rate. Cyanosis gradually appears and arterial blood gases initially show the typical changes of an interstitial pneumonia with hypoxaemia and a low carbon dioxide level (<4 kPa, 30 mmHg) in the presence of a normal pH. As the infection progresses the $P\text{a}_{CO_2}$ rises as in any other type of severe respiratory failure. Auscultation of the chest reveals no added breath sounds and no evidence of wheezing or rhonchi present. This 'silent chest' is typical of the illness.

Chest X-ray (Fig. 6.6) shows widespread granular shadowing, initially perihilar but spreading throughout both lung fields as the disease progresses. The patient is typically unable to take deep breaths because of the decreased lung compliance and the film is often described as 'expiratory' in nature, although this is in fact due to the low lung volume caused by the underlying disease.

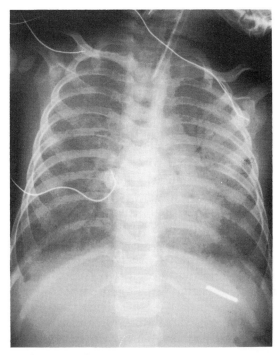

Fig. 6.6 Pneumocystis pneumonia.

Treatment of pneumocystis pneumonia consists of high dose trimethoprim and sulphamethoxazole (20 mg/kg and 100 mg/kg per 24 hours respectively) for a period of 10–14 days. This should be given by the intravenous route initially although it is also effective orally. Resolution on this regime can be expected in up to 75% of cases (Winston et al 1980). This is started empirically before lung biopsy is undertaken. In the acute illness, if high dose co-trimoxazole fails to produce a response within 48 hours, broncho-alveolar lavage or lung biopsy is performed to confirm the diagnosis and the patient is then started on pentamidine, a much more toxic drug which has to be given by the intramuscular route in a dose of 4 mg/kg/day. It has a number of side-effects including hypoglycaemia, liver and renal toxicity, thrombocytopenia and hypotension in up to 50% of cases. Response to this can, however, be quite dramatic. Those with the worst disease will require ventilation but it is often difficult to achieve adequate oxygenation because of the alveolar block to gas transfer. The pressures required frequently result in air leak from the lung including pneumothorax, pneumomediastinum and subcutaneous emphysema. Mortality is high but those who do survive the illness can make a complete recovery.

Pneumocystis infection is common in patients with HIV infection and there has been a recent report of the successful use of pentamidine by aerosol for adults with this condition (Montgomery et al 1987).

Many patients with malignant disease on chemotherapy or immune deficiency are given low dose co-trimoxazole as prophylaxis against this form of pneumonia (Hughes 1977).

Measles

Measles virus in the normal host can produce an acute bronchitis, bronchiolitis or pneumonia similar to other viral infections. The prognosis for this form of illness is extremely good, providing that any bacterial pathogens found at the same time are treated appropriately (Gremillion & Crawford 1981). A few children have been recorded as having adenovirus obliterative bronchiolitis after this form of measles and this can cause permanent lung damage (Sly et al 1984).

A much rarer form of infection in the lungs is so called measles giant cell pneumonia which is seen in children who have a defect of cell mediated immunity. The presenting features of this illness are very similar to pneumocystis pneumonia but the diagnosis can be confirmed by viral immunofluorescence of nasopharyngeal secretions. These children do not show the other usual features of measles and the typical rash is absent. This is a reflection of the fact that they are unable to mount the usual immune response to the virus. There is however an acute interstitial reaction in the lung including the development of the typical giant cells. The chest X-ray shows hazy shadowing in both lungs but this has a more patchy appearance than that seen in pneumocystis pneumonia, at least in the initial stages.

Similar blood gas changes to those found in pneumocystis pneumonia are also seen. Treatment is diffcult. Supportive measures including ventilation can be tried but are usually associated with a high rate of air leak including pneumothorax, pneumomediastinum and subcutaneous emphysema. The disease is usually fatal with progressive respiratory failure continuing despite intensive support. At present there is no other specific therapy.

Cytomegalovirus (CMV)

CMV infection is quite common in otherwise healthy children where it produces an upper respiratory illness with transient cervical adenopathy. As many as one-third of children have serum antibodies present by the age of 10 (Yow et al 1987).

CMV pneumonitis is seen in otherwise normal infants. Perinatally ac-quired CMV is not uncommon (Peckham et al 1983). This can subsequently colonise the lungs resulting in a low grade inflammatory response which gives rise to a pattern of respiratory disease manifested by episodes of wheeze which are typical of persistent or recurrent bronchiolitis. Children who present in this way should be screened for other conditions such as immune deficiency or cystic fibrosis. It is relatively easy to grow the virus from the urine and sometimes from respiratory secretions in these cases. The long term prognosis for infants with this type of CMV infection, if they are otherwise normal, is excellent.

Severe pneumonia due to CMV is seen in the immunocompromised host and presents with similar clinical features to pneumocystis pneumonia or measles giant cell pneumonitis. It may be rapidly progressive and is often fatal. This infection is a serious problem in patients undergoing any form of transplantation as the virus can be acquired from donated tissue including bone marrow, kidney, heart or lung. Evidence for the presence of CMV should first be sought by culture of respiratory secretions and urine and by specific antibodies in blood if the host can mount a response. Definitive diagnosis is by lung biopsy when the typical intracellular 'owl's eye' appearance is seen on microscopy. Treatment is with high concentration specific immunoglobulin therapy (Nicholls et al 1983, Blacklock et al 1985). A number of antiviral agents active against CMV are currently under trial.

Rubella pneumonitis

Rubella infection acquired late in pregnancy classically produces generalised disease at birth. A low grade interstitial pneumonitis is sometimes seen during the first few months of life and presents with bilateral hazy shadow-ing on the chest X-ray in the presence of low grade respiratory symptoms including persistent cough, tachypnoea and respiratory muscle indrawing. The condition is usually diagnosed following open lung biopsy which is also used to exclude other conditions such as pneumocystis pneumonia and idiopathic interstitial pneumonitis. Patients with rubella pneumonitis respond to steroid therapy (Boner et al 1983).

Fungal pneumonia

The major organisms causing fungal pneumonia in children are *Candida albicans* and aspergillus. These infections usually occur in malnourished preterm infants who have had extended courses of broad spectrum antibiotics or in immunocompromised patients with reduced cell mediated immunity including those with chronic granulomatous disease. Colonisation may begin in the trachea but rapid spread into the lung and the surrounding chest wall is not uncommon. Systemic spread beyond these boundaries also occurs when it is often rapidly progressive and fatal. Auscultation elicits variable changes from little or no added sounds to the presence of coarse bilateral crepitations. Chest X-ray shows bilateral patchy consolidation sometimes with cystic cavities present. Diagnosis is difficult, particularly in the case of *Candida albicans* since this organism is commonly present in the upper respiratory tract and specimens taken from this area for culture may merely be contaminated. The presence of candida antigen in the blood is more indicative of acute infection.

Chest X-ray usually shows fluffy bilateral shadowing or discrete circular lesions comprising the typical 'fungal ball' of invasive bronchopulmonary aspergillosis. Localised change is also seen where there is an underlying congenital abnormality such as a lung cyst. Either of these organisms can rapidly disseminate throughout the body if not treated early and aggressively. Treatment includes the use of antifungal agents such as intravenous amphotericin, 5-flucytosine, ketoconazole (Roberton 1985) or newer compounds such as itraconazole.

Aspergillus also occurs in the lung as allergic bronchopulmonary aspergillosis (ABPA). This is seen in cystic fibrosis and is discussed in Chapter 9.

PERSISTENT COUGH

The child with persistent cough is a very common problem in paediatric practice. This may arise for a number of reasons and these may be subdivided into several groups shown in Table 6.4.

Investigation of the child with this problem can be simple or complicated depending on the underlying cause. A careful history including a full review of relevant family, social and environmental factors is often very helpful in elucidating the cause. This is followed by a detailed physical examination looking for further clues as to the underlying process and its effects on the respiratory system. Further investigations which should be considered are shown in Table 6.3. The number of these undertaken depends on how easy it is to establish the cause. It is preferable to begin with the simpler and less

Table 6.4 Causes of persistent cough

Chronic or recurrent upper or lower respiratory tract infection	Bronchiectasis
Asthma/allergy	Immune deficiency
Bronchial hyper-reactivity	Cilia abnormality
Aspiration	Tracheal compression — extrinsic
Foreign body inhalation	Cardiac failure
Pertussis	Smoking
Tracheo-oesophageal fistula	Psychogenic
Cystic fibrosis	

invasive tests and to proceed to the more complicated and expensive procedures only if the symptoms warrant it.

Treatment is obviously related to the underlying condition which fortunately can be elucidated in most cases. In those with the most complicated problems there may be more than one pathological process at work. Once the mechanism is understood an appropriate plan of treatment and support can be developed. The vast majority of patients can then be relieved of their symptoms over a period of time.

REFERENCES

Barry W, Cockburn F, Cornall R, Price J F, Sutherland G, Vardag A 1986 Ribavirin aerosol for acute bronchiolitis. Archives of Disease in Childhood 61: 593–597
Bass J W, Klenk E C, Kothheimer J B et al 1969 Antimicrobial treatment of Pertussis. Journal of Pediatrics 75: 768–781
Blacklock H A, Griffiths P, Stirk P, Prentice H G 1985 Specific hyperimmune globulin for cytomegalovirus pneumonitis. Lancet II: 152–153
Boner A, Wilmott R W, Dinwiddie R et al 1983 Desquamative interstitial pneumonia and antigen antibody complexes in two infants with congenital rubella. Pediatrics 72: 835–839
Buchdahl R M, Reiser J, Ingram D, Rutman D, Cole P, Warner J O 1988. Ciliary abnormalities in respiratory disease. Archives of Disease in Childhood 63: 238–243
Cautrell R W, Bell R A, Morioka W T 1978 Acute epiglottitis: intubation versus tracheostomy. The Laryngoscope 88: 994–1005
Clarke S K R, Gardner P S, Poole P M, Simpson H, Tobin J O'H 1978 Respiratory syncytial virus infection — admissions to hospital industrial, urban and rural areas. Report to the Medical Research Council Subcommittee on RSV vaccines. British Medical Journal 2: 796–798
Colley J R T 1976 The epidemiology of respiratory disease in childhood. In: Hull D (ed) Recent advances in paediatrics. Churchill Livingstone, Edinburgh, pp 221–258
Communicable Disease Report 1987 Whooping cough: England and Wales. No: 86/27 p 4
Conrad D A, Christenson J C, Waner J L, Marks M I 1987 Aerosolised ribavirin treatment of respiratory syncytial virus infection in infants hospitalised during an epidemic. The Pediatric Infectious Disease Journal 6: 152–158
Cumming G R, MacPherson R I, Chernick V 1971 Unilateral hyperlucent lung syndrome in children. Journal of Pediatrics 78: 250–260
Dinwiddie R 1981 Pertussis. Journal of Maternal and Child Health 6: 307–309
Drug and Therapeutics Bulletin 1984 The management of acute otitis media 22: 53–55
Enders J F, McCarthy K, Mitus A, Cheatham W J 1959 Isolation of measles virus at autopsy in cases of giant cell pneumonia without rash. New England Journal of Medicine 261: 875–881

Freeland A P 1987 Acute laryngeal infections in childhood. In: Evans J N G (ed) Scott
    Brown's otolaryngology, 5th edn, vol 6. Paediatric Otolaryngology. Butterworths,
    London, pp 449–465
Godfrey S 1984 The wheezy infant. In: Meadow R (ed) Recent advances in paediatrics.
    Churchill Livingstone, Edinburgh, pp 137–153
Gordon I, Dinwiddie R, Matthew D J 1987 Respiratory system. In: Gordon I (ed)
    Diagnostic Imaging in Paediatrics. Chapman and Hall, London, pp 27–57
Gremillion D H, Crawford G E 1981 Measles pneumonia in young adults: an analysis of 106
    cases. American Journal of Medicine 71: 539–542
Hibbert J 1987 Tonsils and adenoids. In: Evans J N G (ed) Scott-Brown's otolaryngology,
    5th edn, vol 6 Paediatric Otolaryngology. Butterworths, London, pp 368–383
Hughes W T 1977 Pneumocystis carinii pneumonia. New England Journal of Medicine
    297: 1381–1383
Jaffe J P, Maki D G 1981 Lung biopsy in immunocompromised patients: one institutions's
    experience and an approach to management in the compromised host. Lancet
    48: 1143–1153
Johnston I D A, Anderson H R, Lambert H P, Patel S 1983 Pertussis long term
    morbidity. Lancet ii: 1104–1108
Kaul A, Scott R, Gallagher M, Scott M, Clement J, Ogra P L 1978 Respiratory syncytial
    virus infection: rapid diagnosis in children by use of indirect immunofluorescence.
    American Journal of Diseases of Children 132: 1088–1090
Kovacs J A, Gill V, Swan J C et al 1986 Prospective evaluation of a monoclonal antibody in
    diagnosis of Pneumocystis carinii pneumonia. Lancet II: 1–3
Lancet Editorial 1985 Acute respiratory infections in under fives: 15 million deaths a year.
    Lancet II: 699–701
Lancet Editorial 1988 Pneumonia in childhood. Lancet I: 741–743
Lang W R, Howden C W, Laws J, Burton J F 1969 Bronchopneumonia with serious
    sequelae in children with evidence of adenovirus type 21 infection. British Medical
    Journal i: 73–79
Mitchell D P, Thomas R L 1980 Secondary airway support in the management of croup.
    Journal of Otolaryngology 9: 419–422
Montgomery A B, Debs J R, Luce J M et al 1987 Aerosolised pentamidine as sole therapy for
    Pneumocystis carinii pneumonia in patients with acquired immunodeficiency syndrome.
    Lancet II: 480–483
Nicholls A J, Brown C B, Edward N, Cuthbertson B, Yap P L, McLelland D B L 1983
    Hyperimmune globulin for cytomegalovirus infections. Lancet I: 532–533
Olsen A L, Klein S W, Charney E et al 1978 Prevention and therapy of serous otitis media by
    oral decongestant. Pediatrics 61: 679–684
Peckham C S, Chin K S, Coleman J C, Henderson K, Hurley R, Preece P M 1983
    Cytomegalovirus infection in pregnancy: preliminary findings from a prospective study.
    Lancet I: 1352–1355
Pifer L L, Hughes W T, Stagno S, Woods D 1978 Pneumocystis carinii infection: evidence
    for high prevalence in normal and immuno-suppressed children. Pediatrics 61: 35–41
Pukander J, Luotoren J, Siplia M, Timonen M, Karma P 1982 Incidence of acute otitis
    media. Acta Oto-Laryngologica 93: 447–453
Roberton D M 1985 The lung in immunological disease. In: Milner A D, Martin R J (eds)
    Neonatal and pediatric respiratory medicine. Butterworths, London, pp 126–160
Royal College of General Practitioners — Swansea Research Unit 1987 Study of intellectual
    performance of children in ordinary schools after certain serious complications of
    whooping cough. British Medical Journal 295: 1044–1047
Silverman M 1984 Bronchodilators for wheezy infants. Archives of Disease in Childhood
    59: 84–87
Simpson H, Mok J Y Q 1985 Outcome of respiratory disease in childhood. In: Milner A D,
    Martin R J (ed) Neonatal and pediatric respiratory medicine. Butterworths, London,
    pp 211–235
Simpson H 1987 Management of whooping cough. Journal of Maternal and Child Health
    12: 168–171
Sly P D, Soto-Quiros, Landau L I, Hudson I, Newton-John H 1984 Factors predisposing
    to abnormal pulmonary function after adenovirus type 7 pneumonia. Archives of Disease
    in Childhood 59: 935–939

Styles W McN 1985 Caring for children in General Practice. In: Harvey D, Kovar I (eds) A textbook for the DCH. Churchill Livingstone, Edinburgh, pp 42–58

Takala A K, Alphen L V, Eskola J, Palmgren J, Bol P, Makela P H 1987 *Haemophilus influenzae* type B strains of outer membrane subtypes 1 and 1c cause different types of invasive disease. Lancet II: 647–650

Turner J A P, Corkey C W B, Lee J Y C, Levison H, Sturgess J 1981 Clinical expressions of immotile cilia syndrome. Pediatrics 67: 805–810

Winston D J, Lau W K, Gale R P, Young L S 1980 Trimethoprim-sulfamethoxazole for the treatment of *Pneumocystis carinii* pneumonia. Annals of Internal Medicine 92: 767–769

Yow M D, White N H, Taber L H et al 1987 Acquisition of cytomegalovirus infection from birth to ten years: a longitudinal serological study. Journal of Pediatrics 110: 37–42

7. Immune disease and the lung

The interactions between the body's immune system and the lungs are vital in the general defence against infection and in the aetiology of a number of allergic conditions affecting the respiratory system. A variety of serious pulmonary infections can occur when there is a breakdown or deficiency in the immune defences.

PRINCIPLES OF IMMUNITY

In order to understand the role of the immune system in the development of lung disease it is important to have a knowledge of the normal mechanisms by which this part of the body defends itself from attack by outside agents. The defence mechanisms of the immune system may be divided into three major components as elsewhere in the body. These comprise the non-specific initial responses and the specific responses which can be sub-divided into those which function either through the cell mediated or humoral immune systems.

Initial defences

The initial defence systems are mainly structural but with important general secretory antimicrobial and anti-allergic components. Examples of this include the anatomical structure of the nasal passages and the external ear canal which are designed to trap invading bacteria and foreign substances. The secretions in the nose and ears contain substances which are generally bactericidal as well as other specific immunologically active agents such as immunoglobulin A. The airways themselves are lined by pseudostratified columnar epithelium with ciliated cells and goblet cells down to the terminal bronchioles. Beyond this level the alveoli are lined by thin squamous type I pneumocytes across which gas exchange takes place, type II surfactant secreting pneumocytes which are more cuboidal in shape (Breeze & Wheeldon 1977) and alveolar macrophages. The goblet cells of the larger airways have a major secretory function and produce the respiratory mucus which forms the mucociliary blanket on top of the cilia. This also contains a number of important non-specific antimicrobial substances which inhibit adherence of organisms to the lining of the airways. Other substances present in this mucus include lysozyme, lactoferrin and alpha-1-antitrypsin (Roberton 1985). There is also a cellular component to this form of defence which includes freely moving lung macrophages reinforced by polymorphonuclear neutrophils during the initial inflammatory response. These cells have non-specific bactericidal properties and act as an important barrier to infection until the specific immune mediated system mounts its slower but more prolonged response (Kirkwood & Lewis 1983).

Larger particulate matter entering the airways is caught in the nose although smaller particles of 2–3 μm descend further down the respiratory tree and are trapped by the ciliary mechanism. The cilia are found throughout the respiratory tract down to the terminal bronchioles and are approximately 6–7 μm in length although they become shorter the deeper they are in the respiratory system. They beat at 12–16 Hz (Buchdahl et al 1988), mainly in an upward direction and in a coordinated way called metachronal waves which stimulate the flow of mucus out of the lungs; this mechanism is assisted by the normal cough reflex.

Cilia have a specific ultrastructural appearance called the '9+2' pattern (Lancet 1988). This consists of nine double armed tubules, 'doublets', peripherally and a central core of two single tubules, 'singlets', (Figs 7.1 and 7.2). Attached to each of the double tubules are inner and outer dynein arms which are ATPase containing. These are thought to be responsible for the ciliary movements which are so important to their function. The frequency with which the cilia beat is variable and is probably more rapid in the larger airways (Rutland et al 1982). Ciliary beat frequency may be diminished by structural abnormalities and by external influences such

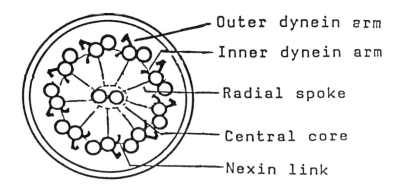

Fig. 7.1   Structure of normal cilia.

as intercurrent respiratory infection, accidentally inhaled chemicals, aspirin ingestion and possibly cigarette smoke (Roberton 1985). Ciliated epithelial cells are present down to the terminal bronchioles and beyond this level the defence against the smallest particles is mediated via the mucus secretions and the freely wandering alveolar macrophages which can directly ingest invading organisms.

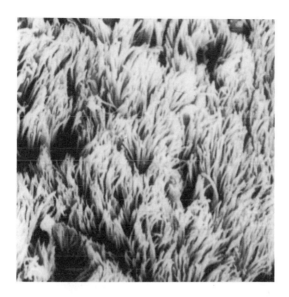

Fig. 7.2   Electron photomicrograph of normal human cilia. × 50 000. Courtesy of Dr G Gau, Queen Charlotte's Hospital, London.

Primary ciliary dyskinesia/immotile cilia syndrome

A number of conditions in which there is either an absence or a severely reduced ciliary motility have been reported (Roberton 1985, Buchdahl 1988). Children with classical symptoms have recurrent sinusitis, bronchiectasis and situs inversus; this triad comprises Kartagener's syndrome. The classical syndrome is an autosomal recessive condition with incomplete penetrance occurring in approximately 1 in 15 000 births (Rott 1983). Males with this syndrome are usually infertile because of reduced ciliary motility of the sperm tails. A wide variety of ciliary defects have now been reported and the condition has been renamed primary ciliary dyskinesia (Sleigh 1981). Nowadays only about 50% of patients presenting with ciliary defects actually have classical Kartagener's syndrome.

Cilia can be obtained by a special nasal brushing technique and examined immediately for motility by a photometric method (Rutland & Cole 1982).

Electron microscopy reveals a variety of structural defects which must be present in at least 50% of the cilia examined to be significant. The abnormalities reported include defective dynein arms, defective or missing radial spokes, microtubular abnormalities, compound cilia, abnormally long cilia and complete ciliary aplasia (Sturgess et al 1980). Cilia dysfunction may be present even in structurally normal cilia (Greenstone et al 1983). Some motility defects are secondary to viral or bacterial infection and return to normal after treatment.

As the condition is present from birth it can produce symptoms of respiratory distress in the neonatal period (Whitelaw et al 1981, Ramet et al 1986). Many children present later with chronic upper and lower respiratory tract disease. There is a strong correlation with secretory otitis media and conductive hearing loss. Lower respiratory tract infection is almost universal. All 18 affected children reported by Buchdahl et al (1988) had developed chronic lower respiratory tract problems although this population was highly selected because of the frequency and severity of their symptoms. These children represented 11% of a larger group investigated for chronic respiratory tract disease. Thirteen of the 18 had chronic upper respiratory problems and all had had some neonatal respiratory difficulty. The typical appearance on chest X-ray is shown in Fig. 7.3.

As most of these abnormalities are structural they are therefore irreversible so therapy is directed to vigorous treatment of intercurrent infection

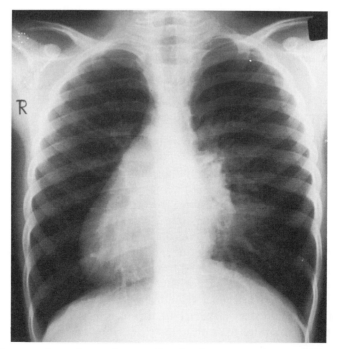

Fig. 7.3 Kartagener's syndrome: dextrocardia, situs inversus, persistent collapse and consolidation of left mid-zone.

with antibiotics and physiotherapy to delay the onset and progression of bronchiectasis. Appropriate ENT intervention can alleviate some of the recurrent upper respiratory tract problems. Particular attention should be paid to the detection and treatment of conductive hearing loss. Adult males will require appropriate testing and counselling in regard to infertility.

Cell mediated immunity

The major functions of the immune system are carried out at the tissue level by certain types of lymphocytic cell. These are found as two major subtypes known as T and B lymphocytes. T lymphocytes or thymus dependent lymphocytes are programmed by passage through the thymus gland to produce specific responses such as antigen recognition, graft rejection, tumour surveillance, and delayed hypersensitivity to foreign protein such as tuberculoprotein. The T cells and macrophages initially process antigen following which it is presented to the circulating pool of B lymphocytes. Lymphocytes are particularly important in protection against viral and some fungal infections.

T lymphocytes are also responsible for immunological memory and for the production of cell mediators such as lymphokines affecting other lymphocytes and macrophages. They are divided into major groups such as helper or suppresser cells which are important in the immune response (Fig. 7.4) and also cytotoxic cells which direct antigens (class II antigens) onto the surface of foreign cells. These cells therefore function either through the production of substances such as lymphokines or they may be directly cytotoxic — killer cells. Lymphokines attract neutrophils and macrophages to areas of local inflammation where they are directly aimed at the ingestion and killing of invading organisms. Cytotoxic killer T cells can respond directly to specific receptors (class I antigens) on the surface of foreign cells and cause direct cell lysis. The killer cell is not itself destroyed and is then available to attack further invading foreign material. Macrophages also have a role in the preparation of foreign material for presentation mainly to helper T cells. This is an example of the important cooperation between the different cell types which facilitates the effective function of the system as a whole.

A number of specific diseases involving abnormalities of cell mediated immunity have been described which can lead to chronic respiratory disease and permanent lung damage. Some conditions affecting the cell mediated immune system can result in acute infection of the lungs by specific opportunistic organisms; these are described later.

Humoral immunity

The other major arm of the immune system which is important in the pathogenesis of respiratory disease is the humoral immune system. Although classified separately it is also regulated via the T cell system. Humoral immunity functions mainly through the production of specific immunoglobulin

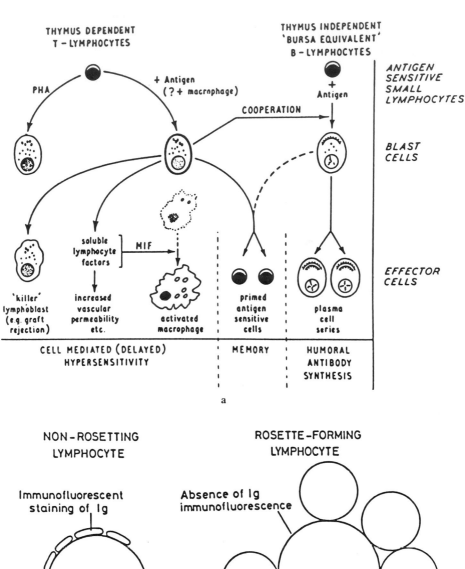

THYMUS DEPENDENT
T – LYMPHOCYTES

THYMUS INDEPENDENT
'BURSA EQUIVALENT'
B – LYMPHOCYTES

ANTIGEN
SENSITIVE
SMALL
LYMPHOCYTES

PHA

+ Antigen
(? + macrophage)

+
Antigen

COOPERATION

BLAST
CELLS

soluble
lymphocyte
factors

MIF

EFFECTOR
CELLS

'killer'
lymphoblast
(e.g. graft
rejection)

increased
vascular
permeability
etc.

activated
macrophage

primed
antigen
sensitive
cells

plasma
cell
series

CELL MEDIATED (DELAYED)
HYPERSENSITIVITY

MEMORY

HUMORAL
ANTIBODY
SYNTHESIS

a

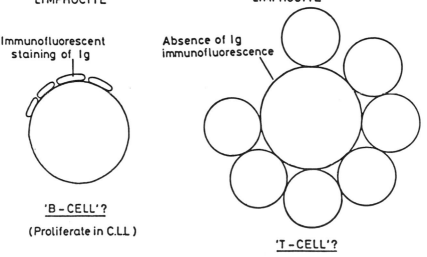

NON – ROSETTING
LYMPHOCYTE

ROSETTE – FORMING
LYMPHOCYTE

Immunofluorescent
staining of Ig

Absence of Ig
immunofluorescence

'B – CELL'?

(Proliferate in C.LL)

'T – CELL'?

b

Fig. 7.4 (a) The cells of the immune system. (b) Some characteristics of T and B lymphocytes. B cells have immunoglobulin on the cell surface. T cells form spontaneous rosettes with sheep erythrocytes. (Reproduced with permission of Dr M de Swiet and the Editor of the Lancet.)

from B lymphocytes. These are programmed in avian species through the Bursa of Fabricus, the primary lymphoid organ. This organ is not specifically found in humans; however, the equivalent is the bone marrow which serves a similar function, hence the retention of the term 'B' lymphocyte. These cells are involved in the production of specific antibody or immunoglobulin in response to stimulation by foreign protein. When this happens they increase their metabolic rate and divide further to become plasma cells. The plasma cells and their associated immunoglobulin secretions are particularly important in the body's resistance to bacterial infection.

Immunoglobulins are found in five main classes each with a very specific chemical structure and defined biological role in life. The immunoglobulin classes are IgG, IgA, IgM, IgD and IgE. Although a great deal remains to be learnt about them, the role of each within the immune system is quite different, especially in the lung.

IgG is relatively small with a molecular weight of 150 000 — this enables it to cross easily into the interstitial tissues. The IgG antigen–antibody interaction leads to the formation of immune complexes, stimulating the release of complement and enhancing the local phagocytic responses of neutrophils and macrophages. IgG levels do rise initially during acute infection but the major response occurs 3–4 weeks later as this immunoglobulin forms the principal part of the secondary phase of the immune response. Phagocytosis is also enhanced by the attachment of IgG to the invading cell. IgG is the major immunoglobulin transferred from mother to baby in utero protecting the infant from infection in the early months of life. Much of this transfer occurs near to term so preterm babies miss out on a great deal of this important protective mechanism.

IgG subclasses

Four IgG subclasses are recognised. The genes for the expression of these subclasses lie on the long arm of chromosome number 14 (Flanagan 1982). Their biological properties are still under investigation but they appear to be involved in a wide variety of disease states including many in the respiratory system (Schur 1987).

The normal values for IgG and the IgG subclasses are shown in Table 7.1. There is a wide range at all ages with a gradual increase during childhood (Morell et al 1972, Schur et al 1979). Serum IgG1 and IgG3 levels rise more rapidly to adult values than IgG2 and IgG4. Low levels of IgG2 and IgG4 should therefore be interpreted with caution in children under two years of age. In the normal adult the percentage contribution of each subclass to the total IgG level is IgG1 65%, IgG2 25%, IgG3 7% and IgG4 3% (Morgan & Levinsky 1988a).

IgG1 and IgG3 are the most efficient complement binders especially to platelets and monocytes; they are also found in the cystoplasm of B lymphocytes. IgG2 and IgG4 are poor complement binders and are found on

Table 7.1   Total serum IgG and IgG subclasses in mg/dl for age (from Schur 1987)

Age(yr)	IgG*	IgG1	IgG2	IgG3	IgG4†
0–1	420	340	59	39	19
	(250–690)	(190–620)	(30–140)	(9–62)	(6–63)
1–2	470	410	68	34	13
	(270–810)	(230–710)	(30–170)	(11–98)	(4–43)
2–3	540	480	98	28	18
	(300–980)	(280–830)	(40–240)	(6–130)	(3–120)
3–4	600	530	120	30	32
	(400–910)	(350–790)	(50–260)	(9–98)	(5–180)
4–6	860	540	140	39	39
	(440–1000)	(360–810)	(60–310)	(9–160)	(9–160)
6–8	890	560	150	48	81
	(580–1400)	(280–1120)	(30–630)	(40–250)	(11–620)
8–10	1000	690	210	85	42
	(530–1900)	(280–1740)	(80–550)	(22–320)	(10–170)
10–13	910	590	240	58	60
	(500–1680)	(270–1290)	(110–550)	(13–250)	(7–530)
13–Adult	910	540	210	58	60
	(580–1450)	(280–1020)	(60–790)	(14–240)	(11–330)

* Geometric means are presented for each immunoglobulin at every age. The normal ranges, given in parentheses, are obtained by taking the mean logarithm ± twice the S.D. of the logarithms and then taking the antilogs of the results.
† 10% of individuals appear to have absent IgG4 levels.

the surface of B lymphocytes. IgG1 and IgG3 are involved in antibody production to protein antigens and IgG2 to carbohydrate antigens including bacterial capsular polysaccharides. IgG4 appears to be involved in allergic reactions since various foods and inhaled antigens can induce IgG4 specific antibodies. The precise role of these antibodies in relation to allergic reactions and to the more common IgE reaginic antibodies is not yet clear.

In childhood there is a 3:1 male to female ratio for those with reduced levels of one or more IgG subclass (Morgan & Levinsky 1988a), with IgG2 deficiency being the most common. IgG subclass deficiency can occur even in the presence of a normal total serum IgG.

Specific correlations of IgG subclass deficiency and respiratory disease have been observed in children. Those with low IgG2 levels appear to be particularly prone to otitis media (Oxelius 1984) and lower respiratory tract infection (Smith et al 1984). This may be because the IgG2 deficiency leads to a poor response to the polysaccharide capsular antigens of bacteria such as pneumococcus and *Haemophilus influenzae* (Ambrosino et al 1985). There is also an association between IgG1 deficiency, low total IgG or IgA and recurrent or severe respiratory infection in children (Beard et al 1986). IgA deficiency has also been seen in relation to IgG2 with or without Ig4 subclass deficiency. This may be because the genes for these immunoglobulins lie close together on the long arm of chromosome 14 (Flanagan et al 1982). Atopic disease is particularly common among those who have IgG3 deficiency in whom IgG4 levels may be reduced or significantly elevated (Morgan et al 1986). About 10% of the population appear to have absence of IgG4 yet the vast majority are asymptomatic (Schur 1987).

The treatment of patients with IgG subclass deficiency depends on the presence of significant symptoms as a result. Those who have frequent or recurrent serious bacterial infection should have antibiotics early during the course of any such illness and may require continuous low dose prophylactic antibiotics such as cotrimoxazole once daily. A few will require intravenous replacement with immunoglobulin infusion at 3–4 week intervals.

IgA (molecular weight 170 000) is the major secretory immunoglobulin and is found in all mucosal surface secretions at high levels. In this phase it adopts a dimeric form where two molecules are joined by a third called the 'secondary piece'. This substance is produced by the mucosal lining cells and is thought to protect the IgA from digestion by other enzymes. It is the most important immunoglobulin in the protection of respiratory mucosal surfaces from initial attack by foreign proteins which may be involved in either infective or allergic reactivity with the host. IgA is relatively deficient at birth and in the first few months of life, but is present in large quantities in colostrum and breast milk. Hence the importance of breast feeding in the prevention of early infection.

IgM is a large molecule consisting of five basic units with a molecular weight of 900 000; it is mainly confined to the intravascular space because of its size. It is the first antibody to be produced against infection and so forms part of the primary response. Measurement of specific IgM is often used to diagnose acute infection by a particular organism.

IgD is found in very small amounts in the serum and its role in the immune system is not yet understood.

IgE has a molecular weight of 200 000 and is the principal immunoglobulin involved in the response to allergen exposure from outside. High levels of IgE are commonly found in asthmatic or atopic patients. Cells in the body which are involved in the acute allergic response include mast cells and basophils and these may have allergen specific IgE antibodies attached to them. This means that on contact with the relevant allergen a specific reaction occurs with the mast cell or basophil releasing histamine and other locally vasoactive substances which cause allergic symptoms such as bronchospasm or localised tissue oedema. Leukotrienes and prostaglandins are also involved in these reactions. Very high levels of IgE are associated with recurrent infection and are discussed on pages 141 and 142.

IMMUNE DEFICIENCY SYNDROMES

A number of conditions occur in which there are major abnormalities of the immune system leading to serious infections of the lung with the potential for long term damage. The major conditions are shown in Table 7.2.

Severe combined immune deficiency (SCID)

This condition is usually characterised by a profound deficiency of both cell mediated and humoral immunity. Affected children have very poorly functioning T cells which may or may not be present in normal numbers

Table 7.2 Cell mediated or combined immune deficiency

Severe combined immune deficiency (SCID)
Adenosine deaminase (ADA) deficiency (SCID)
Purine nucleoside phosphorylase deficiency (SCID)
Reticular dysgenesis (SCID)
Neutrophil mobility defect
Malnutrition
Measles
Treatment for malignant disease
Di George's syndrome
Human immunodeficiency virus (HIV) infection

---

in the peripheral blood. The T cell numbers are assessed by sheep red cell rosette formation or other techniques such as monoclonal antibodies and are found to be grossly deficient. Their response to phytohaemagglutinin (PHA) is very low or undetectable. There is an associated panhypogamma-globulinaemia so that antibody formation is also severely impaired. The great variety of SCID syndromes probably represent a range of disorders of lymphoid maturation arrest varying from totally defective lymphoid maturation involving all bone marrow derived cells, such as in reticular dysgenesis, to specific enzyme disorders of the purine salvage pathway such as adenosine deaminase deficiency. Other milder variants are seen such as those with normal levels of immunoglobulins but very poor antibody production.

The classical presentation of an immune deficiency occurs between 3 and 6 months of age when maternal antibody protection has worn off. The child presents with the insidious onset of chronic respiratory infection in association with failure to thrive and quite often recurrent loose stools. This condition clearly has to be distinguished from cystic fibrosis which may present in a very similar way. The lung infection is frequently caused by unusual 'opportunistic' organisms such as Cytomegalovirus, *Candida albicans*, *Pneumocystis carinii*, measles, varicella, adenovirus or tuberculosis. Evidence of chronic or recurrent low grade infection elsewhere such as persistent candidiasis, recurrent herpes of the skin or a previous history of a more serious infection such as meningitis should alert one to this possible diagnosis. Physical examination can also yield important clues that there could be an immune deficiency. There may be a paucity of lymph nodes despite chronic infection and the tonsils are very small or absent. Chest X-ray reveals either a small or absent thymic shadow.

Treatment of the underlying lung disease depends on the causative organism. As this may be of an unusual type it is important to be aggressive in the search for the diagnosis. Open lung biopsy is frequently required in such cases within 48–72 hours of admission if initial treatment with broad spectrum antibiotics and high dose trimethoprim-sulphamethoxazole (for *Pneumocystis carinii*) has failed to produce a satisfactory response. Specific treatment for the offending organism, be it viral, bacterial or fungal, is given in high dosage. It may be supplemented by intravenous pooled human immunoglobulin to replace this part of the immunodeficiency (Winston et al 1982). It is very important to give these patients irradiated blood products since live lymphocytes can cause a graft-versus-host reaction which is usually fatal. If the child recovers from the initial illness it is useful to use cotrimoxazole as a prophylaxis against pneumocystis infection.

Children with SCID syndromes usually die within the first 2 years of life. Their only hope of successful treatment is to have a bone marrow transplant, preferably matched from a histocompatible sibling. If the affected child is the first born or if the immediate family is small suitable donors may prove difficult to find; haploidentical bone marrow transplant is then the treatment of choice. The treatment is not only extremely complex and expensive but 30–40% of patients succumb to associated complications before, during or after the transplant. If the graft does take properly and any graft versus host disease is controlled then the chances of longer term continuing engraftment and survival are as high as 80%.

Adenosine deaminase deficiency (ADA deficiency) and purine nucleoside phosphorylase deficiency

These conditions are examples of inherited forms of SCID in which there is a specific enzyme defect (Giblett et al 1972, 1975). The lymphocytes are damaged by the accumulation within them of abnormal metabolites such as deoxyadenosine (Simmonds et al 1978). These children suffer from lung disease which is similar to other forms of SCID; their only hope of long term cure is by successful bone marrow transplant. Those with ADA deficiency can present early in life with mixed T and B cell defects whereas those with the very rare nucleoside phosphorylase deficiency present later in childhood, principally with T cell defects, neurological symptoms and autoimmune haemolytic anaemia. These forms of SCID are inherited as autosomal recessive disorders and antenatal diagnosis is possible (Linch et al 1984).

Reticular dysgenesis

Reticular dysgenesis is a rare recessively inherited severe immune deficiency arising in the bone marrow. These children present with profound deficiency of the myeloid precursors in bone marrow and neutropenia — T and B cell numbers are extremely low. They usually succumb to intercurrent infection very early in life. The only available treatment is bone marrow transplant.

Neutrophil mobility defects

A number of children have been described who have frequent infections, particularly of the upper and lower respiratory tract, in whom defective neutrophil mobility is a factor. In vitro these cells move sluggishly and show diminished ingestion of opsonised yeast particles although in a number of cases they can be stimulated by ascorbic acid (vitamin C) or cimetidine. Administration of ascorbic acid is useful therapeutically.

Recently an inherited syndrome with specific enzyme defects has been described in a number of children presenting with delayed umbilical cord separation, recurrent pyogenic infection, diminished pus formation and granulocytosis. These patients had profound abnormalities of neutrophil mobility and phagocytosis of opsonised particles. They were found to have severe deficiency of adhesive surface glycoproteins, especially Mac-1 and LFA-1. This deficiency results in excessive cell stickiness, especially in neutrophils, which may explain their reduced mobility (Anderson et al 1985).

Di George's syndrome

This is due to a developmental anomaly of the third and fourth branchial arches. In its complete form there is absence of the thymus and parathyroid glands and an abnormality of the great vessels, especially a double aortic arch. These children can present with neonatal tetany and develop recurrent respiratory infection particularly due to viruses, fungi or pneumocystis. They have deficient lymphoid maturation with low T cell numbers and although the total immunoglobulin levels are often normal specific antibody formation is poor. They have a high mortality from their cardiac and lung disease. Treatment with fetal thymic tissue has occasionally been successful (Thong et al 1978) and some infants with partial Di George syndrome have shown spontaneous improvement with time (Asherson & Webster 1980). Successful bone marrow transplant has also been reported (Goldsobel et al 1987).

Malnutrition

Patients with severe malnutrition suffer from frequent respiratory infection because they have reduced cell mediated immunity and hypoproteinaemia. As they may be unable to mount a satisfactory response to such infections they are more liable to develop permanent lung damage such as bronchiectasis or obliterative bronchiolitis.

Measles

After measles there is a transient immune suppression which may allow secondary infection with other viruses such as adenovirus (Sly et al 1984) or precipitate a recurrence of previous tuberculous infection as sensitivity to tuberculoprotein is often diminished. This is particularly likely to happen in those who are already malnourished. Whenever possible children should be protected from measles by immunisation. Measles vaccine is however a live vaccine and in this context cannot be given to those with major immune deficiency.

Children with significant immune suppression who acquire infection with measles virus are likely to develop a specific and usually fatal form of giant cell interstitial pneumonia which is described in more detail on pages 121 and 122.

Malignant disease on chemotherapy

Patients with underlying malignant disease on chemotherapy often have depressed cellular immunity. They are unusually prone to opportunistic infection with organisms such as cytomegalovirus, measles, *Pneumocystis carinii* and fungi such as candida or aspergillus.

Chronic granulomatous disease

Chronic granulomatous disease is an X-linked recessive disorder in which there is an inability of the neutrophils and monocytes to kill ingested bacteria. This is thought to be due to an intrinsic cellular deficiency of cytochrome B. These cells also fail to reduce the dye nitroblue tetrazolium (NBT) — this forms the basis of the NBT test which is used for diagnosis. Children with this problem present with recurrent bronchopneumonia, empyema and hilar adenopathy. They often have persistent skin infection and cervical adenopathy. There is an associated hypergammaglobulinaemia. Treatment is by prolonged and aggressive antibiotic therapy and early drainage of any empyema. Despite very active treatment this disease continues to carry a high mortality in the first few years of life.

DISORDERS DUE TO HUMORAL IMMUNE DEFICIENCY

The other major group of disorders affecting the lung are those due to defects of the humoral immune system. These are principally manifested as a deficiency of antibody production. The more commonly seen types are shown in Table. 7.3

IgA deficiency

There is a physiological deficiency of serum IgA in the early months of life until the infant develops his or her own intrinsic levels. During this period

Table 7.3 Defects of humoral immunity

Immunoglobulin A deficiency
Common variable immune deficiency
X-linked agammaglobulinaemia
Transient hypogammaglobulinaemia
Decreased IgG and IgA with increased IgM (hyper IgM syndrome)
Hyper IgE syndrome
Immunoglobulin subclass deficiency

protection is by maternal IgA in breast milk. As IgA is the principal immunoglobulin of mucosal surfaces these low levels in early life are one reason why infants are particularly prone to respiratory infections.

Persistent selective IgA deficiency after this period is the commonest primary immune deficiency in the population affecting approximately 1 in 500 (Hanson et al 1983). The clinical effects of IgA deficiency are extremely variable and most individuals are asymptomatic. Those who have persistently low or absent IgA are however clinically more prone to chronic upper and lower respiratory tract infection and middle ear infection. Those with low concentrations (<0.05 g/l) have a higher incidence of pneumonia and are more likely to have permanent deficiency than those with less reduced levels; in a very small proportion this may lead to serious lung damage such as bronchiectasis (Morgan & Levinsky 1988b). In patients with atopic disorders including asthma the incidence of IgA deficiency is considerably higher approaching 1 in 100 individuals (Hanson et al 1983). The mechanism by which this occurs is not fully understood but it is thought that the decreased surface immunity might allow access to the circulation of inhaled antigenic substances to which the child may become allergic.

IgA deficiency may be a temporary phenomenon especially in children (Plebani et al 1986). During the development of the immune system IgA is the latest of the immunoglobulins to develop and IgA deficiency may merely be the expression of delayed maturation of this part of the humoral immune system. The reasons why most individuals are asymptomatic are also not clear; the rest of the immune system is thought to compensate in other ways, for example by an increase is mucosal IgM secretion (Brandtzaeg et al 1987). There is also an association with other subtle immune deficits such as IgG subclass deficiency (Beard et al 1986) which may further predispose the individual to respiratory infection.

Management of the child with symptomatic IgA deficiency includes early antibiotic therapy during intercurrent infection, control of associated allergic symptoms, prophylactic antibiotics such as cotrimoxazole and rarely immunoglobulin infusions for those with significant lung damage (Morgan & Levinsky 1988b). Most symptomatic children with IgA deficiency improve with age and at least 50% can expect to become asymptomatic by the time they reach adult life.

Common variable immunodeficiency

This is an ill defined form of immune deficiency in which there is a variable degree of hypogammaglobulinaemia. It tends to present after the first year of life and results in illness of varying severity depending on the degree and type of deficiency. There may be a partially reduced cell mediated response as well. These children suffer from recurrent respiratory tract infections. In some cases chronic bacterial infection leads to permanent lung damage with resultant bronchiectasis. Treatment is with intravenous immunoglobulin replacement at monthly intervals in those with significant symptoms.

X-linked agammaglobulinaemia (Bruton's disease)

This condition is an X-linked recessive disorder seen only in males. Immunoglobulin levels are extremely low although T cell numbers and non-specific immunity are normal. Affected infants develop recurrent upper and lower respiratory tract bacterial infections during the second part of the first year of life when transferred maternal antibody has worn off. On examination they have virtually absent tonsils and adenoids and this may be a clue to the diagnosis. They tend to have recurrent pulmonary infection because they fail to produce antibody after exposure to an organism. Treatment nowadays consists of physiotherapy, appropriate antibiotics and life-long monthly intravenous immunoglobulin replacement to keep the chest clear and to avoid or delay the onset of bronchiectasis (Roberton 1985).

Decreased IgG and IgA with increased IgM (hyper IgM syndrome)

Children with this problem are usually male again suggesting an X-linked recessive inheritance. IgG and IgA are low or absent while IgM is high. There may be an associated neutropenia. These patients are prone to infection of the lungs with *Pneumocystis carinii*.

Transient hypogammaglobulinaemia of infancy

All neonates are initially protected by transferred maternal IgG during late fetal life. Throughout the first 6 months the infant starts to produce his own immunoglobulins in increasing quantities so that by the time maternal antibody has disappeared these will provide adequate protection. A small number of infants show a delay of up to a year or more in the onset of this natural process. During this period they are specially prone to bacterial respiratory tract infection. If these are severe then intravenous immunoglobulin replacement and antibiotic prophylaxis is necessary until maturation has occurred, at the most by 4–5 years of age.

Hyper IgE syndrome

Although this syndrome is characterised by very high levels of IgE (>2000 IU/ml), children who have this condition suffer from severe recurrent infections, especially staphylococcal. There is also a marked eosinophilia in the blood. T and B cell numbers are normal as are the levels of the other immunoglobulins. IgG antibody response is, however, poor. The lymphocyte response to common antigens is also depressed as is the neutrophil chemotactic response.

These children suffer from repeated skin infection and episodes of pneumonia, particularly with staphylococci. Other Gram-positive and Gram-negative bacteria and fungi such as candida and aspergillus can be a major problem. Large pneumatoceles are found in almost all cases with pulmonary involvement. These may be very difficult to manage since they are often recurrent and because they may harbour persistent infection which the patient finds hard to clear. Lobectomy is often required to deal with this problem. Vigorous treatment of any lung infection is always indicated and these patients should receive continuous antistaphylococcal antibiotics throughout life.

Other conditions

There are a number of other rare conditions in which immune deficiency is associated with recurrent respiratory infection. These include Wiskott-Aldrich syndrome which is X-linked and where there is also eczema, thrombocytopenia and recurrent loose stools; Chediak-Higashi syndrome in which there is a neutrophil mobility defect correctable by ascorbic acid, at least in vitro; ataxia telangiectasia which is an autosomal recessive disease associated with immunoglobulin A and E deficiency; reduced cell mediated immunity; absent tonsils and lymph nodes; cerebellar degeneration and recurrent pneumonia. A number of abnormalities of the complement system have also been described (Roberton 1985).

SPECIFIC INFECTIONS

Pneumocystis carinii

Many normal children have asymptomatic contact with this organism and 48–60% have antibodies to it by mid-childhood (Pifer et al 1978, Gerrard et al 1987). It is also one of the most common causes of opportunistic lung infection in the immunocompromised host. The clinical aspects are reviewed in Chapter 6. In the susceptible host it can cause severe progressive pneumonia which is fatal if not treated aggressively from an early stage. As the organism is susceptible to cotrimoxazole many clinics use this in low dose as prophylaxis to prevent infection in high risk patients.

Cytomegalovirus (CMV)

Immune suppressed patients are prone to a number of viral infections in the lung. These may occur in combination with bacteria or fungi in the susceptible host. One of the most common viruses is CMV. Infection in normal children is common, one-third having antibodies by the age of 10 (Yow et al 1987); it usually causes little systemic upset. In the immunocompromised however it causes a much more severe illness. The organism is acquired nosocomially, via blood products or through transplanted tissue such as bone marrow, kidney, heart or lungs. Reactivation of previous infection also occurs as a result of immunosuppressive therapy.

The clinical signs are very similar to those seen with pneumocystis infection and are reviewed in Chapter 6, pages 121 and 122. At present treatment is difficult but pooled hyperimmune globulin is helpful (Nicholls et al 1983, Blacklock et al 1985). The condition still carries a high mortality in the immune suppressed.

Measles

Measles virus causes an unusual form of giant cell pneumonitis in the immune suppressed patient, this is more common in those with defects of cell mediated immunity. The disease presents in a similar way to infection with pneumocystis or cytomegalovirus. The clinical signs are reviewed in Chapter 6. There is as yet no specific treatment for this type of infection and it is usually fatal in the immunocompromised patient. It is far better to prevent the risk of this infection by previous immunisation in early childhood.

Aspergillus fumigatus

Severe and sometimes overwhelming infection of the lungs with this fungus occurs in those with reduced cell mediated immunity especially in chronic granulomatous disease. The clinical features are reviewed in Chapter 6. The infection may begin in the tracheobronchial tree but can spread rapidly to the lung and the surrounding chest wall. Systemic spread beyond these boundaries is not uncommon when it is often rapidly progressive and usually fatal. Treatment is with antifungal agents such as amphotericin and 5-flucytosine.

Candida albicans

This organism commonly causes oral infection, especially in those who are already on broad spectrum antibiotics because of bacterial infection. It is thus a frequent contaminant of sputum specimens taken for culture. It can however spread down into the lungs or invade the bloodstream resulting in rapidly progressive, widespread multiorgan disease. This is seen in extremely preterm infants and in the immune suppressed patient. Lung infection is especially likely in the neutropenic child (Roberton 1985). The physical signs are variable but similar to those seen with aspergillus. The clinical features and treatment are reviewed in Chapter 6.

Human Immunodeficiency Virus (HIV)

Increasing numbers of children infected with this virus are now being reported. As many as 10% of patients with primary immune deficiency may have HIV infection (Ammann 1985). Vertical transmission from affected mother to child will be seen increasingly as the number of cases infected through unscreened blood products diminishes (Pawha et al 1986). The specific pattern of abnormality seen initially appears to be one of panhypergammaglobulinaemia and T cell deficiency (Ammann et al 1985). Sooner or later all will become HIV antibody positive. These children may present with any opportunistic lung infection including all of those already described. HIV antibodies should therefore be sought in any child who presents with an unusual or indolent lung infection, especially those whose parents are in high risk groups for HIV acquisition.

Apart from the opportunistic infections to which these patients are prone a specific pneumonic pattern of lymphoid interstitial pneumonitis (LIP) has been described in HIV positive children (Joshi et al 1985). This is typified by diffuse infiltration of the alveolar septae and peribronchial areas by lymphocytes, plasma cells and immunoblasts. This can occur in the presence or absence of opportunistic organisms such as pneumocystis or CMV. Epstein-Barr virus DNA has also been found in a number of lung biopsy specimens from children with LIP (Andiman et al 1985). There is as yet no specific treatment.

It is advisable to immunise symptomatic HIV infected children and those carrying HIV antibodies from their mother, themselves asymptomatic, with diphtheria, tetanus, pertussis, measles and polio vaccine although not with BCG (Campbell 1988) since there is a significant risk of systemic dissemination due to the underlying T cell abnormality. Children who are symptomatic because of HIV infection but who are unimmunised should also be given appropriate immunoglobulin to measles or varicella if they are in direct contact with those who are suffering from active infection with either of these viruses. Children whose parents or other household members are immunocompromised for any reason, such as HIV infection, should be given inactivated polio vaccine. The subject of childhood acquired immunodeficiency syndrome is well reviewed by Barbour (1987).

REFERENCES

Ambrosino D M, Schifman G, Gotschlich E C et al 1985 Correlation between G2 m(n) immunoglobulin allotype and human antibody response and susceptibility to polysaccharide encapsulated bacteria. Journal of Clinical Investigation 75: 1935
Ammann A J 1985 The acquired immunodeficiency syndrome in infants and children. Annals of Internal Medicine 103: 734–737
Ammann A J, Kaminsky L, Cowan M, Levy J A 1985 Antibodies to AIDS-associated retrovirus distinguish between pediatric primary and acquired immunodeficiency diseases. Journal of the American Medical Association 253: 3116–3118
Anderson D C, Schmalsteig F C, Finegold M J et al 1985 The severe and moderate phenotypes of heritable Mac-1, LFA-1 deficiency: their quantitative definition and relation to leukocyte dysfunction and clinical features. The Journal of Infectious Disease 152: 668–689
Andiman W A, Martin K, Rubinstein et al 1985 Opportunistic lymphoproliferation associated with Epstein-Barr viral DNA in infants and children with AIDS. Lancet II: 1390–1393

Asherson G L, Webster A D B (eds) 1980 Di George Syndrome. In: Diagnosis and treatment of immunodeficiency diseases. Blackwell Scientific, London, pp 175-179

Barbour S D 1987 Acquired immunodeficiency syndrome of childhood. Pediatric Clinics of North America 34: 247-268

Beard L J, Ferrante A, Oxelius V A, Maxwell G M 1986 IgG subclass deficiency in children with IgA deficiency presenting with recurrent or severe respiratory infections. Pediatric Research 20: 937-942

Blacklock H A, Griffiths P, Stirk P, Prentice H G 1985 Specific hyperimmune globulin for cytomegalovirus pneumonitis. Lancet II: 152-153

Brandtzaeg P, Karlsen G, Hansen G et al 1987 The clinical condition of IgA deficient patients is related to the proportion of IgD and IgM producing cells in their nasal mucosa. Clinical and Experimental Immunology 67: 626-636

Breeze R G, Wheeldon E B 1977 The cells of the pulmonary airways. American Journal of Respiratory Disease 116: 705-707

Buchdahl R M, Reiser J, Ingram D, Rutman D, Cole P, Warner J O 1988 Ciliary abnormalities in respiratory disease. Archives of Disease in Childhood 63: 238-243

Campbell A G M 1988 Immunisation for the immunosuppressed child. Archives of Disease in Childhood 63: 113-114

Flanagan J G, Rabbitts T 1982 Arrangement of immunoglobulins heavy chain constant region genes implies evolutionary duplication of a segment containing gamma, epsilon and alpha genes. Nature 300: 709

Gerrard M P, Eden O B, Jameson B, Craft A W 1987 Serological study of *Pneumocystis carinii* infection in the absence of immunosuppression. Archives of Disease in Childhood 1987: 177-779

Giblett E R, Anderson J E, Cohen F, Pollara B, Meuwissen H J 1972 Adenosine deaminase deficiency in two patients with severely impaired cellular immunity. Lancet 2: 1067-1069

Giblett E R, Amman A J, Wara D W, Sandman R, Diamond L K 1975 Nucleoside phosphorylase deficiency in a child with severely defective T cell immunity and normal B cell immunity. Lancet 1: 1010-1013

Goldsobel A B, Haas A, Stiehm E R 1987 Bone marrow transplantation in DiGeorge syndrome. Journal of Pediatrics 111: 40-44

Greenstone M A, Dewar A, Cole P J 1983 Ciliary dyskinesia with normal ultrastructure. Thorax 38: 875-876

Hanson L A, Bjorkander J, Oxelius V-A 1983 Selective IgA deficiency. In: Chandra R K (ed) Primary and secondary immunological disorders. Churchill Livingstone Edinburgh, pp 64-84

Joshi V V, Oleske J M, Minnefor A B 1985 Pathological pulmonary findings in children with acquired immunodeficiency syndrome. A study of ten cases. Human Pathology 16: 241-246

Kirkwood E, Lewis C (eds) 1983 Section A, basic principles. In: Understanding medical immunology, Wiley, Chichester, pp 3-36

Lancet 1988 Editorial. Ciliary dyskinesia and ultrastructural abnormalities in respiratory disease. Lancet I: 1370-1372

Linch D C, Levinsky R J, Rodeck C H, MacLennan K A, Simmonds H A 1984 Prenatal diagnosis of three cases of severe combined immunodeficiency severe T cell deficiency during the first half of gestation in fetuses with adenosine deaminase deficiency. Clinical and Experimental Immunology 56: 223-232

Morell A, Skarvil F, Hitzig W H et al 1972 IgG subclasses: development of the serum concentrations in 'normal' infants and children. Journal of Pediatrics 80: 960-964

Morgan G, Levinsky R, 1988a Clinical significance of IgG subclass deficiency. Archives of Disease in Childhood 63: 771-773

Morgan G, Levinsky R 1988b Clinical significance of IgA deficiency. Archives of Disease in Childhood 63: 579-581

Morgan G, Seymour N D, Turner M W, Strobel S, Levinsky R J 1986 Heterogenicity of clinical syndromes associated with selective IgG subclass deficiency. Progress in Immunodeficiency Research and Therapy 11: 229-233

Nicholls A J, Brown C B, Edward N, Cuthbertson B, Yap P L, McClelland DBL 1983 Hyperimmune immunoglobulin for cytomegalovirus infections. Lancet i: 532-533

Oxelius V A 1984 Immunoglobulin G (IgG) subclasses and human disease. American Journal of Medicine 76: 7–18

Pawha S, Kaplan M, Fikrig S et al 1986 Spectrum of human T-cell lymphotophic virus type III infection in children. Recognition of symptomatic, asymptomatic and seronegative patients. Journal of the American Medical Association 255: 2299–2305

Pifer L L, Hughes W T, Stagno S, Woods D 1978 *Pneumocystis carinii* infection: evidence for high prevalence in normal and immunosuppressed children. Pediatrics 61: 35–41

Plebani A, Ugazio A G, Monafo V, Burgio G R 1986 Clinical heterogeneity and reversibility of selective immunoglobulin A deficiency in 80 children. Lancet I: 829–831

Ramet J, Byloos J, Delree M, Saepe L, Clement P 1986 Neonatal diagnosis of the immobile cilia syndrome. Chest 90: 138–140

Roberton D M 1985 The lung in immunological disease. In: Milner A D, Martin R J (eds) Neonatal and pediatric respiratory medicine. Butterworths, London, pp 126–160

Rott H D 1983 Genetics of Kartaganer's syndrome. European Journal of Respiratory Disease 64 (Supp 127): 1–4

Rutland J, Cole P J 1982 Non-invasive sampling of nasal cilia for measurement of beat frequency and study of ultrastructure. Lancet II: 564–565

Rutland J, Griffin W M, Cole P J 1982 Human ciliary beat frequency in epithelium from intrathoracic and extrathoracic airways. American Review of Respiratory Diseases 125: 100–105

Schur P H 1987 IgG subclasses, a review. Annals of Allergy 58: 89–99

Schur P H, Rosen F, Norman M E 1979 Immunoglobulin subclasses in normal children. Pediatric Research 13: 181–183

Simmonds H A, Panayi G S, Corrigall V 1978 A role for purine metabolism in the immune response: adenosine deaminase activity and deoxyadenosine catabolism. Lancet 1: 60–63

Sleigh M A 1981 Primary cilia dyskinesia. Lancet II: 476

Sly P D, Soto-Quiros, Landau L I, Hudson I, Newton-John H 1984 Factors predisposing to abnormal pulmonary function after adenovirus type 7 pneumonia. Archives of Disease in Childhood 59: 935–939

Smith T F, Morris E C, Bain R P 1984 IgG subclasses in non-allergic children with chronic chest symptoms. Journal of Pediatrics 105: 896–900

Sturgess J M, Chao J, Turner J A P 1980 Transposition of ciliary microtubules — another cause of impaired ciliary motility. New England Journal of Medicine 303: 318–322

Thong Y H, Robertson E F, Rischbieth H G et al 1978 Successful restoration of immunity in DiGeorge syndrome with fetal thymic epithelial transplant. Archives of Disease in Childhood 53: 580–584

Whitelaw A, Evans A, Corrin B 1981 Immobile cilia syndrome: a real cause of neonatal respiratory distress. Archives of Disease in Childhood 56: 432–435

Winston D J, Ho W G, Rasmussen L E et al 1982 Use of intravenous immune globulin in patients receiving bone marrow transplants. Journal of Clinical Immunology 2: 42S–47S

Yow M D, White N H, Taber L H et al 1987 Acquisition of cytomegalovirus infection from birth to ten years: a longitudinal serologic study. Journal of Pediatrics 110: 37–42

RECOMMENDED READING

Rossman C M, Newhouse M T 1988 Primary cilia dyskinesia: evaluation and management. State of the art review. Pediatric Pulmonary 5: 36–50

8. Asthma

Asthma is a common disease in children which has often been underdiagnosed in the past because there has been confusion about definition. Recently it has been realised that the spectrum of asthma in children covers a wide variety of symptoms, from those who have only occasional wheeze in response to respiratory tract infection to others who have daily symptoms with chronic airway obstruction, precipitated by a wide variety of extrinsic and intrinsic factors. Asthma can be defined as 'increased responsiveness of the airways to various stimuli manifested by widespread narrowing, changing in severity spontaneously or in response to treatment' (American Thoracic Society 1966). This would include infants who in the past were labelled as having 'wheezy bronchitis'. The disease follows a natural remitting and relapsing course and is very variable in severity, the symptoms seen varying from intermittent cough and wheeze only in association with intercurrent respiratory infection to a much more labile state precipitated by a wide variety of other triggers including contact with inhaled or ingested allergens, exercise, excitement, laughing, emotional upset, atmospheric pollutants such as cigarette smoke or dust, and changes in environmental temperature and humidity. There is also a hereditary predisposition and those in whose family there is already evidence of atopic disease are undoubtedly at greater risk.

The primary problem for the asthmatic child is a state of bronchial hyper-reactivity in which the bronchial smooth muscle over-reacts to the many normal stimuli with which it is in contact throughout daily life. The present concept of asthma is of a spectrum of bronchial hyper-reactivity varying from the normal, through mild over-reaction with stimulation to situations of increasing severity, ultimately leading to a state of continuous bronchospasm with airway obstruction and chronic overinflation in those who are most severely affected.

EPIDEMIOLOGY OF ASTHMA IN CHILDREN

A number of studies in the 1960s and 1970s documented the prevalence of wheezing in the United Kingdom at rates of 11–24.7% (Fry 1961, Horn & Gregg 1973, Leeder et al 1976, Davis 1976, Peckham & Butler 1978). Dawson et al (1969) quoted a prevalence rate for classical asthma in children aged 5–16 of 4.8%. If however those who were classified as having recurrent wheeze during infections or 'wheezy bronchitis' are included, the figure rises to 11.5%. Williams & McNicoll (1969) were not able to separate wheezy bronchitis as a distinct entity from asthma. They noted that children with both problems had a similar incidence of underlying allergic features and those with wheezy bronchitis did not always actually have good evidence of a respiratory infection initiating each wheezy episode. They thus regarded both conditions as part of a spectrum of the same disease — asthma. Sibbald et al (1980) studied the family histories of children with a history of asthma and wheezy bronchitis (defined as wheezing only occurring during respiratory infection). They found a significantly higher incidence of classical asthma in the families of both groups of children when compared to controls. In both the asthmatic and wheezy bronchitis groups this increase was confined to children who were atopic as defined by a positive reaction to one of a number of skin tests. They took this as evidence to suggest that there was a common genetic defect present in both illnesses.

Despite the frequency with which this condition is known to occur there has been widespread under-recognition of the disease in children (Speight et al 1983). Lee et al (1983) found a prevalence of wheezing in 7 year old schoolchildren of 11%. They concluded that all wheezy children had symptoms of a common basic disorder and that they should be treated as having asthma. Although these studies appear to show a rather similar incidence of wheezing in the childhood population, other evidence has suggested that there is a genuine increase in frequency during the last four decades (Lancet 1986a). Asthma was diagnosed in 6.2/1000 firstborn children in a 1946 cohort but in 18.9/1000 of the firstborn offspring of these parents when their children were aged 0–4 years (Wadsworth 1985). Overall asthma mortality in England and Wales has also risen by an average annual rate of 4.7% in the years 1974–1984, particularly in the 5–34 age group (Burney 1986). Anderson (1989) has however recently provided evidence to suggest that this increase is not occurring in the 5–14 age group, and that mortality in the 0–4 age group has fallen steadily over the last 30 years. He points out that there has been an impressive rise in hospital admission rates for asthma during this period, possibly because of the availability of nebulisers and a parental expectation of hospital care for the acutely wheezy child. There are at present 40–45 childhood deaths each year in England and Wales from asthma (Silverman 1985). An annual mortality rate of 0.47/100 000 children less than 15 years of age was reported by Carswell (1985). This is similar to the rate of 0.59/100 000 among children of European origin reported from New Zealand by Sears et al (1986). Carswell also states that approximately 1 in 21 000 asthmatic children die from the disease each year. Both authors stress the role of under-recognition and under-treatment of severe asthma among those who died. There was also a high incidence of psychosocial problems among the families in whom the deaths occurred. The majority of those who died had had their first asthmatic symptoms in early childhood, usually before the age of 4 years.

The cause for this persistent mortality remains unclear but recent interest has centred on the role of environmental factors such as airborn allergens, parental smoking (Kershaw 1987, Andrae et al 1988), atmospheric pollution with agents such as sulphur dioxide and the role of food colourings including sodium metabisulphate (Baker et al 1981) and monosodium glutamate (Allen & Baker 1981). Changes in the weather including thunderstorms can also precipitate attacks in some cases (Egan 1985, Packe & Ayres 1985). It may well be that many outbreaks are caused by a number of factors acting together in a susceptible host.

Hereditary factors are also important in asthma and there is a greatly increased frequency of other atopic manifestations in both the patients and their immediate relatives. As many as 90% of children with asthma have other atopic features including allergic rhinitis, urticaria, eczema and food allergy (Godfrey 1984). A child with asthma is twice as likely to have an atopic mother than an atopic father (Montgomery-Smith 1974). Konig & Godfrey (1973) reported that children with asthma were three times more likely to have atopic relatives or relatives with a positive exercise test than children of unaffected control families and that skin test positivity amongst relatives was twice as common as in the control population. Kuzemko (1980) reported a family history of asthma in 59%, hay fever in 29%, food allergy in 19% and atopic dermatitis in 18% of 676 asthmatic children. Despite these hereditary factors many children with asthma are born into families with no close history of any similar problem. Clifford et al (1987) looked at the children of asthmatic parents and found that those with one asthmatic parent have double the chance of developing the symptoms of asthma compared to the general population. They also found a high incidence of bronchial hyper-reactivity to methacholine challenge in 93% of the asthmatic parents and 45% of the children. All atopic children were positive to this test as were 50% of the non-atopics. They therefore concluded that there was a link between atopic status and bronchial hyper-reactivity.

The overall ratio of males to females in childhood asthma is of the order of 2:1 with a higher ratio of males to females as disease severity increases. In those with chronic asthma the ratio of boys to girls varies from 2:1 in the first 2 years of life to 1.5:1 aged 7 and reaches 1:1 at the time of adolescence; in adult life the ratio is reversed and there are more females than males. Boys generally tend to have more severe asthma than girls and in those with the worst chronic perennial asthma the ratio of boys to girls is 4:1.

PATHOPHYSIOLOGY

The typical changes in the lung include a variable degree of airway obstruction and an exaggerated bronchoconstrictor response to various stimuli; this is associated with a hypersecretory state involving excess mucus production and inflammation of the epithelial lining of the airway, all of which contribute to the airflow obstruction which is seen. The walls of the airways are lined with a spiral layer of smooth muscle which when stimulated causes narrowing of the lumen. It is thought that in the normal person this mechanism is a protective response on the part of the lower respiratory tract against invasion by unwanted extraneous substances such as atmospheric pollutants, viruses or bacteria. The asthmatic child has an abnormal bronchial hyper-responsiveness to these stimuli which is associated with an excess of mucus production and oedema of the airway lining, a process which is mediated by a number of different mechanisms.

Allergic state

The allergic state may be defined as an altered reactivity to allergens or antigens to which the subject has been previously exposed. One of the most important of these mechanisms is the response to allergens which act by direct stimulation of the immune system causing an associated alteration of neural control mechanisms which function through the autonomic nervous system. The allergic reactions which are seen can be divided into four categories (Coombs & Gell 1953).

Type 1: Immediate hypersensitivity or anaphylactic reaction

This is an immediate reaction brought on within a few minutes of exposure when the allergen reacts with tissue cells previously sensitised by reaginic (IgE) antibody produced elsewhere but fixed onto the surface of mast cells and basophils. This results in the release of pharmacologically active substances such as histamine and prostaglandins. An example of this is allergic rhinitis.

In its most severe form this type of reaction results in acute anaphylaxis in which there is a massive release of vasoactive substances resulting in hypotension, shock, airway oedema and difficulty in breathing which can be fatal. This occurs in a previously sensitised person, for example, following stresses such as contact with certain foods, a bee sting, a penicillin injection or an anti-tetanus booster.

Type 2: Cytotoxic reaction

This reaction is seen when circulating antibody combines with a host cell or is attracted to a cell by an antigen fixed to it. It can occur due to cross reacting antibodies but the final result is tissue damage to the host. Examples of this in the blood are: ABO incompatibility, autoimmune haemolytic anaemia or rhesus sensitisation. An example of this in the lung would be Goodpasture's syndrome in which tissue antigens are found in the lung and kidney — this reaction leads to haemoptysis and haematuria.

Type 3: Arthus or immune complex mediated reaction

This reaction develops over a few hours and is the result of the production of immune complexes which are made of combined antibody activated compliment and antigen which is present in excess. Immune complexes are normally formed during the reaction to infectious disease but are usually removed quickly from the circulation and do not normally cause problems. In this disease state excessive immune complexes persist and tissue damage results. The polymorph neutrophils are attracted to the area of the reaction following activation of the compliment system. These cells then become involved in local tissue damage by release of their intrinsic lysosomal enzymes. This can occur in the form of a vasculitis involving blood vessels such as systemic lupus erythematosis or as an extrinsic allergic alveolitis in the lung.

Type 4: Delayed or cell mediated hypersensitivity

This is a reaction which takes at least 24 hours to develop and which is mediated by sensitised T-lymphocytes and does not involve antibody and compliment, unlike the other types of hypersensitivity reaction. When the T-lymphocytes contact the antigen lymphokines are released which cause local inflammatory changes and encourage further cellular infiltration with other lymphocytes and macrophages. Examples of this include the tuberculin hypersensitivity reaction, contact dermatitis, rejection of grafts following organ transplantation and some types of autoimmune disease such as rheumatoid arthritis.

Allergy and the inflammatory response

Many of the changes in the airway of the asthmatic child are due to a local inflammatory response; the most important pathway for this is mediated through IgE. The surfaces of mast cells and basophils in the airway lining have receptor sites for specific IgE antibodies which recognise its 'Fc' component. When the appropriate allergen arrives at the cell surface it bridges two adjacent IgE molecules, a process which then destabilises the cell membrane resulting in the release of preformed mediators including histamine, neutrophil and eosinophil chemotactic factors, proteases and platelet activating factor (PAF). Some of these substances such as histamine and PAF are direct bronchoconstrictors and also result in an increase in mucus secretion; others such as the chemotactic factors attract inflammatory cells including neutrophils, mononuclear cells, macrophages and eosinophils—an inflammatory response is thus triggered through the mast cell and by activation of the alveolar macrophages. These inflammatory cells release substances such as lysozymes and basic proteins which also contribute to the local tissue reaction and mucosal oedema (Barnes 1983).

The inflammatory changes result in activation of cell membranes; this process produces arachidonic acid which is then metabolised by one of two enzyme pathways utilising either lipoxygenase or cyclo-oxygenase (Table 8.1). The end products of the lipoxygenase pathway include various leukotrienes, some of which, for example leukotrienes C and D, are capable of producing local bronchoconstriction and plasma exudation (these substances were previously known as slow reacting substance of anaphylaxis —

Table 8.1   Arachidonic acid metabolism

Lipoxygenase pathway	Cyclo-oxygenase pathway
1. Arachidonic acid	1. Arachidonic acid
2. Leucotriene A4	2. Thromboxane
3. Leucotriene B4	3. Prostaglandin F2, E2
4. Leucotrienes C4, D4, E4	4. Prostacyclin

SRSA). The end products of the cyclo-oxygenase pathway include prostaglandins of various types and thromboxane. Prostaglandin F_2 produces bronchoconstriction and prostaglandin E_2 bronchodilates, thromboxane A_2 bronchoconstricts. Some young adults develop wheezing after taking aspirin and this is thought to be due to a blocking effect on the cyclo-oxygenase pathway so enhancing metabolism by the lipoxygenase route which results in excess leukotriene production.

The result of these processes is that bronchial challenge to the airways in asthma results in an early and a late reaction (Fig. 8.1) with acute bronchoconstriction occurring in the first 2 hours which then resolves but can be followed by a late reaction 4–6 hours later. This challenge also precipitates a more prolonged general increase in bronchial irritability which can last for up to 10 days after exposure to the offending agent (Cockroft 1983). It is thought that the immediate reaction is probably due to an acute release of histamine and prostaglandin PGD_2 (Lewis et al 1981); neutrophil chemotactic factor is also active at this stage. A more chronic role for the mast cell in which it is thought to release mediators by slow leakage over a longer period of time rather than by acute degranulation is also under investigation. During the late reaction there appears to be a considerable amount of oedema of the airway. In this phase there are increased numbers of eosinophils present which subsequently degranulate releasing PAF and various proteases which cause bronchoconstriction and local tissue damage resulting in further oedema and airway narrowing.

Autonomic nervous system

The role of the autonomic nervous system is very important in the pathogenesis of asthma — it is known that in the parasympathetic system vagal nerve stimulation produces bronchoconstriction, a response which can be blocked by atropine. In the sympathetic system alpha adrenergic stimulation results in bronchoconstriction and beta-adrenergic stimulation in bronchodilation. A balance is thought to occur between the influence of vagal induced resting bronchoconstrictor activity and circulating catecholamines acting on cell membrane beta-2-adrenergic receptors; it is also known that beta blocking agents can cause bronchoconstriction (Zied & Beall 1966). When the balance of dual control is disturbed acute wheezing results. Alpha-adrenergic over-reactivity may be important in this im-

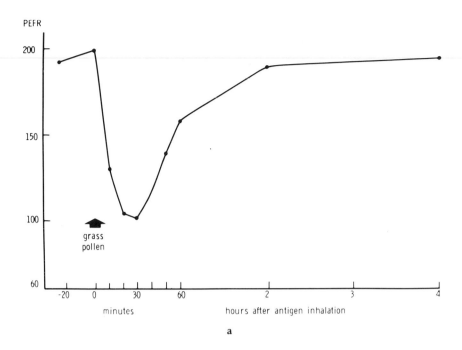

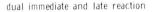

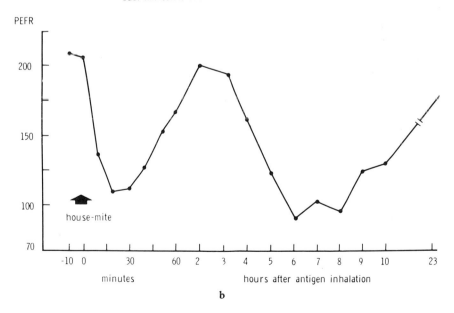

Fig. 8.1   Peak expiratory flow rate after bronchial challenge with specific allergen: (a) Immediate reaction, (b) Immediate and late reaction.

balance and is known to result in bronchoconstriction when stimulated by histamine, possibly through a change in calcium iron flux (Barnes et al 1983); this response to histamine is used as a standard test of bronchial lability.

The histamine challenge test (Fig. 8.2) is a relatively simple and reproducible method of testing for bronchial hyper-reactivity. The aim of the test is to produce a response curve of changes in airway obstruction against the inhalation of doubling concentrations of histamine. As the pharmacological effects of this agent last for only a few minutes it is safe to use in routine clinical practice. In children the tidal breathing method is used in which the patient inhales a number of test solutions of doubling concentration for 2 minutes each via a nebuliser. The response to a control diluent solution and to each doubling concentration of histamine given at 5 minute intervals is then measured over a period of 3 minutes (Silverman & Wilson 1985). The test is continued until there is a 30% drop in lung function (either PEF or FEV_1). The concentration which produces a fall of 20% is then calculated (Fig. 8.2), this is known as the provocation concentration of 20% or PC_{20}. Methacholine and carbachol have also been utilised as bronchial challenging agents using similar techniques.

A third neurogenic pathway is also thought to exist, this is called the non-adrenergic non-cholinergic (NANC) pathway (Barnes 1984). This pathway appears to exert an inhibitory influence on airway tone, mucus secretion and bronchial blood flow (Lancet 1986b). The system appears to act mainly

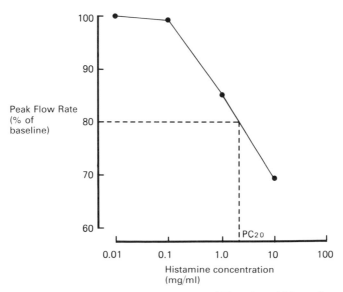

Fig. 8.2 Determination of PC_{20}, the concentration of histamine which produces a 20% fall in respiratory function.

in the larger airways and possibly through the influence of vaso-active intestinal peptide (VIP) which is the most potent relaxant of human bronchi in vitro so far discovered (Palmer et al 1986). There does not however appear to be an effect in the peripheral airways and this is compatible with their observation that the necessary receptors are not present in the bronchiolar smooth muscle. The exact role of this system in both the normal and in the asthmatic person has yet to be clarified but it is likely to be of particular importance in the asthmatic in whom an underlying inflammatory response has already occurred.

Exercise

The role of exercise in asthma is very important, particularly in children who are expected to take part in regular games at school. It has been known for a very long time that exercise produces breathlessness in the asthmatic patient (Floyer 1698). This phenomenon, which is known as exercise induced asthma (EIA), is another manifestation of bronchial hyper-reactivity. The typical response is shown in Chapter 2 (Fig. 2.4). During a standard exercise test the subject undertakes a period of free running for 6 minutes—this should be sufficient to produce a heart rate in excess of 180 beats/minute. A more precise test can be performed using a treadmill at an angle of 10–15% at a rate of 5–8 km/h (Silverman & Anderson 1972). Initially there is bronchodilation but after 3–5 minutes bronchoconstriction begins. This reaches its maximum level 5 minutes post-exercise following which gradual recovery occurs.

It has also been known for many years that some types of exercise produce significantly more or less EIA than others, for example swimming and cycling produce less, and free running produces more than treadmill running which causes most of all (Fitch & Morton 1971, Anderson et al 1971). After the exercise is completed there is a refractory period for about 2 hours (Edmunds et al 1978). This period may be used to 'run through' the EIA over the next hour or so (Schnall & Landau 1980). The temperature and humidity of the inspired air also affect the reproducibility of the test (McFadden 1983) so for research purposes an air conditioned laboratory is required for testing.

The simplest method of interpreting the exercise test is to accept a fall of 15% or more from baseline PEF or FEV_1 as indicating a positive response (Silverman & Anderson 1972). Burr et al (1974) found that 98% of healthy, non-asthmatic children had a fall in PEF of less than 15% post-exercise. Kattan et al (1978) found EIA with a fall in FEV_1 of greater than 15% in 84% of asthmatic children. Verity et al (1984) found a higher incidence of positive exercise tests in non-asthmatic male rather than female siblings of known asthmatics aged under 15 years. They concluded that this could be one reason for the apparent increased incidence of asthma in pre-adolescent boys who tend to be more physically active than girls of the same age and which therefore highlights their greater intrinsic bronchial lability at this age.

The pathophysiology of EIA is complex and is not yet fully understood. Godfrey (1983a, b) has reviewed the current hypotheses. A great deal of work has been undertaken by various groups looking at the relative roles of heat loss from the airway, humidity of inspired gas and exercise itself, and he suggested that various mechanisms may be working in EIA. One of these could be the release of chemical mediators from mast cells which result in bronchoconstriction; this is supported by Lee et al (1982) who found that neutrophil chemotactic factor, a mast cell derived compound, was released during exercise which preceded EIA. This release and the EIA were inhibited by pretreatment with sodium cromoglycate. A further mechanism put forward by Deal et al (1979, 1987) is that EIA is a response to airway cooling either by hyperventilation or the exercise itself, mediated through a neural response. Godfrey and his colleagues (Bar-Yishay et al 1982) have also shown that even under identical conditions of heat loss running still caused 39% more EIA than swimming; this is evidence for a specific effect in EIA which is related purely to the exercise itself.

The overall view of Godfrey (1983a) is that mediator stores (probably within mast cells) are found in large central temperature-dependent airways and in small temperature independent airways in most asthmatics. Hyperventilation with or without exercise liberates mediator by cooling large airway mast cells. In most asthmatics exercise releases mediator in the small temperature-independent airways. The mediator from either source causes bronchoconstriction via changes in bronchial smooth muscle whose resting tone is set by vagal reflexes originating in the large temperature dependent airways in which cool air increases resting muscle tone and results in reduced small airway calibre and where warm air causes low resting tone.

EIA continues throughout the duration of the asthmatic state with no direct correlation to the severity of the asthma and persists until at least 6 months after the child has become totally symptom free (Balfour-Lynn et al 1980). The current status of exercise testing in children has recently been reviewed by Nixon & Orenstein (1988).

CLINICAL EVALUATION

Clinical evaluation of the asthmatic child involves taking a careful history, a full physical examination and the use of appropriate investigations in each individual case. The history should pay particular attention to: age of onset, frequency and severity of attacks, seasonal variation and precipitating factors. Specific questions should be asked regarding the role of the following in causation: respiratory tract infection, exercise, changes in environmental temperature and humidity, atmospheric pollution, parental smoking habits, allergens both inhaled and ingested, excitement and emotional upset. It is also important to enquire about other atopic problems such as allergic

Table 8.2 Causes of wheezing

Acute viral bronchiolitis	Vascular ring
Asthma	Enlarged paratracheal glands including TB
Recurrent aspiration (reflux)	Mediastinal cysts and tumours
Chronic infective bronchiolitis	Tracheomalacia
Cystic fibrosis	Bronchogenic cyst
Immune deficiency	Bronchial stenosis
Obliterative bronchiolitis	Congenital lobar emphysema
Bronchopulmonary dysplasia	Left ventricular failure
Foreign body	

rhinitis, eczema, food allergy, urticaria and changes in behaviour related to allergen exposure.

It has been stated that 'all that wheezes is not asthma and all that's asthma does not wheeze'. When taking the history it is important to consider the possibility that the wheezing might be due to other causes (Table 8.2). Particular attention should be paid to history of vomiting, especially in infants who may have gastro-oesophageal reflux with aspiration into the lungs; evidence of chronic sputum production and the presence of a large appetite in conjunction with pale fatty offensive stools which would suggest cystic fibrosis; or evidence of frequent infections elsewhere which could suggest immune deficiency. A previous history of severe respiratory infection, either viral or bacterial, suggests chronic lung damage, as could a history of pre-term birth and neonatal respiratory problems which have caused chronic lung disease or bronchopulmonary dysplasia. Infants and young children who have had acute adenovirus bronchiolitis can develop a form of obliterative bronchiolitis with permanent damage to the small airways (Lange et al 1969, Sly et al 1984).

When clinically indicated, appropriate investigations should be undertaken to exclude these other causes. It should also be remembered that some children with asthma present only with a persistent cough (Konig 1981) which may be amenable to the appropriate anti asthma therapy.

School

Particular enquiry should also be made about the amount of school absence which is occurring due to the illness. Storr et al (1987) reported that 5% of children attending local primary schools were receiving inhalation treatment with bronchodilator agents. On average they had missed seven school days in the previous year. School absence may be happening for one of two reasons. Firstly there may be genuine absence due to the severity of the symptoms; this is an indication that the asthma is being undertreated and the child therefore needs a thorough review and probably more vigorous and continuous medication. Secondly, serious absenteeism may be happening for psychological reasons; this can be due to direct manipulation by the patient of the symptoms, a reflection of poor academic progress which will worsen as the time off school increases or secondary to serious psychosocial disturbance within the family. All these aspects need to be reviewed in each individual case.

The growth pattern should also be carefully reviewed since many children with severe asthma grow slowly, particularly in middle childhood and most of these have a delayed bone age. The vast majority however will ultimately reach normal adult height (Balfour-Lynn 1986, Shohat et al 1987).

A full family history is extremely important, both in relation to asthma and other atopic features but also to elucidate possible inherited conditions causing chronic chest disease such as cystic fibrosis, alpha-1-antitrypsin deficiency or immune deficiency.

The home environment should also be discussed, including the child's bedroom and the presence of possible allergens including house dust, house dust mites, animal danders from household pets and plants. A dietary history is useful, including not only foods but which drinks the child prefers as these too can stimulate bronchial hyper-reactivity, especially cold iced drinks and those containing citrus fruits, colourings, additives and cola (Silverman & Wilson 1985). In those with severe attacks, especially in infancy, the possibility of gastro-oesophageal reflux and recurrent aspiration should be considered. The possibility of foreign body inhalation should also be remembered.

Parental smoking habits should also be reviewed. Kershaw (1987) found that passive smoking from parents contributed significantly to the onset of recurrent wheeze in the first 5 years of life, especially in those without elevated serum IgE levels. He also found that there was a preponderance of males and that clinical overinflation of the chest was more common in this group. Parental smoking should of course be discouraged at all times, especially during pregnancy and after the arrival of children in the family.

Exercise

The role of exercise induced asthma (EIA) in the child's day to day activities and in the precipitation of acute symptoms should be elucidated since many children are inhibited from normal physical activities due to the onset of EIA. The degree of bronchospasm varies with different types of exercise, being greatest with running, less with cycling and less still with swimming. EIA can easily be blocked by appropriate medication such as sodium cromoglycate or a beta-agonist before the exercise begins or by a small number of warm up periods so that the exercise induced wheeze becomes refractory (Schnall & Landau 1980).

Severity

Asthma in childhood is recognised in varying degrees of severity. Recognition of these may be useful from the point of view of clinical assessment. The important work of McNicoll & Williams (1973) has emphasised the usefulness of this approach in long term studies which have examined the natural history of this disease. They recognised four grades of illness classified as A, B, C and D at the age of 14 years. Grade A children have had no more than five attacks, usually beginning after the age of 3 years and having ceased by 8 years. Grade B patients had mild episodic asthma usually with three to four attacks annually for 4–5 years with remission by age 10–12 years (mild episodic asthma). Grades C and D had continuing asthma to the age of 14 years and usually commenced before the age of 2 years; all had evidence of chronic airway obstruction between episodes. Grade C patients had wheezed in the 12 months prior to their 14th birthday. Grade D children had severe unremitting asthma (Williams & Phelan 1975); this type of asthma was more commonly seen in boys than girls at this age in a ratio of 4:1.

Recent work from this group has given a much clearer understanding of the longer term prognosis for asthma in adult life (Martin et al 1980a, b, Kelly et al 1987). These studies showed that 55% of those whose wheezing began before the age of 7 years who had stopped by adolescence remained wheeze free. Fewer than 20% of those with persistent symptoms throughout childhood became wheeze free at adolescence and also that the male to female ratio had equalised in the more severe grades by the age of 21. Sixty-eight per cent of those with frequent wheezing at 14 years still suffered from this at 28 years; of those with infrequent wheezing at 21 years, 44% had worsened by 28 years.

As far as the day to day clinical management of asthma is concerned it is useful to divide it into three grades of severity as described by Canny & Levison (1987): mild infrequent asthma with less than one attack every 2 months (75% of asthmatic children), frequent episodic asthma with more than one attack every 2 months (20% of asthmatic children) and chronic severe asthma with persistent daytime and nocturnal symptoms, exercise limitation and persistent lung function abnormalities (5% of asthmatic children).

Apart from the history a careful physical examination is vital. Particular attention should be paid to height and weight (plotted on centile charts), presence or absence of finger clubbing (not usually seen in asthma), state of ears, nose, throat and tonsils and the presence and size of lymph nodes. Children with significant immune deficiency often have small shotty lymph nodes, absence of tonsils and no thymic shadow on the chest X-ray. Immune competent children with chronic upper respiratory infection may have persistent cervical lymphadenopathy. The shape of the chest is also important; it may reveal chronic overinflation from persistent small airway disease with air trapping or pectus excavatum secondary to chronic upper airway obstruction from enlarged tonsils and adenoids. Auscultation may reveal widespread rhonchi or crepitations depending on the patient's asthmatic state at the time. The heart sounds should be checked to exclude any concommitant heart disease. Blood pressure should be measured, especially in those who have had or are likely to have steroid therapy. If frequent steroid therapy has been given the eyes should be checked for cataract. The skin should be examined for other allergic features such as eczema and urticaria.

Investigation

The investigations commonly used in asthma are shown in Table 8.3. The number of tests undertaken on each individual will vary according to the frequency and severity of symptoms.

Those with mild infrequent symptoms need little more than simple pulmonary function tests including measurement of forced vital capacity (FVC), forced expiratory volume in 1 second (FEV_1), peak expiratory flow rate (PEF), and a flow–volume curve before and after inhalation of a bronchodilator (Fig. 8.3). Depending on the severity of the asthma, further investigation may be required including more sophisticated lung function tests. Exercise testing can be useful in the evaluation of games-related wheezing at school. Other investigations such as skin tests and chest X-ray are sometimes indicated in this group. Those with frequent episodic or chronic severe asthma require more detailed investigation with full lung function tests, an exercise test when indicated, a chest X-ray to assess overinflation and to rule out other causes of wheezing and skin tests to investigate specific allergic factors.

The correlation between skin tests and allergic bronchial hyper-reactivity is of the order of 80%. This means that 20% of allergens causing a sig-

Table 8.3   Investigation of asthma

Lung function tests	Barium swallow
Skin tests	Sweat test
Chest X-ray	Specific IgE antibodies (RAST test)
Full blood count (eosinophils)	Full immunology
Immunoglobulins (+ total IgE)	Histamine or methacholine challenge
Exercise test	Respiratory viral antibodies
	Oesophageal pH study

The number of tests performed will vary from one or two to all of them depending on the individual

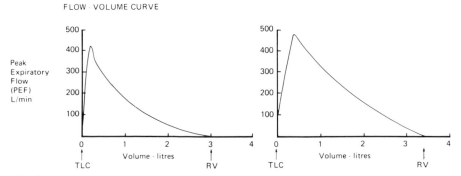

Fig. 8.3   Flow–volume curve before (left) and after (right) bronchodilator; note increase in peak flow, flow at low lung volumes and vital capacity (TLC to RV).

nificant bronchial response could be missed. The skin test reflects the presence of an IgE type I hypersensitivity response. It is best performed by the intraepidermal introduction of the test solution into the skin by a very fine needle. Ninety per cent of those with positive tests will be detected by using the following allergens: house dust mite, grass pollen, *Aspergillus fumigatus* and any furry pet in the house (Rees 1984). A positive reaction is counted as a weal of 3 mm or greater than any reaction to an inert control solution.

Other investigations, including full blood count (for eosinophilia) and immunoglobulin levels to detect IgA deficiency are helpful in the young child who has frequent and severe wheezing attacks. Measurement of total IgE is sometimes useful in those under 2–3 years of age where skin tests are more often negative. Overall, however, the measurement of total IgE is not very predictive in determining the incidence or severity of asthma. In clinical practice, skin tests can be performed from the age of 18 months onwards as immediate and useful information is gained by this method. The measurement of radioallergosorbent tests (RASTs) for allergen specific IgE antibodies in the blood is not in widespread use in UK asthma clinics as it is more expensive and it takes longer to obtain the results than a simple skin test. RASTs are however often used in other countries and have as good a correlation with allergic bronchial hyper-reactivity as skin tests.

Those with severe asthma require more detailed investigation to exclude other causes of recurrent wheezing such as a sweat test for cystic fibrosis and full immunology screen (including IgG subclass measurement) for other forms of immune deficiency. A barium swallow to exclude gastro-oesophageal reflux and hiatus hernia as contributory factors to wheezing episodes is useful, especially in the infant or young child who has frequent or severe attacks. If there is still doubt about the degree of reflux continuous oesophageal pH monitoring may be necessary during an overnight stay in hospital.

The role of psychogenic and emotional factors in the pathogenesis of asthma can be very important. This is particularly relevant in children who fail to respond to appropriate medical therapy and in whom there is evidence of behaviour disturbance or difficulty in the home or school environment. These families often need referral for psychiatric evaluation and family counselling as part of their overall review (Lask & Matthew 1979).

TREATMENT

The major components of treatment for the child with asthma are shown in Table 8.4.

The amount of treatment is varied according to the individual and the severity of disease. A discussion of the causative factors, an explanation of the severity, and reassurance regarding the long term outcome, which is usually good, should be given to the child and to his or her parents. This can often be coupled with discussion of the various investigations which are

Table 8.4   Management of asthma

1. Education of child and family
2. Recognition of precipitating factors and their avoidance — especially allergens
3. Drug therapy
   Beta-agonists — Salbutamol or Terbutaline
   Theophylline
   Sodium cromoglycate (Intal)
   Ipratropium bromide (Atrovent)
   Steroids — inhaled or oral
4. Treatment of associated disorders
   Chronic infection
   Gastro-oesophageal reflux
5. Psychological — family support

to be performed in each case and their usefulness in delineating the various factors involved in the patient's symptoms. A review of the role of allergic factors where these are thought to be important is useful and can be aided by the performance of skin prick tests. An assessment of the role of inhaled allergens in the environment should be carried out and the use of avoidance measures for house dust, house dust mites, feathers and furry pets should be explained. The role of seasonal variation of inhaled allergens such as pollens and fungi should be reviewed. Lung function tests which reveal exercise induced wheezing then require an explanation of the role of prophylactic drugs such as beta-agonists or sodium cromoglycate in the prevention or alleviation of these symptoms. An understanding of the role of emotional upset and excitement in the provocation of an asthma attack should also be given to the parents and the child.

Asthmatic symptoms in children induced by food and drink have recently been investigated by Wilson (1985) and Wilson & Silverman (1985). They found that 73% of asthmatic children surveyed reported symptoms in response to individual foods or drinks. The most common offending agents were cola drinks, ice, orange squash, nuts and chocolate. There was a significantly higher incidence in Asian than non-Asian children of symptoms from cola drinks, ice, nuts and foods cooked in oil. Many children noticed these symptoms during the night following ingestion of the particular food or drink. These workers also pointed out that it was difficult to confirm increased bronchial reactivity by measurement of PEF alone and that a formal histamine challenge test was required to elucidate this response. Where necessary advice about the avoidance of particular foods or drinks can be a useful preventive measure.

Drug treatment

The advent of highly effective drug therapy for most children with asthma and the development of appropriate delivery systems has greatly improved the day to day management of this illness, particularly in the younger child. The pharmacological aim of current therapy is to increase the tissue levels

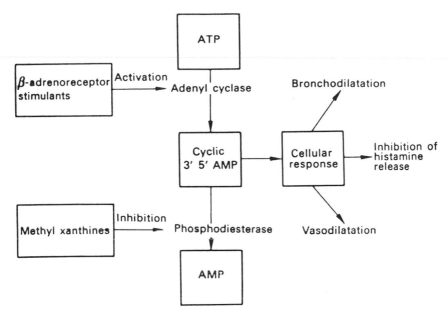

Fig. 8.4 Mode of action of beta-stimulants and methylxanthines in asthma (with kind permission from Kuzemko 1980).

of cyclic AMP which inhibits the release of mast cell mediators and also causes relaxation of the bronchial smooth muscle. The mechanism by which this comes about is shown in Fig. 8.4.

Children with occasional episodic asthma can usually be satisfactorily treated with beta-agonists such as salbutamol or terbutaline. These become particularly effective during the second year of life (Lenney & Milner 1978), although more recently this group has been able to demonstrate a protective effect of salbutamol against the bronchoconstriction produced in response to the inhalation of nebulised water in infants under 1 year of age (O'-Callaghan et al 1988). The delivery system is very important and the young child will usually require either oral medication for the milder case (Dinwiddie et al 1983) or a home nebuliser for those with more severe or recurrent disease. Greenough et al (1986) showed a significant improvement in lung compliance and FRC after the inhalation of nebulised salbutamol in children aged 2–8 years. It has been suggested that the anticholinergic agent ipratropium bromide (Atrovent) is a more effective bronchodilator for infants, however the evidence for this is conflicting (Henry et al 1984). Hodges et al (1981) showed that a single dose produced a reduction in airway resistance, but the same group did not show clinical benefit during a controlled trial in acute bronchiolitis (Henry et al 1983). Prendiville et al (1987) studied the effects of nebulised ipratropium bromide in wheezy infants aged 4–15 months; they found a significant reduction in specific airway resistance (TGV × initial inspiratory airway resistance), a measure of central airway narrowing, after treatment but no change in peripheral airway resistance as measured by a partial expiratory flow volume curve (Vmax FRC).

These findings suggest that ipratropium has its maximum effect on the larger central airways, it is therefore not surprising that it is relatively ineffective in conditions such as bronchiolitis where the increased resistance is more peripheral.

The pre-school child and school aged child will often benefit from the use of powdered preparations such as salbutamol rotacaps or terbutaline turbohaler since their synchronisation with a pressurised aerosol is not always good at this age. There are now available a number of other delivery systems such as the nebuhaler or volumatic plastic cone into which the aerosol preparation can be sprayed which have significantly improved the delivery of the appropriate dose to the younger child. Pool et al (1988) found that repeated 'huffs and puffs' into the nebuhaler were as effective as a single deep inhalation in young asthmatics. O'Callaghan et al (1989) have shown that addition of a face mask to the spacer provides an effective delivery system for ipratropium bromide even in the first year of life. Although in clinical practice most paediatricians tend to favour the inhaled to the oral route, Dawson et al (1986) have suggested that a combination of inhaled powder and oral salbutamol is the most effective way of delivering this agent. In the patient on long term treatment compliance with this regime could be a problem especially when the asthma is stable and the child is less symptomatic. One of the most important aims of asthma treatment is: 'to deliver the right amount of the right medicine to the right place at the right time'.

Oral theophylline (methylxanthine) therapy has enjoyed a resurgence in popularity during recent years. This has occurred because of the availability of improved preparations, particularly delayed release compounds allowing twice or even once daily dosage (Tabachnick et al 1982). The ability to measure whole blood theophylline on capillary samples has also facilitated titration of the appropriate dose for each child (Elias-Jones et al 1987). Intermittent theophylline during acute attacks is a useful addition to the beta-agonists (McKenzie 1986); it has also been used successfully as prophylaxis (Furakawa et al 1984) where it has been shown to be as effective as sodium cromoglycate. All theophylline preparations have a narrow therapeutic index and the potential for toxicity is always present. Side-effects such as nausea, vomiting and abdominal pain are not uncommon. Maintenance of the serum level within the therapeutic range of 5–20 μg/ml (28–110 μmol/l) (Nerminathan & McKenzie 1984) should reduce the incidence of these complications. Theophylline metabolism is also delayed by a number of factors including acute respiratory viral infection (especially influenza), during antibiotic treatment with erythromycin, and with the simultaneous use of cimetidine. Theophyllines can also cause relaxation of the gastro-oesophageal sphincter (Stein et al 1980) and this can facilitate reflux which of itself may exacerbate wheezing (Silverman 1985). This is an important factor to consider when using these agents in wheezy infants with bronchopulmonary dysplasia. There is also evidence to suggest that theophylline can affect schoolwork and behaviour in children (Sattin 1984,

Springer et al 1985). There is no doubt that this group of compounds has a significant role to play in the management of childhood asthma; their use however, particularly on a regular basis, must be closely supervised both clinically and by measurement of blood levels when appropriate.

The oral antihistamine ketotifen is widely used outside the United Kingdom for asthma prophylaxis. Clinical trials to date have not shown convincing efficacy for this compound in children so its use is relatively uncommon in asthma clinics in this country.

Inhaled sodium cromoglycate has been used for a number of years in the prophylaxis of asthma; it is a remarkably safe drug having virtually no side effects. As it is only effective by inhalation it must be delivered from a capsule, a pressurised aerosol or via a nebuliser for the young child. Cogswell & Simpkiss (1985) found a significant improvement in night time cough, day activity, number of symptom free days and asthma severity when its use was studied in pre-school children under 5 years of age. It did not affect wheeze score after acute respiratory tract infection or the number of acute hospital admissions. This agent thus has a frequent role in the prophylaxis of asthma especially in young children to whom it is given via nebuliser. Sodium cromoglycate is also effective in the prophylaxis of exercise induced asthma (EIA), (Corkey et al 1982). It is best given 10–15 minutes before the exercise begins. The new mast cell stabilising agent nedocromil sodium is also effective in the prevention of EIA (Chudry et al 1987).

Steroids

The role of oral steroids in the treatment of severe asthma should not be underestimated; they are particularly useful during acute exacerbations in those with chronic severe asthma. They function by inhibition of the enzyme phospholipase A2 which is important in the production of membrane mediated bronchoconstrictors such as leukotrienes and thromboxane. These are produced by mast cells and other inflammatory cells within the lung. Steroids also increase the responsiveness of the beta-adrenergic receptors so improving the efficacy of the beta-agonists which are usually being given simultaneously. The need for continuous oral steroid therapy as prophylaxis has however greatly diminished with the advent of the inhaled steroids, which can be given even to quite young children. Most children who require this form of treatment will be well controlled with beclomethasone dipropionate (becotide) either in the aerosol form or as a powdered rotacap (Edmunds et al 1979). Budesonide is a suitable alternative (Field et al 1982). Nebulised beclomethasone has been successfully used in young children aged 20 months to 5.6 years (Storr et al 1986) although clinically it is not as effective as the capsule or aerosol preparations are in older children. It is important that the nebulised solution is adequately delivered to the lungs either by a close fitting face mask or, preferably, through a mouth piece. In conventional doses inhaled steroids do not cause adrenal suppression but this may occur at high dosage in excess of 20 $\mu g/kg/day$. They do not usually have any adverse effects on growth.

The use of continuous oral prednisolone for prophylaxis is unusual nowadays; this form of treatment is only required in 1–2% of children attending a hospital clinic. It is important to check the patient's blood pressure, eyes for cataracts and urine for glycosuria before and at regular intervals during treatment. It is preferable to give the steroids on alternate days if possible as side-effects including inhibition of growth are less frequent on this regime. The response to treatment can usefully be monitored by the use of diary cards to record symptoms in conjunction with daily peak flow measurements in suitable cases.

Hyposensitisation

The use of desensitising injections has never really gained popularity among hospital practitioners in the United Kingdom. Recent reports of a small but significant mortality in relation to this treatment when used parenterally will undoubtedly remove this approach further from clinical practice (Committee of Safety of Medicines 1986). Despite this there is still a need for further research into the role of immunotherapy of this kind in asthma (Warner & Kerr 1987).

TREATMENT OF ACUTE ASTHMA

The child who has relentless unremitting or very severe acute asthma, particularly if it is exacerbated by anxiety, is in a potentially life threatening situation. An attack of this severity is also more likely to occur where maintenance treatment is not being taken properly. This happens in situations where there is poor compliance with medication, inadequate inhalation technique, overuse of beta-agonists, undermedication or lack of parental supervision of the child and his illness.

When an acute episode occurs it is important to assess its severity by taking a careful history, by physical examination and appropriate investigation. Enquiry should be made as to its mode of onset and the duration of the present episode; it is very important to establish how much medication has been taken recently — this particularly applies to beta-agonists and especially to theophylline in the last 4 hours. If steroids have already been given the dose and time should be noted. Children with significantly impaired respiratory function will demonstrate signs such as inability to talk in sentences, restlessness, confusion, duskiness or cyanosis. There will be obvious respiratory distress with sweating, and increased work of breathing in the presence of a relatively slow respiratory rate with marked expiratory difficulty. Wheezing may or may not be a prominent feature; if there is severe airway obstruction this may not be heard — the so-called 'silent chest'. This is particularly seen in the adolescent with severe perennial asthma who has chronic airway obstruction and mucus plugging — 'the silent overinflated asthmatic'. The chest is usually markedly hyperinflated and auscultation reveals high pitched rales and rhonchi bilaterally with markedly reduced air entry over both lung fields. The usual appearance on chest X-ray in severe asthma is shown in Fig. 8.5.

There is often a pulsus paradoxus in excess or 15 mmHg. PEF or FEV_1 is either unrecordable or severely reduced to less than 30% predicted for height. Oxygen saturation is reduced, arterial blood gases demonstrate hypoxaemia and a normal or slightly elevated carbon dioxide. Those with the most severe symptoms will show signs of impending exhaustion.

A scheme of treatment is shown in Fig. 8.6. Initially, further nebulised beta-agonists such as salbutamol or terbutaline are given. If a rapid response to this is not obtained then intravenous theophylline is started; a loading dose is given over 20 minutes if the patient has not had any in the previous 4 hours otherwise treatment is commenced with the maintenance dose. Theophylline not only bronchodilates but improves respiratory muscle contractility, especially the diaphragm (Aubier et al 1981) and it also acts as a respiratory stimulant. Oxygen is given by face mask or nasal cannula to maintain saturation at 90–95% if possible. Intravenous fluids are initially provided at a rate sufficient to overcome any dehydration which is commonly present in the early stages. This usually happens because of poor oral

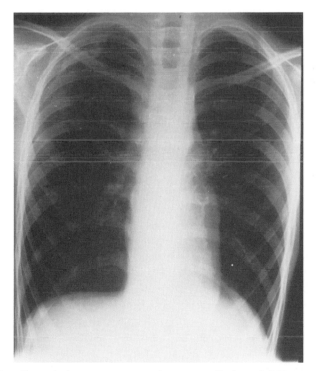

Fig. 8.5 Chest X-ray during severe acute asthma: generalised overinflation, no focal consolidation.

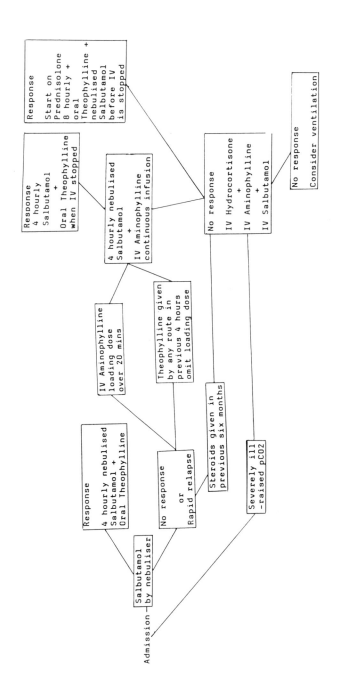

Fig. 8.6 Suggested treatment plan for acute asthma.

Table 8.5 Drug dosage in asthma

Salbutamol
Nebulised
1 nebules (2.5 mg in 2.5 ml) up to 4-hourly
or 0.5–1.5 ml 0.5% nebuliser solution made
up to 2–4 ml with normal saline up to
4-hourly.
Inhaled
2 puffs metered aerosol (100 μg/puff) 3–4
times daily or pre-exercise. May be given
by 750 ml Volumatic plastic cone. Less
than 30 kg body weight, 1 rotacap, 200 μg;
over 30 kg 1 rotacap, 400 μg, 3–4 times
daily.
Oral
0.6 mg/kg/day in 3–4 divided doses,
maximum 16 mg/day.
Intravenous
Loading dose 1 μg/kg/min given slowly
over 10 minutes. Maintenance
0.2 μg/kg/min increasing by 0.1 μg/kg/min
if necessary. Maximum dose 4 μg/kg/min.
Only to be used in intensive care (Bohn et
al 1984).

Terbutaline
Nebulised
1 respule 5 mg in 2 ml up to 4-hourly.
0.2–0.5 ml (2–5 mg) respiratory solution
diluted to 2–4 ml with normal saline 4–6
hourly.
Inhaled
2 puffs (0.25 mg/puff) 3–4 times daily by
metered aerosol. May be given via 750 ml
Nebuhaler plastic cone.
Oral
0.15–0.75 mg/kg/day in 4 divided doses
(maximum dose 20 mg/day).
Injection (sc im iv)
0.01 mg/kg/dose (maximum 0.3 mg) single
dose.

Ipratropium bromide (Atrovent)
0.4–2 ml (100–500 μg) nebuliser solution
diluted to 2–4 ml with normal saline up to
4-hourly.

Theophylline
Oral
20–24 mg/kg/day in divided doses.
Intravenous
Loading dose 5 mg/kg given slowly over 20
minutes. Maintenance dose 0.9 mg/kg/hour
by continuous infusion.

Sodium cromoglycate (Intal)
Inhaled
Metered aerosol 5 mg/puff 1–2 puffs 3–4
times daily. 1 spincap (20 mg), via
halermatic 3–4 times daily. 1 nebule (20 mg
in 2 ml) 3–4 times daily.

Beclomethasone (Becotide)
Inhaled
4 puffs (50 μg/puff) twice daily or 2 puffs
3–4 times daily using metered aerosol; may
be given by 750 ml plastic cone. Less than
30 kg body weight, 1 rotacap 100 μg; over
30 kg, 1 rotacap 200 μg 3–4 times daily
Nebulised (50 μg/ml)
Under 1 year 50 μg diluted to 2 ml, 2–4
times daily; over 1 year 100 μg diluted to
2–4 ml, 2–4 times daily.

Budesonide (Pulmicort)
Inhalation
2–4 puffs metered aerosol Pulmicort LS
(50 μg/puff) twice daily; may be given by
750 ml plastic cone Nebuhaler or collapsible
spacer device

Hydrocortisone
Intravenous
4 mg/kg 2-hourly, reduce to 4 mg/kg
4–6-hourly after response occurs

Prednisolone
1–2 mg/kg/day reducing gradually over
5–7 days

intake, fluid loss due to vomiting, sweating and hyperventilation. After correction of dehydration iv fluids are given at 75% of daily maintenance in order to avoid the complication of inappropriate antidiuretic hormone (ADH) secretion which can lead to cerebral oedema, especially in those who subsequently require ventilation. Almost all children who come to intravenous therapy will need a short course of steroids beginning with iv hydrocortisone at 2-hourly intervals. If there is a significant metabolic acidosis small quantities of sodium bicarbonate should be given. If the response to this therapy is inadequate then intravenous salbutamol should

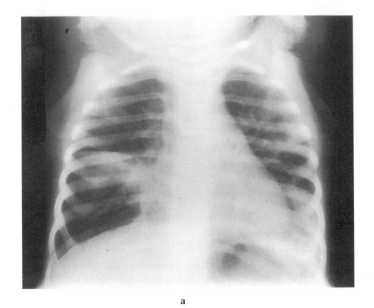

a

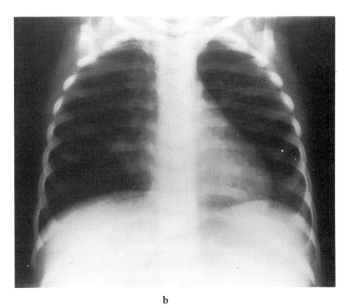

b

Fig. 8.7   (a) Mucous plugging causing atelectesis in acute asthma. (b) The same patient after 24 hours on standard treatment (antibiotics not used). Courtesy of Dr G Fischer.

be given; doses as high as 4 μg/kg/min may be necessary (Bohn et al 1984). This form of treatment should only be carried out in an intensive care unit where full and continuous cardiac, respiratory and blood pressure monitoring facilities are available.

Ventilation is required for those few children who fail to respond to the measures described. The usual indications are exhaustion, impairment of conscious level, significant hypoxia ($Pa_{O_2}<8$ kPa/60 mmHg) and hypercarbia ($Pa_{CO_2}>10$ kPa/75 mmHg). Those who do require ventilation should be fully paralysed and sedated; a volume cycled ventilator should be used. The opportunity is then taken to carry out physiotherapy in order to clear lung secretions and mucus plugs. It is important to emphasise that this should not be performed during acute wheezy episodes in the conscious unventilated asthmatic as this will only worsen the bronchospasm. During ventilation relatively slow rates with prolonged expiratory times are used to allow adequate time for expiration (Canny & Levison 1987). In the early phase of ventilation hypoxaemia should be corrected but a higher than normal Pa_{CO_2} level (up to 8 kPa/60 mmHg) is acceptable in order to reduce the risk of pneumothorax at this time (Darioli & Perret 1984).

When the patient has recovered sufficiently for the ventilation to be weaned the paralysis is stopped in order to encourage an adequate cough reflex which then further assists in the clearance of lung secretions by natural means. As recovery proceeds extubation occurs and there is a gradual change from intravenous to oral and nebulised medication with an eventual return to baseline prophylaxis.

CONCLUSION

Despite the many problems which children with asthma face in day to day life, the majority can expect a great deal of improvement in their symptoms with age. Although much remains to be learnt about the basic pathophysiology of the asthmatic process there is now available an increasing range of effective medication for the control of symptoms. Most children with asthma can be returned to a normal life style, especially those with mild to moderate disease. This makes asthma one of the most challenging but rewarding diseases to treat in childhood.

REFERENCES

Allen D H, Baker G J 1981 Asthma and MSG. Medical Journal of Australia ii: 576
American Thoracic Society 1966 Thorax 1: 762
Anderson H R 1989 Is the prevalence of asthma changing? Archives of Disease in Childhood 64: 172–175
Anderson S D, Connolly N, Godfrey S 1971 Comparison of bronchoconstriction induced by cycling and running. Thorax 26: 396–401
Andrae S, Axelson O, Bjorksten B, Fredriksson M, Kjellman N-IM 1988 Symptoms of bronchial hyperreactivity and asthma in relation to environmental factors. Archives of Disease in Childhood 63: 473–478
Aubier M, De Troyer A, Sampson M 1981 Aminophylline improves diaphragmatic contractility. New England Journal of Medicine 305: 249–252
Baker G J, Collett P, Allen D H 1981 Bronchospasm induced by metabisulphite-containing foods and drugs. Medical Journal of Australia ii: 614
Balfour-Lynn L, Tooley M, Godfrey S 1980 A study comparing the relationship of exercise-induced asthma to clinical asthma in childhood. Archives of Disease in Childhood 56: 450–454

Balfour-Lynn L 1986 Growth and childhood asthma. Archives of Disease in Childhood 61: 1049–1055

Barnes P J 1983 Pathogenesis of asthma: a review. Journal of Royal Society of Medicine 26: 580–586

Barnes P J 1984 The third nervous system of the lungs: physiology and perspectives. Thorax 39: 561–567

Barnes P J, Skoogh B E, Brown J K, Nadel J A 1983 Activation of alpha adrenergic response in smooth muscle: a post receptor mechanism. Journal of Applied Physiology 54: 1469–1476

Bar-Yishay E, Gur L, Inbar Q, Neuman I, Dlin R A, Godfrey S 1982 Difference between swimming and running as stimuli for exercise-induced asthma. European Journal of Applied Physiology 48: 387–397

Bohn D, Kalloghlian A, Jenkins J, Edmonds J, Barker G 1984 Intravenous salbutamol in the treatment of status asthmaticus in children. Critical Care Medicine 10: 892–896

Burney P G J 1986 Asthma mortality in England and Wales: evidence for a further increase 1974–1984. Lancet ii: 323–326

Burr M L, Eldridge B A, Borysiewicz L K 1974 Peak expiratory flow rates before and after exercise in schoolchildren. Archives of Disease in Childhood 49: 923–926

Canny G J, Levison H 1987 The modern management of childhood asthma. Pediatric Review and Communication 1: 123–162

Carswell F 1985 Thirty deaths from asthma. Archives of Disease in Childhood 60: 25–28

Chudry N, Correa F, Silverman M 1987 Nedocromil sodium and exercise induced asthma. Archives of Disease in Childhood 62: 412–414

Clifford R D, Pugsley A, Radford M, Holgate S T 1987 Symptoms, atopy, and bronchial response to methacholine in parents with asthma and their children. Archives of Disease in Childhood 62: 66–73

Cockroft D W 1983 Mechanism of perennial allergic asthma. Lancet ii: 253–256

Cogswell J J, Simpkiss M J 1985 Nebulised sodium cromoglycate in recurrently wheezy preschool children. Archives of Disease in Childhood 60: 736–738

Committee of Safety of Medicines 1986 CSM Update Desensitising Vaccines. British Medical Journal 293: 948

Coombs R R A, Gell P G H (eds) 1953 Clinical aspects of allergy. Blackwell Scientific, Oxford, p 575

Corkey C, Mindorff C, Levison H, Newth C 1982 Comparison of three different preparations of disodium cromoglycate in the prevention of exercise induced bronchospasm. American Review of Respiratory Diseases 125: 623–626

Darioli R, Perret C 1984 Mechanical controlled hypoventilation in status asthmaticus. American Review of Respiratory Diseases 129: 385–387

Davis J B 1976 Asthma and wheezy bronchitis in children. Clinical Allergy 6: 329–338

Dawson D, Horobin G, Illsley R, Mitchell R 1969 A survey of childhood asthma in Aberdeen. Lancet i: 827–830

Dawson K P, Unter D E M, Deo S, Fergusson D M 1986 Inhalation powder and oral salbutamol combination. Archives of Disease in Childhood 61: 1111–1113

Deal E C, McFadden E R, Ingram R H, Jaeger J J 1979 Hyperpnea and heat flux: initial reaction sequence in exercise-induced asthma. Journal of Applied Physiology 46: 476–483

Deal E C, McFadden E R, Ingram R H, Strauss R H, Jaeger J J 1987 Role of respiratory heat exchange in the production of exercise induced asthma. Journal of Applied Physiology 46: 467–475

Dinwiddie R, Gewitz M, Van der Laag H, Frame M H 1983 Plasma terbutaline levels in asthma. Archives of Disease in Childhood 58: 223–224

Edmunds A T, Tooley M, Godfrey S 1978 The refractory period following exercise induced asthma, its duration and its relation to exercise. American Review of Respiratory Disease 117: 247–254

Edmunds A T, McKenzie S, Tooley M, Godfrey S 1979 A clinical comparison of beclomethasone dipropionate delivered by pressurised aerosol and as a powder from a rotahaler. Archives of Disease in Childhood 54: 233–235

Egan P 1985 Weather or not. Medical Journal of Australia 142: 330

Elias-Jones A C, Cottle A L, Leakey T E B, Larcher V F 1987 Whole blood assay of theophylline concentrations using immunochromatographic stick at the bedside. Archives of Disease in Childhood 62: 836–837

Field H V, Jenkinson P M A, Frame M H, Warner J O 1982 Asthma treatment with a new corticosteroid aerosol, budesonide, administered twice daily by spacer inhaler. Archives of Disease in Childhood 57: 864–866

Fitch K D, Morton A R 1971 Specificity of exercise in exercise induced asthma. British Medical Journal iv: 577–581

Floyer J 1698 A treatise of the asthma, 3rd edition. Wilkins, London

Fry J 1961 'Acute wheezy chests': clinical patterns and natural history. British Medical Journal i: 227–232

Furakawa C T, Shapiro G G, Bierman W et al 1984 A double blind study comparing the effectiveness of cromolyn sodium and sustained release theophylline in childhood asthma. Pediatrics 74: 453–459

Godfrey S 1983a Exercise induced asthma. In: Clark T J H, Godfrey S (eds) Asthma. Chapman and Hall, London, pp 57–78

Godfrey S 1983b Exercise induced asthma. Archives of Disease in Childhood 58: 1–2

Godfrey S 1984 The wheezing infant. In: Meadow R (ed) Recent advances in paediatrics. Churchill Livingstone, Edinburgh, pp 137–153

Greenough A, Loftus B G, Pool J, Price J F 1986 Response to bronchodilators assessed by lung mechanics. Archives of Disease in Childhood 61: 1020–1023

Henry R L, Milner A D, Stokes G M 1983 Ineffectiveness of ipratropium bromide in acute bronchiolitis. Archives of Disease in Childhood 58: 925–926

Henry R L, Hiller E J, Milner A D, Hodges I G C, Stokes G M 1984 Nebulised ipratropium bromide and sodium cromoglycate in the first two years of life. Archives of Disease in Childhood 59: 54–57

Hodges I G C, Groggins R C, Milner A D, Stokes G M 1981 Bronchodilator effect of inhaled ipratropium bromide in wheezing toddlers. Archives of Disease in Childhood 56: 729–732

Horn M E C, Gregg I 1973 The role of viral infection and host factors in asthma and chronic bronchitis. Chest 32 (Suppl 4): 44–48

Kattan M, Keens T G, Mellis C M, Levison H 1978 The response to exercise in normal and asthmatic children. Journal of Pediatrics 92: 718–721

Kelly W J W, Hudson I, Phelan P D, Pain M C F, Olinsky A 1987 Childhood asthma in adult life: a further study at 28 years of age. British Medical Journal 294: 1059–1062

Kershaw C R 1987 Passive smoking potential atopy and asthma in the first five years of life. Journal of the Royal Society of Medicine 80: 683–688

Konig P 1981 Hidden asthma in children. American Journal of Diseases in Children 135: 1053–1055

Konig P, Godfrey S 1973 The prevalence of exercise induced bronchial lability in families of children with asthma. Archives of Disease in Childhood 48: 513–518

Kuzemko J A (ed) 1980 Incidence, prognosis and mortality. In: Asthma in children. Pitman Medical, Tunbridge Wells, Kent, pp 3–15

Lancet 1986a Editorial. Bronchial asthma and the environment. Lancet ii: 786–787

Lancet 1986b Editorial. NANC nerves in airways. Lancet ii: 1253–1254

Lange W R, Howden C W, Laws J, Burton J F 1969 Bronchopneumonia wih serious sequelae in children with evidence of adenovirus type 21 infection. British Medical Journal i: 73–79

Lask B, Matthew D J 1979 Childhood asthma — a controlled trial of family psychotherapy. Archives of Disease in Childhood 54: 116–119

Lee T H, Nagy L, Nagakura T, Walport M J, Kay A B 1982 Identification and partial characterization of an exercise-induced neutrophil chemotactic factor in bronchial asthma. Journal of Clinical Investigation 69: 889–899

Lee D A, Winslow N R, Speight A N P, Hey E N 1983 Prevalence and spectrum of asthma in childhood. British Medical Journal 286: 1256–1258

Leeder S R, Corkhill R T, Irwig L M, Holland W W, Colley J R T 1976 Influence of family factors on asthma and wheezing during the first five years of life. British Journal of Preventive and Social Medicine 30: 213–218

Lenney W, Milner A D 1978 At what age do bronchodilator drugs work? Archives of Disease in Childhood 53: 532–535

Lewis R A, Holgate S T, Roberts L J, Oates J A, Austen K F 1981 In: Becker E L (ed) Biochemistry of the acute allergic reaction. Allan R Liss, New York, pp 239–245

McFadden E R 1983 Respiratory heat and water exchange: physiological and clinical implications. Journal of Applied Physiology 54: 331–336

McKenzie S 1986 Current state of theophylline in asthma. Archives of Disease in Childhood 61: 1046–1048

Martin A J, Landau L I, Phelan P D 1980a Lung function in young adults who had asthma in childhood. American Review of Respiratory Disease 122: 609–616

Martin A J, McLennan L A, Landau L I, Phelan P D 1980b The natural history of childhood asthma to adult life. British Medical Journal 280: 1397–1400

McNicoll K N, Williams H E 1973 Spectrum of asthma in childhood I clinical and physiological components. British Medical Journal iv: 7–11

Montgomery-Smith J 1974 Incidence of atopic disease. Medical Clinics of North America 58: 10

Nerminathan V, McKenzie S 1984 Once a day theophylline: serum concentrations. Archives of Disease in Childhood 59: 762–765

Nixon P A, Orenstein D M 1988 Exercise testing in children. Pediatric Pulmonology 5: 107–122

O'Callaghan C, Milner A D, Swarbrick A 1988 Nebulised salbutamol does have a protective effect on airways in children under 1 year old. Archives of Disease in Childhood 63: 479–483

O'Callaghan C, Milner A, Swarbrick A 1989 Spacer device with face mask for giving bronchodilators to infants with asthma. British Medical Journal 298: 160–161

Packe G E, Ayres J G 1985 Asthma outbreak during a thunderstorm. Lancet ii: 199–204

Palmer J B, Cuss F M C, Barnes P J 1986 VIP and PHM and their role in non-adrenergic inhibitory responses in isolated human airways. Journal of Applied Physiology 61: 1322–1328

Peckham C, Butler N 1978 A national study of asthma in childhood. Journal of Epidemiology and Community Health 32: 79–85

Pool J B Greenough A, Cleeson J G A, Price J F 1988 Inhaled bronchodilator treatment via the nebuhaler in young asthmatic patients. Archives of Disease in Childhood 63: 288–291

Prendiville A, Green S, Silverman M 1987 Ipratropium bromide and airways function in wheezy infants. Archives of Disease in Childhood 62: 97–100

Rees P J 1984 Immunology, pathology and physiology. In: Cochrane G M (ed) Asthma. Update Medical Publications, London, pp 15–24

Sattin A 1984 Behavioural problems in children taking theophylline. Lancet i: 958

Schnall R P, Landau L I 1980 The protective effects of short sprints in exercise induced asthma. Thorax 35: 828–832

Sears M R, Rea H H, Fenwick J et al 1986 Deaths from asthma in New Zealand. Archives of Disease in Childhood 61: 6–10
Disease in Childhood 61: 6–10

Shohat M, Shohat T, Kedem R, Mimouni M, Danon Y L 1987 Childhood asthma and growth outcome. Archives of Disease in Childhood 62: 63–65

Sibbald B, Horn E C, Gregg I 1980 A family study of the genetic basis of asthma and wheezy bronchitis. Archives of Disease in Childhood 55: 354–357

Silverman M 1985 Asthma in childhood. Current Medical Literature, London, pp 3–36

Silverman M, Anderson S D 1972 Standardisation of exercise tests in asthmatic children. Archives of Disease in Childhood 47: 882–889

Silverman M, Wilson N 1985 Bronchial responsiveness in children: a clinical review. In: Milner A D, Martin R J (eds) Neonatal and pediatric respiratory medicine. Butterworths, London, pp 161–189

Sly P D, Soto-Quiros, Landau L I, Hudson I, Newton-John H 1984 Factors predisposing to abnormal pulmonary function after adenovirus type 7 pneumonia. Archives of Disease in Childhood 59: 935–939

Speight A N D, Lee D A, Hey E N 1983 Underdiagnosis and under treatment of asthma in childhood. British Medical Journal 286: 1253–1256

Springer C, Goldenberg B, Bendov I, Godfrey S 1985 Clinical, physiologic, and psychologic comparison of treatment by cromolyn or theophylline in childhood asthma. Journal of Allergy and Clinical Immunology 76: 64–69

Stein M R, Towner T C, Weber R W 1980 The effect of theophylline on the lower esophageal sphincter pressure. Annals of Allergy 45: 238–241

Storr J, Lenney C A, Lenney W 1986 Nebulised beclomethasone diproprionate in preschool asthma. Archives of Disease in Childhood 61: 270–273

Storr J, Barrell E, Lenney W 1987 Asthma in primary schools. British Medical Journal 295: 251–252

Tabachnik E, Scott P, Correia J et al 1982 Sustained release theophylline: a significant advance in the treatment of childhood asthma. Journal of Pediatrics 100: 489–492

Verity C M, Vanheule B, Carswell F, Hughes A O 1984 Bronchial lability and skin reactivity in siblings of asthmatic children. Archives of Disease in Childhood 59: 871–876

Wadsworth M 1985 Intergenerational differences in child health. In: Measuring socio-demographic change. London OPCS occasional paper 34: 51–58

Warner J O, Kerr J W 1987 Hyposensitisation. British Medical Journal 294: 1179–1180

Williams H E, McNicoll K N 1969 Prevalence, natural history and relationship of wheezy bronchitis and asthma in children. An epidemiological study. British Medical Journal 4: 321–325

Williams H E, Phelan P D (eds) 1975 Asthma. In: Respiratory illness in children. Blackwell Scientific, Oxford, pp 106–181

Wilson N M 1985 Food related asthma: a difference between two ethnic groups. Archives of Disease in Childhood 60: 861–865

Wilson N M, Silverman M 1985 The diagnosis of food sensitivity in childhood asthma. Journal of the Royal Society of Medicine 78 (Suppl 5): 11–16

Zied G, Beall G N 1966 Bronchial response to beta-adrenergic blockade. New England Journal of Medicine 275: 580–584

9. Cystic fibrosis

Cystic fibrosis (CF) is an autosomal recessive disease which is most commonly found in Caucasian peoples. In the United Kingdom it affects about 1 infant in 2500 and it is estimated that 300–350 new cases will be born in this country each year. The prevalence of CF in the UK in mid-1985 was about 5000 cases (Dodge et al 1988). The gene for cystic fibrosis has now been specifically identified (Kerem et al 1989, Riordan et al 1989, Rommens et al 1989). Previous to this major advances in the techniques of DNA analysis including the use of restriction endonucleases (enzymes which cleave DNA at specific sites dependent upon local base sequences) resulted in the identification of a number of discrete polymorphic DNA fragments which lie close to the CF gene and which have been used as probes in the analysis of genetic material from CF patients. These techniques localised the CF gene to the long arm of chromosome number 7 (Wainwright et al 1985) and the gene was shown to be very closely linked to 2 particular DNA probes, the met oncogene and pJ3.11 which are situated in the region of 7q31 (Wainwright et al 1985, White et al 1985). New techniques such as pulse field electrophoresis and chromosome mediated gene transfer were used to identify the position of the CF gene more precisely (Buchwald et al 1988). A large collaborative study of families in Europe and North America showed that in all informative cases, the CF gene was linked to the chromosome 7 markers. It seems likely that most northern European families have inherited the same mutant allele from aa single ancestor (Beaudet et al 1986, Brock 1988).

Recent evidence has also suggested that there may be genetic differences between CF with and without meconium ileus. Mornet et al (1988) found different haplotypes for the CF gene with respect to the probe pJ3.11 suggesting the possibility of multiallelism (different mutations at the same site) which might code for presentation with or without meconium ileus; these findings have yet to be confirmed by others. The availability of relatively specific DNA probes has led to increasingly reliable prenatal diagnosis (Farrell et al 1986).

The basic defect of CF has not yet been clearly established — it will become much better understood now that the gene has been isolated. Studies have shown that there is a profound abnormality in the transport of chloride ions across the membranes of affected cells (Quinton 1983). This abnormality also causes a high transcellular epithelial potential difference which can be blocked by amiloride. This elevated transepithelial potential difference is also expressed in the nasal mucosa and it has been used as a possible diagnostic test for the disease (Sauder et al 1987).

The major clinical and diagnostic features arise almost entirely from the abnormalities affecting the exocrine glandular system (Fig. 9.1). The areas most affected clinically are the respiratory system and the digestive tract. As age increases other problems occur with increasing frequency; these include diabetes, hepatic cirrhosis and reproductive problems. The sweat typically shows high levels of sodium and chloride and the patient often tastes salty when kissed. These sweat electrolyte abnormalities form the basis of the most specific diagnostic test so far available (Gibson & Cooke 1959).

The disease is life-long and eventually results in premature death. Most patients develop chronic pulmonary disease because of progressively deteriorating lung function and also nutritional problems secondary to pancreatic insufficiency.

When the condition was originally described in the 1930s (Anderson 1938), life expectancy was less than 2 years. The disease itself shows very considerable variation between one patient and another; some infants die within the first few months of life from severe disease while others do not present with significant symptoms until adult life. The majority, however, do present in infancy and early childhood. Over the past 30 years, there has been an increasing recognition of the disease, especially in its milder forms. Large CF clinics have also developed where particular expertise has been gained in the care of children with the disease. All of these factors

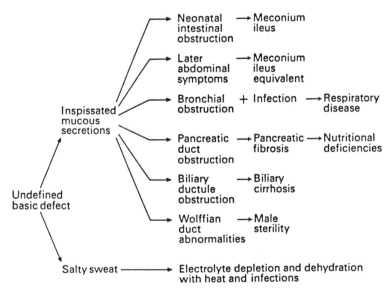

Fig. 9.1 Clinical features of cystic fibrosis (from Anderson & Goodchild 1976 with permission).

Table 9.1 Incidence of cystic fibrosis in different countries and races

Race	Country	Incidence	Reference
Caucasians	United Kingdom	1/2500	Dodge et al 1988
Caucasians	Italy	1/2600	Righetti et al 1976
Caucasians	Sweden	1/8000	Selander 1962
Caucasians	Denmark	1/4800	Nielson et al 1988
Caucasians	United States	1/2400	Kram et al 1962
Jewish	Israel	1/5000	Levin 1963
Afro-American	United States	1/17 000	Kulzycki & Shauf 1974
Mongoloid	Hawaii	1/90 000	Wright & Morton 1966

have resulted in a significant increase in life expectancy such that there is now a median survival of 27–30 years (Batten 1988).

The incidence of CF varies from one racial group to another (Table 9.1), from one country to another and even within different regions of the same country (Roberts et al 1988). The incidence among Caucasians in the United States is similar to that in Europe; it is much less common, although not rare, among Afro-Americans. It is probably not uncommon among the peoples of Arabia and the Indian subcontinent but it is very rare in the Chinese and Japanese. There are several problems about ascertaining the prevalence of CF in the population (Raeburn 1983). If data is collected from CF clinic registers or from abnormal sweat test results in reference laboratories, this will only indicate the incidence of symptomatic disease which was sufficient to raise suspicion of the diagnosis. This will underestimate the prevalence of CF unless there is a higher level of awareness amongst the community as a whole. A number of siblings of CF patients are also found to have abnormal sweat tests; some of them are virtually asymptomatic and a few are clinically normal. CF neonatal screening programmes should ultimately give a better estimate of the disease prevalence throughout the population but even these are not yet proving to be 100% reliable.

GENETIC FACTORS

The current incidence in the UK suggests a heterozygote carrier rate for the gene of 1 in 20 of the Caucasian population. As carriers are entirely healthy and since there is, as yet, no reliable detection test, this is only an estimate. The reason for the persistence of the gene at such a level is not understood since there appears to be no obvious heterozygote advantage at present. It is possible that the carrier might have a high resistance to a disease which was present in the past such as pulmonary tuberculosis. Meindl (1987) has suggested that this could occur because CF heterozygotes may produce excessive amounts of hyaluronidase in the fibro-

Table 9.2   Predicted risk of cystic fibrosis by parental genotype

Parental genotype	Risk
Both parents unknown (no family history of CF)	1/1600
Both parents heterozygote	1/4
One parent has CF One parent heterozygote	1/2
One parent heterozygote One parent unknown	1/80
One parent has CF One parent unknown	1/40
One parent's sibling has CF One parent unknown	1/120
One parent's first cousin has CF One parent unknown	1/320
One parent's step sibling has CF One parent unknown	1/160

Based on an assumed carrier rate in the population of 1 in 20

blasts. These cells are important in the successful isolation of virulent pathogens such as *Mycobacterium tuberculosis* and this could be one reason why the gene has persisted with such high frequency in the population. It can be calculated on the basis of the present estimates of carriage rate that in the countries of the European Community and the USA there must be approximately 25 million carriers of the CF gene. As more and more CF patients survive to adult life it is important to know the likely occurrence rate with other genotypes: these are shown in Table 9.2 (which assumes the parents are Caucasian).

PRENATAL DIAGNOSIS

Prenatal diagnosis has become increasingly reliable. It is currently available by one of two techniques; either by chorionic villus sampling (CVS) at 8–10 weeks gestation or by amniocentesis at 16–18 weeks. The CVS method relies on the use of DNA markers closely linked to the cystic fibrosis gene, which is known to lie on the long arm of chromosome number 7. Using restriction endonucleases, the DNA in this area can be broken into discrete fragments which can then be separated by gel electrophoresis into bands according to their molecular weight. Further radioisotope probes are used to mark bands containing the genes and by comparing the patterns obtained from each parent and the affected child it is possible to identify the specific bands which contain the CF gene (Farrell et al 1986). At present 98% of families are fully or partially informative by these tests. The test can only be performed where genetic material has already been obtained from an affected child; this will usually be from a blood sample taken during life but successful prenatal diagnosis has also been performed using retrospective analysis of standard blood spot (Guthrie) tests routinely used for phenylketonuria screening. Occasionally, it is possible to test an extended family on the paternal or maternal side utilising genetic material from an affected child for the DNA analysis (Brock et al 1986). The present tests therefore can only be performed on families where there is already an affected child and are not available for the 80% of cases presenting with no prior family history of CF (MacLusky et al 1987).

Recently it has become possible to amplify DNA itself by the use of the polymerase chain reaction (PCR) without the use of radioactivity. This will facilitate the rapid identification of the presence of the CF gene in genetic material (Feldman et al 1988). Williams et al (1988a) have also described same day, first trimester antenatal diagnosis for CF by gene amplification; this procedure also utilises the polymerase chain reaction. This has the advantage of allowing the test to be performed on a tiny quantity of genetic material, such as half of a single chorionic villus. The same group has also described a similar technique applied to the analysis of buccal epithelial cells which offers a non-invasive method for future screening of immediate family members. All of these techniques allow tracking of the gene through affected families and prediction of fetal genotype. If the test is positive it is highly reliable with a 95% chance that the baby will have CF. If the test indicates a carrier fetus, the risk of the baby having CF is 2%. If the test is negative, the risks for the baby having CF are 0.04% (these figures are based on the assumption that the spontaneous crossover rate of the gene within the chromosome is less than 1%). The additional fetal loss rate after CVS is approximately 2% which is added to the 4–5% spontaneous rate of fetal loss at this early gestation (Hoggs et al 1985, Super et al 1987).

If early prenatal diagnosis is unsuccessful or the family is uninformative using the present DNA probes, a further prenatal test is available at 16–18 weeks gestation. This involves measurement of fetal gut microvillar enzymes in amniotic fluid particularly intestinal alkaline phosphatase, which is significantly less inhibited in the presence of phenylalanine than in normals (Brock 1983). This abnormality reflects changes in the fetal digestive system which is one of the earliest abnormalities detectable in the disease. The results are usually available within 48 hours of the amniocentesis. If the test proves positive there is a 92% chance of an affected infant (Brock et al 1985) and if negative the chances of the baby having CF is 3%. The excess fetal loss rate after amniocentesis is 1–2%. This test is again most useful for affected families but it is theoretically possible to use it in families with no previous history of CF where the parental genotype is unknown.

NEONATAL SCREENING

Neonatal screening for CF is now available utilising the fact that the fetal pancreas is damaged in utero and this results in a leakage of trypsin into the circulation before birth. This results in elevated levels of immunoreactive trypsin (IRT) which are detectable in the first few weeks of life (Crossley et al 1979). This method has been applied practically by the measurement of IRT on dried blood spots routinely collected for the neonatal screening of other diseases such as phenylketonuria or hypothyroidism (Kuzemko & Heeley 1983). The incidence of CF varies from one part of the UK to another, but in East Anglia is 1 : 2130 (Kuzemko 1986). This group found an elevated IRT level in the first 2 weeks of life in 0.5% of 93 000 infants sampled, but after retesting at the age of 2–4 weeks, 38 infants remained positive and only two were subsequently proven not to have CF. A similar incidence has been reported from Australia by Wilcken et al (1983) who screened 75 000 infants and who also had a retest rate of 0.6%. The false negative rate in both studies was extremely low. Roberts et al (1988) found an incidence of CF in Northern Ireland of 1:1807 live births. The IRT test is unreliable in neonates with meconium ileus tested after surgery (Heeley & Heeley 1987).

As yet there is no conclusive evidence that early diagnosis by neonatal screening significantly improves long term survival. There is some evidence to suggest that screened infants have improved growth in early years of life and that they initially have fewer symptoms (Wilcken & Chalmers 1985); with increasing age however the differences become less marked. The psychological disturbance of families where a false positive diagnosis is made must also be considered carefully before mass screening programmes are implemented. On the other hand, one advantage to families with an affected child is that appropriate genetic counselling and early prenatal diagnosis can be offered for subsequent pregnancies. Where screening programmes are in practice, the average age of diagnosis of cystic fibrosis is reduced even amongst infants who are not detected by screening, indicating a heightened awareness among clinicians of the condition generally.

One of the major problems in confirming the diagnosis is the reliability of the sweat test in the young child, firstly because of the difficulty in obtaining sufficient sweat but also because the result may be within normal levels even though the child has CF (Roberts et al 1988). Further detailed studies of the advantages and disadvantages of neonatal screening are being undertaken, the results of which will need to be carefully reviewed before mass screening for the entire population can be recommended.

DIAGNOSIS

The sweat test remains the most reliable specific diagnostic test for CF. This is performed by the use of pilocarpine iontophoresis to stimulate sweat

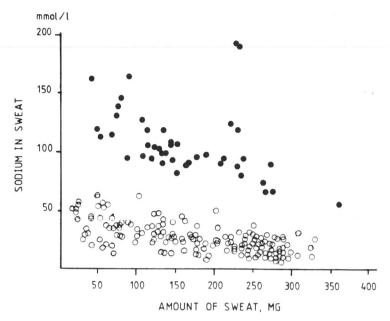

Fig. 9.2 Sweat sodium concentration related to weight of sweat sample obtained in children with (●) and without cystic fibrosis (○) (from Hjelm et al 1986 with permission).

production and its analysis for sodium levels (Gibson & Cooke 1959). The measurement of the chloride level in the sweat is an equally reliable diagnostic test (Schwachman et al 1981). Classically levels of sodium or chloride in excess of 70 mmol/l on a sample weighing over 100 mg are diagnostic. The diagnosis may be made on smaller quantities of sweat in children under 8 years of age if the data of Hjelm et al (1986) for sodium levels are used (Fig. 9.2). Others have used the measurement of sweat osmolality as a test for CF; this appears to be reliable in experienced hands (Carter et al 1984).

It is very important that the sweat test is performed by a person skilled in the procedure as false positive results can easily be obtained and may be misinterpreted (Littlewood 1986). In cases of difficulty the relation of the sodium to the chloride level is also useful. In normal individuals the sodium is usually higher than the chloride and the sum of the sodium plus chloride usually lies below 140 mmol/l (Littlewood 1986). In patients with CF, the chloride is usually higher than the sodium and the sum of sodium plus chloride is usually greater than 140 mmol/l (Green et al 1985). Sweat sodium levels increase with age and 5–10% of normal adolescents and adults have values greater than 60 mmol/l. There is also a higher than average level in those with severe asthma. Other causes of an elevated sweat sodium level are shown in Table 9.3.

These findings can make the interpretation of the sweat test very difficult in the older patient. In cases where there is particular difficulty a fludrocortisone test can be performed. This involves repeating the sweat test after giving oral 9-alpha fludrocortisone 3 mg/m^2/day for 2 days. The sweat

Table 9.3   Causes of elevated sweat sodium or chloride in children

Cystic fibrosis	Fucosidosis
Adrenal insufficiency	Mucopolysaccharidosis
Ectodermal dysplasia	Severe malnutrition
Hypothyroidism	Hypopitutarism
Nephrogenic diabetes insipidus	HIV infection
Glycogen storage disease type 1	

electrolytes fall towards the normal range in unaffected individuals but not in those with CF (Hodson et al 1983). Should the sweat test fail to give adequate diagnostic information then evaluation of pancreatic function is quired (Wang et al 1982). These tests usually also show very low or absent bicarbonate levels and the presence of small quantities of viscid duodenal secretions. The gut enzyme stimulation tests reveal very low levels of trypsin, amylase and lipase (Hadorn et al 1968). The respiratory epithelium in CF has an increased transmembrane potential difference (Knowles et al 1981, 1983) and this measurement is also under investigation as a possible diagnostic test for CF (Hay and Gedder 1985, Sauder et al 1987).

PRESENTATION

Cystic fibrosis can present in many different ways because of its effect on various organ systems. The common modes of presentation in the neonatal period are shown in Table 9.4. The currently available tests for prenatal diagnosis in families with an affected child are becoming increasingly reliable and most pregnancies where the fetus has CF will be terminated. However a small number of parents do not wish to undertake termination even though the fetus has been confirmed as having the disease. There will also be a small number of cases in which the tests have predicted a 'carrier' fetus who does in fact have the disease. The risk of this at present is of the order of 2% (Dinwiddie 1987).

Fetal ultrasound sometimes reveals a hyperechogenic mass in the fetal abdomen indicating intrauterine meconium ileus at 14–18 weeks (Muller et al 1985). This would indicate the high likelihood of CF in a family where there is already an affected child (Papp et al 1985), but there is a consider-

Table 9.4   Neonatal presentation of cystic fibrosis

Prenatal diagnosis (Chrionic villus sample, amniocentesis, meconium ileus on ultrasound)

Meconium ileus

Meconium perforation and peritonitis

Obstructive jaundice

Elevated immunoreactive trypsin

Positive sweat test (sibling known to have CF)

able risk of false positive diagnosis on the basis of microvillar enzyme studies when there is no close family history of CF ((Sharples et al 1988).

Meconium ileus

Meconium ileus is the commonest presentation immediately after birth; about 10–15% of cases will present in this way (Donnison et al 1966). The infant classically fails to pass meconium after birth because the bowel is obstructed by sticky inspissated intestinal contents. In milder cases, there may only be delayed passage of meconium, therefore sometimes the diagnosis is missed. In the more obvious case, there is marked abdominal distension with visible peristalsis increasing over the first 2 days of life and associated with bile-stained vomiting. Other complications are seen including intrauterine perforation and meconium peritonitis, volvulus or gut atresia (Mabogunje et al 1982). There is usually little doubt about the diagnosis if there is a family history of CF but otherwise the differential diagnosis includes Hirschsprung's disease, small bowel atresia, other causes of congenital intestinal obstruction and idiopathic meconium ileus in the absence of CF. Abdominal X-ray (Fig. 9.3) will show distended loops of bowel and often a mottled appearance indicating inspissation of meconium. If there has been perforation prenatally calcified material may also be seen in the peritoneal cavity.

Treatment is directed towards correction of dehydration and disturbed acid–base balance and relief of the bowel obstruction. It is also important to perform a chest X-ray as a base line, particularly as the baby may need ventilation postoperatively. In some cases the meconium ileus responds to a gastrografin enema, especially if it is used early in the course of the illness (Waggett et al 1970). Gastrografin is water soluble and radio-opaque; it has a high osmolality and acts by withdrawing fluid from the circulation into the bowel lumen so softening the meconium mass and allowing it to pass. It is very important that the infant has sufficient intravenous fluid at this time because of the risk of dehydration as the fluid moves into the gut lumen. It is important that this procedure is carried out in a paediatric surgical unit so that operative intervention can be undertaken if necessary. The progress of the enema should be observed radiologically; many cases do not respond to this procedure and still require surgical intervention. The original procedure utilised resection of the non-viable bowel, removal of meconium plugs and the creation of an end-to-side defunctioning ileostomy (Bishop & Koop 1957). As the ileostomy fluid losses can contribute to postoperative dehydration and malnutrition, most surgeons now prefer to perform primary end-to-end or end-to-side anastomosis after resection of the necrotic bowel; this has become easier because of improved surgical techniques. Infants treated in this manner feed earlier, regain birth weight more quickly and do not appear to have any increase in postoperative complications.

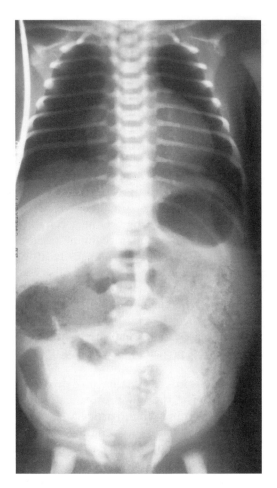

Fig. 9.3 Meconium ileus in the neonate: distended abdomen, dilated loops of bowel, inspissated meconium and clear lung fields.

All infants with meconium ileus should have a sweat test which can be reliably performed at the age of 3–4 weeks. Meconium ileus does occur spontaneously in infants who do not have CF (Rickham & Boeckman 1965), although this is uncommon. Postoperatively intensive support is often required including intravenous feeding when necessary, physiotherapy to the chest and antibiotics when appropriate. Breast feeding should be encouraged whenever possible and is frequently successful. Pancreatic enzymes should be given in all cases. Those who are unable to breast feed should be fed on any standard infant formula with added pancreatic enzymes. A number of infants have postoperative malabsorption and require predigested milk such as Pregestemil or Nutramigen with enzyme supplements. Infants with meconium ileus used to have a worse prognosis than those presenting later but this early mortality has been decreasing in recent years (Wilmott et al 1983, Dodge et al 1988).

INFANCY

CF most commonly presents in infancy and usually takes the form of poor weight gain, large appetite, loose bulky offensive stools and recurrent or persistent respiratory tract infection (Goodchild & Dodge 1985a). Despite these features, the infant is usually alert and, unless significantly malnourished, development is normal. The diagnosis is often missed initially because the child is thought to have some other malabsorptive condition such as coeliac disease, disaccharide intolerance or food allergy. The typical CF stools are pale and oily, they tend to float in water because of their high fat content, are difficult to flush away and have a particular pungent penetrating odour which is virtually diagnostic for the disease. Infants who present with any of these features must have a sweat test in order to exclude this condition. Respiratory tract infections are extremely common in the first year of life, particularly bronchiolitis (Abman et al 1988), and many infants with CF are indeed first detected when they present with persistent respiratory tract signs. Those who have severe bronchiolitis requiring intensive care, symptoms which do not resolve, or significant X-ray shadowing should always have a sweat test performed to exclude CF.

The lungs in CF are normal at birth (Reid & de Haller 1964) but with the onset of infection they become colonised with bacteria which result in increasingly viscid sputum production, obstruction of the small airways (Phelan et al 1969) and impaired clearance of lung secretions; these changes produce the typical respiratory signs which are seen in the infant (Table 9.5). These may take the form of a persistent moist or sharp barking cough often associated with the presence of purulent secretions seen in the pharyngeal area. This is easy to miss since infants usually swallow sputum at this stage. More ominous signs are the presence of a persistently raised respiratory rate, wheezing, hyperinflation of the chest and intercostal muscle retraction and cyanosis. Some infants with CF also have a parox-

Table 9.5   Presentation of cystic fibrosis in infancy

Failure to thrive

Recurrent loose stools — steatorrhoea

Persistent or recurrent respiratory tract infection

Anaemia and oedema

Pseudo-Bartter's syndrome

Rectal prolapse

Heat exhaustion

ysmal cough rather similar to that seen in pertussis and these spasms often lead to vomiting with loss of the nutritional intake. Finger clubbing can occur at an early stage and marked finger wrinkling in water is another diagnostic pointer.

A few infants present in other less common ways. Some develop persistent hyponatraemia and hypokalaemia secondary to excessive sweat electrolyte loss. This is known as pseudo-Bartter's syndrome and these children often require large quantities of supplemental sodium and potassium during the first few months of life. Other infants present at this age with anaemia, oedema and hypoproteinaemia which is secondary to malnutrition caused by the underlying pancreatic deficiency (Neilson & Larsen 1982). The sweat test itself was developed after it was noted that infants with apparent malabsorption often developed heat exhaustion in hot climates. This is due to excess sodium loss and the relationship of this to CF was originally noted by Kessler & Anderson (1951). The observation that the baby 'tastes salty' when kissed should never be taken lightly as more than one parent or nurse has made the diagnosis following this important observation.

Rectal prolapse occurs in about 10% of young children with CF and in some cases it may be the presenting feature. The diagnosis should always be considered in any young child who presents with this problem, especially if there are other suggestive signs such as steatorrhoea or a history of recurrent respiratory infection. This complication usually responds satisfactorily to appropriate dietary management of the disease in conjunction with pancreatic enzyme replacement; surgical treatment is not normally required.

Persistent respiratory symptoms or recurrent respiratory infection are the classical presentations of the illness. Some infants have persistent wheeze, tachypnoea and respiratory indrawing after an episode of bronchiolitis. Auscultation of the chest reveals high pitched rhonchi in association with small airway obstruction and fine and coarse crepitations due to retained pulmonary secretions in patchy areas of bronchopneumonia. Respiratory function tests (Phelan et al 1969) show increased lung volumes and decreased airway conductance indicating small airway obstruction. The simplest test however is the chest X-ray which will often show overinflation with forward bowing of the sternum, depression of the diaphragm and early bronchial wall thickening secondary to chronic infection (Chrispin & Norman 1974). Persistent lobar collapse and bronchiectasis can be seen even in infancy and may affect either the upper or lower lobes (see Fig. 9.5). Any young child who presents with bronchopneumonia, particularly if it is staphylococcal, should have a sweat test. Staphylococcal empyema is another mode of presentation at this age. Other organisms such as *Haemophilus influenzae*, *Escherichia coli* or *Pseudomonas aeruginosa* (*P. aeruginosa*) should also be treated with suspicion and a sweat test requested. CF patients who are first diagnosed at this age because of respiratory disease do not always fare badly, at least initially. This is because the lung is still growing and developing rapidly and there is considerable room for recovery if further chronic infection can be prevented or controlled in the early years.

CHILDHOOD AND ADOLESCENCE

CF can present in later childhood, adolescence or even in adult life. The modes of presentation at this time are shown in Table 9.6.

CF should be suspected at this stage in any patient who has persistent signs of respiratory disease which are difficult to control and which are associated with chronic symptoms such as cough, sputum production or wheezing; some patients only complain of breathlessness particularly on exertion. A chest X-ray shows increased shadowing due to bronchial wall thickening and small mottled areas of chronic pulmonary sepsis. In those with mild disease, the first sign to be detected may be the presence of finger clubbing which should always prompt a sweat test as one of the basic investigations. Rapid and excessive finger wrinkling in water is another clue although it is not diagnostic. Some older patients are discovered during investigation of asthma which is proving difficult to control. They frequently do not have significant digestive problems and often do not need pancreatic supplements. A small number of patients present with evidence of biliary cirrhosis either with an enlarged liver or spleen or with haematemesis.

Another presentation is with recurrent abdominal pain, particularly if abdominal palpation reveals a faecal mass in the caecal area and the abdominal X-ray shows gaseous distension of the gut and evidence of subacute obstruction. Chronic sinusitis is virtually universal in older patients with CF and nasal polyps are also common (Drake-Lee & Pitcher-Wilmot 1982); these can however be an important diagnostic clue and again are an indication for a sweat test. Those who have any chronic disease often have delayed onset of puberty and if this is associated with poor growth other symptoms of CF should specifically be sought. As 99% of adult males with cystic fibrosis are infertile, a few have presented for the first time in infertility clinics because of this problem. Some children are also first detected because a sibling is diagnosed as having CF. A routine sweat test should always be performed on all brothers and sisters of affected cases since the disease may be mild and may not have been detected at this

Table 9.6   Presentation of cystic fibrosis in childhood, adolescence or adult life

Recurrent wheeze, cough and purulent sputum production	Diabetes mellitus
	Heat exhaustion
Persistent 'asthma'	Delayed puberty
Finger clubbing	Male infertility
Nasal polyposis and chronic sinusitis	Haemoptysis
Biliary cirrhosis	Sibling with CF
Meconium ileus equivalent (recurrent abdominal pain — faecal mass)	

stage. These patients are not always entirely symptom free and on close examination will have often had some respiratory or digestive problems in the past, albeit of a mild degree.

MANAGEMENT

Management of the patient with CF has to be comprehensive and life long. Since the disease is multisystem it requires a multidisciplinary approach; some of the important aspects are shown in Table 9.7. Major components of management initially revolve around confirmation of the diagnosis and education of the parents and child in the day to day care which is required for the optimum management of the disease. The realisation that their child has a serious life long and life threating illness naturally comes as a great shock to any family. The degree of stress at the time of diagnosis may be further exacerbated by the acuteness and severity of symptoms at the time of presentation. Alternatively, the parents of a child diagnosed by neonatal screening before there are any clinical signs present have a different but equally stressful problem with which to cope. Whichever group the child falls into a great deal of time and effort needs to be spent in educating the parents about the illness as there is so much for them to understand. Each day appears to bring some new potential problem and in addition there are the important genetic aspects which must be explained. The availability of prenatal diagnosis has also to be reviewed and arranged if necessary. Questions as to long term outcome also have to be addressed although it is always difficult to give more than general guidelines initially.

It is important at this stage to develop good habits of regular care, particularly in respect to the respiratory, nutritional and psychological requirements of the patient and the family. Those who present in infancy or early childhood are also undergoing a period of rapid growth and development and are at a time of life when there is scope to prevent or delay the onset and progress of the more chronic changes, particularly in the lungs. As the child increased in age a number of other complications can occur and these are discussed later. It is also important that the patient is in regular contact with a major general CF centre since it has been shown that life expectancy is significantly increased if this is the case (Warwick 1982, Dodge et al 1988, Nielson et al 1988). Shared care between the district

Table 9.7 Management of cystic fibrosis

Medical
Genetic
Social
Psychological
Educational
Occupational

general hospital, the general practitioner, and the regional CF centre probably provides optimum management.

PULMONARY MANAGEMENT

Pathophysiology

The lungs are essentially normal at birth. During respiratory infections, the CF infant produces abnormal lung secretions which are increasingly sticky and viscid and this leads to impaired mucociliary clearance and an increased incidence of chest infection. By the age of 3 months, 50% of CF infants are symptomatic in one way or another and by the age of 8 months 50% have developed respiratory symptoms (Batten & Matthew 1983). Early pathological changes also include abnormalities of the goblet cells with hyperplasia which suggests an underlying defect in mucus gland secretion. Recurrent infection leads to inflammatory obstruction of the small airways, squamous metaplasia of the bronchial epithelium, mucus plugging and further disruption of the mucociliary lining. More peripherally there tends to be micro-abscess formation especially in the upper lobes. In the longer term these changes become more generalised and there is development of bronchiectasis (Tomashefski et al 1983). As the airways become progressively more damaged there is distortion and collapse; this leads to airway trapping and more persistent infection with further micro-abscess formation and the onset of chronic bronchiectasis. The infective changes in the pulmonary parenchyme are also associated with intrapulmonary vascular shunting, local arteriolar vasoconstriction and eventually the onset of pulmonary hypertension. When there is persistent hypoxia there is structural remodelling of the pulmonary vascular bed which increases the vascular resistance further and ultimately leads to the onset of cor pulmonale and cardiac failure.

The role of allergic reactions in the lung is also important in the development of the pathological process. The interaction of these in relation to the developing infective changes is however difficult to define; the subject has been well reviewed by Wilmott (1985). He reported that only 12% of CF children attending a large clinic had a history of exercise-induced bronchospasm and 7% had pollen asthma. Seasonal allergic rhinitis was reported in 20% and infantile eczema in 10%; by these criteria allergic symptoms are no more common in CF children than in normal children of the same age. Some 53% of the CF children reported wheezing as a symptom but this occurs for a number of reasons other than asthma in this disease. There is a high incidence of positive skin prick tests to common inhaled allergens in CF patients — Wilmott (1985) reported 59% of 123 children showing positive reactions to a battery of 12 allergens including two moulds. Warner et al (1976) had previously shown that 56% of children were positive for *Aspergillus fumigatus* on skin testing. The reason for this high rate of positivity is not clear since although bronchopulmonary aspergillosis is seen in CF, this is an uncommon complication. The prevalence of skin test positivity to other allergens is the same as for normal children. There is however an association with colonisation of the respiratory tract by *P. aeruginosa* and positive skin test reactions but it is thought that the allergic reaction is not an important predisposing factor to Pseudomonas colonisation; it may be a secondary effect from mucosal damage caused by the organism itself (Wilmott et al 1985).

Wheezing is another common feature of lung disease in CF — approximately 50% of patients complain of this symptom (Wilmott 1985). This occurs because of airway narrowing which can result from infection, localised oedema and airway obstruction, asthma or a primary increase in bronchial hyper-reactivity. The responses to bronchial challenge with histamine, methacholine or exercise testing in CF patients have given variable results, especially when performed repeatedly over a period of time (Holtz et al 1981). The clinical implication of this is that the response to bronchodilators such as beta-agonists is variable and a small proportion of patients in fact become worse rather than better after their use (MacLusky et al 1987). A bronchodilator response should be measured to demonstrate benefit before a bronchodilator is prescribed as a regular part of treatment. Another important implication of wheezing is that it may be exercise induced and can limit the ability to partake in normal physical activities and sports. It is often useful to establish by exercise testing those who do show exercise induced wheezing so that it can be blocked by the inhalation of agents such as sodium cromoglycate, salbutamol or terbutaline beforehand, thus improving the patient's exercise tolerance and sense of physical well-being.

The role of respiratory viral infection in the aetiology and progress of the lung disease is still unclear. All young children experience a large number of such infections, particularly during the early years of life. Peterson et al (1981) found evidence of non-bacterial pathogens in 20% of CF cases with acute pulmonary deterioration. The commonest virus isolated was the respiratory syncitial virus (RSV). Stroobant (1985) compared two groups of children with and without *P. aeruginosa* colonisation and found that in all cases where a virus was identified significant pulmonary deterioration had occurred and this was worse in those who had preceding colonisation with *P. aeruginosa*. Abman et al (1988) found RSV in 33% of CF infants admitted to hospital for respiratory distress in the first year of life. These infants had worse symptoms, spent longer in hospital and were more likely to have persistent long term respiratory signs than other CF infants of a similar age. It is also well known that viruses such as RSV can cause considerable local tissue damage during acute infection; it is possible that this could allow access of *P. aeruginosa* to the lower respiratory tract or result in worsening of immune-mediated local tissue damage which can result from infection by this organism and from bacteria such as *Staphylococcus aureus*.

Close and frequent monitoring of lung function is one of the most important aspects of care of the CF patient; regular surveillance helps to

Table 9.8   Respiratory monitoring of the cystic fibrosis patient

Throat/cough swab or sputum	Every visit
Lung function:	
Peak expiratory flow rate	Every visit
Vitalograph FVC	Every visit
FEV 1 second	Every visit
Flow/volume curve	Every visit
Oxygen saturation	Every visit
Full lung function: plethysmography	6 monthly
Chest X-ray: frontal and lateral view	6 monthly
Other tests as indicated clinically:	
Skin tests for allergy	
Full blood count	
Liver function tests/prothrombin time	
Bronchodilator response	
Aspergillus antibodies	
Immunoglobulins	

detect early signs of deterioration often before this is evident clinically. The recommended schedule of monitoring is shown in Table 9.8.

The availability of portable lung function apparatus including a vitalograph and an oxygen saturation monitor make it possible to measure lung function and estimate oxygenation at every visit. A postero-anterior (PA) and lateral chest X-ray are performed every 6–12 months and may be usefully scored according to the system described by Chrispin & Norman (1974).

The frontal and lateral chest X-rays are inspected for the typical abnormalities seen in CF (Fig. 9.4). These include increases in lung volume which result in forward bowing of the sternum (lateral film), spinal kyphosis (lateral film) and a degree of diaphragmatic depression (frontal and lateral films); these changes are due to hyperinflation of the lungs. Each individual item is given a score of: 0, not present; 1, present but not marked; 2, marked, depending on the degree of change. The lung fields are then divided into four zones on the PA film; right upper, right lower, left upper and left lower. Each field is then reviewed for parenchymal lung changes which are a consequence of the bronchial mucus plugging and infection, and which are seen as bronchial wall thickening, mottled shadows, ring shadows and areas of confluent consolidation. A score of 0, 1, or 2 is given according to severity for each zone in relation to each of these changes. The increased bronchial line shadowing indicates thickening of the walls of the airways; these are usually seen as longitudinal shadows with a straight line branching pattern and also as end-on bronchi which show as circular shadows — these are best seen in the lateral view. Mottled shadows indicating sputum collection at the microlobular level show as small rounded opacities with ill-defined edges which are seen as confluent areas of increased radiodensity. Ring shadows are formed by a central area of increased lung radiolucency circumscribed by a discrete shadow of lesser radiancy. These

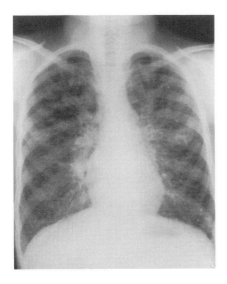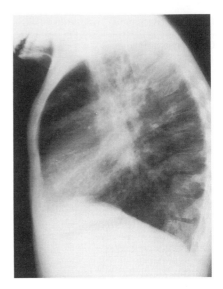

Fig. 9.4   Advanced pulmonary disease in cystic fibrosis: generalised bronchial wall thickening and hyperinflation with mottled shadows and ring formation — typical of CF (Chrispin-Norman score = 16).

shadows are about 0.5 cm in diameter and are predominantly seen in the peripheral lung areas; they represent bronchiectasis at the lobular level. A score is given for the presence and severity of these shadows in each quadrant. Large confluent pulmonary shadows are areas of more generalised lung collapse and consolidation affecting a lobe or a segment within a lobe.

This scoring system is useful in following the development of radiographic changes in the lungs over a period of years and does bear some relationship to the respiratory function tests measured at the same time (Matthew et al 1977). It is advisable that the score is calculated by two observers simultaneously to reduce inter-observer error. In clinical practice scores above 20 indicate advanced pulmonary disease.

The major bacterial pathogens of the lung are *Staphylococcus aureus* (*S. aureus*), *P. aeruginosa* and *Haemophilus influenzae* (*H. influenzae*). Mearns (1980) showed that *S. aureus* is usually the initial pathogen in the lungs but that with increasing age *P. aeruginosa* begins to predominate. Once colonisation of the lung with these organisms has occurred it is very difficult indeed to eradicate them despite intensive specific antibiotic therapy. These organisms then continue to be a potential source of major lung damage throughout life. As the lung disease advances other complications are seen including pneumothorax, haemoptysis and ultimately cor pulmonale. The incidence and management of these problems is discussed later. The specific modes of management for the lung are shown in Table 9.9.

The aim of treatment of the lungs is to minimise the effects of intercurrent infection, clear them of viscid secretions, control any concomitant

Table 9.9   Pulmonary management of cystic fibrosis

Chest physiotherapy and postural drainage

Forced expiration technique (FET)

Antibiotics intermittent or continuous (oral, intravenous or inhaled)

Physical exercise

Bronchodilators

Sodium cromoglycate

Steroids — oral or inhaled

Mucolytics — inhaled

Antifungal agents

bronchial hyper-reactivity and delay the onset and the progression of bronchiectasis (Fig. 9.5) which eventually is inevitable in every case.

Physiotherapy

Physiotherapy with postural drainage on a regular basis is the most important part of treatment aimed at preventing the progression of underlying lung disease (Hodson & Gaskell 1983). The type and frequency should be tailored to the individual's needs so those with minimal lung disease may only need one treatment per day and a fortunate few may indeed manage with none. Regular physiotherapy is however prophylactic in keeping the chest clear

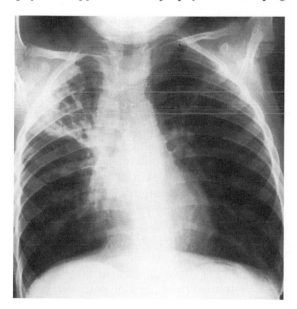

Fig. 9.5   Right upper lobe bronchiectasis in CF: note compensatory left upper zone hyperinflation.

and it also accustoms the patient to this part of their treatment. When they do have an intercurrent chest infection and need this even more then they are able to tolerate it better. This is especially true for children who often resist unfamiliar procedures, particularly when they are feeling unwell. Those who produce sputum regularly should have physiotherapy 2–3 times daily for at least 10–15 minutes. Physiotherapy should be instituted as soon as the diagnosis is made, even in the neonatal period. The technique by which it is performed is extremely important and both parents should be instructed in this by an experienced physiotherapist. During visits to the clinic, the parents' technique and efficacy can be reviewed on a regular basis.

Postural drainage of the chest is an integral part of this treatment and for this the patient is placed in various positions so that with gravity the pulmonary secretions can be drained satisfactorily. The techniques and appropriate positions have been reviewed by Hodson & Gaskell (1983) and Webber (1988). It is important not to undertake vigorous physiotherapy after a meal since a bout of coughing can easily induce vomiting with the loss of vital nutrition. A variety of wedges and special tipping beds are available with the right firmness of mattress and pillows and an appropriate degree of tilt for correct drainage of the lungs.

A useful alternative method for the older child and adult is the use of the forced expiration technique (FET). This is a special method of self-percussion of the chest combined with deep breathing, coughing and postural drainage which is as effective as conventional physiotherapy, once the patient has been taught to do it properly (Prior et al 1979). It involves taking a medium inspiration and then giving a forced and slightly prolonged expiration or 'huff'; this is followed by gentle diaphragmatic breathing and coughing which facilitates the removal of sputum from the lungs. The patient also performs chest compression personally or has help from an assistant. FET can also be used in conjunction with other standard techniques including postural drainage. FET is therefore very helpful for those who wish to perform their own treatment, especially the older patient. In order for FET to work properly it is very important that it is demonstrated to the patient by a physiotherapist trained in this specific technique. FET is as effective as conventional physiotherapy providing the patient undertakes it as part of regular treatment and performs it properly. It does however require full patient co-operation on a day to day basis in order to continue to be effective in the longer term.

The application of positive expiratory pressure to the airway during attempts to clear sputum has been facilitated by the use of a positive expiratory pressure (PEP) mask. This device enables a positive pressure to be maintained throughout expiration while the patient takes deep breaths prior to the expectoration of sputum. The applied pressure prevents early closure of small airways so allowing greater release of retained secretions. This form of treatment when evaluated over a short period does appear to be helpful (Tyrell et al 1986), especially if it is used as an adjunct to regular physiotherapy. It is particularly useful during short trips away from home such as holidays and school camps.

A number of mechanical devices have been developed for use in the treatment of the chest in CF and high frequency oscillation devices have also been tried. However, at present there is no convincing evidence that either technique is a substitute for proper treatment either by conventional physiotherapy or FET.

Physical exercise

Physical exercise is a natural way to stimulate the respiratory muscles and to aid the clearance of lung secretions, especially in CF. Zach et al (1982) found exercise tolerance was increased and respiratory muscles were strengthened at least in the short term if regular exercise was taken. This is usually accompanied by an improved feeling of general well-being. Recent studies have reviewed the benefits of exercise programmes, particularly running (Orenstein et al 1981) and swimming (Edlund et al 1986). These programmes did result in an increase in exercise tolerance and peak oxygen consumption but did not significantly improve lung function in the longer term. Exercise has also been shown to be as effective as conventional physiotherapy in clearing sputum in those with mild disease (Zach et al 1982). The ability to continue sports at any age is both physically and psychologically helpful to the CF patient. Those with mild to moderate lung function abnormality are usually able to undertake normal exercise (Cerny et al 1982, Cropp et al 1982); those with severe lung disease (FEV_1 less than 30% predicted) have significantly reduced capacity for physical work. The use of transcutaneous oxygen saturation monitoring now provides a simple non-invasive method for assessing oxygenation during different levels of exercise in the CF patient (Marcotte et al 1986). It is best to design a programme of submaximal exercise which can be sustained for periods of 10–20 minutes as the patient will find this less uncomfortable and is more likely to persist with the programme on a regular basis. Exercise induced bronchospasm can limit exercise tolerance in those who have bronchial hyperreactivity. In these cases a beta-agonist such as salbutamol or terbutaline or an agent such as sodium cromoglycate taken before the exercise will block this response (Geddes 1984).

Antibiotics

Antibiotics play a major role in the control of lung infection in CF. There are a number of long term regimes in use at the present time, each of which has its advantages and disadvantages and none of which has been shown to be superior to any other. The commonly used policies are as follows:

1. Continuous anti-Staphylococcal antibiotics throughout life from time of diagnosis.

2. Anti-Staphyloccocal antibiotics up to the age of 5 years with intermittent use thereafter.
3. Intermittent therapy initially, changing to continuous therapy when there is evidence of chronic pulmonary infection and daily sputum production.

The aim of any treatment is to delay the onset of persistent lower respiratory tract infection which inevitably occurs as age increases. The two major pathogens involved are *S. aureus* and *P. aeruginosa*. Other organisms such as *Haemophilus influenzae*, *Streptococcus pneumoniae*, haemolytic streptococci, *Klebsiella pneumoniae* and *E. coli* can also cause acute intercurrent infections (Fig. 9.6). The role of viruses and fungi in the production of lung damage is not fully understood but is probably important. Patients with chronic Staphylococcal or Pseudomonas colonisation are more likely to require hospital admission because of exacerbation of lower respiratory tract symptoms from these organisms during upper tract viral infections (Peterson et al 1981, Stroobant 1985). In the young child in particular when such viral infections are so common it is appropriate to cover all but the most trivial respiratory infections with an oral anti-Staphylococcal antibiotic.

Those who favour continuous anti-Staphylococcal therapy in the early years argue that this is the time of rapid lung growth and that the lungs are normal at birth so that colonisation of the young child with *S. aureus* is likely to cause damage. The Staphylococcus is frequently an early

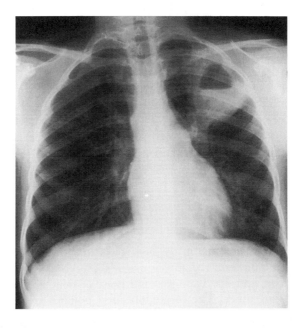

Fig. 9.6 Left upper lobe lung abscess in CF.

pathogen (Mearns 1980) and may be particularly important in the aetiology of lung pathology at this stage of the disease. Continuous treatment of CF patients with an anti-Staphylococcal agent is known to reduce the incidence of anti-Staphylococcal precipitins in the blood. This may be taken as an indication that Staphylococcal growth has been inhibited (Goodchild & Dodge 1985b, Hoiby and Schiotz 1982) and thus the risk of long term damage has been reduced.

Other workers feel that the prolonged use of continuous anti-Staphylococcal therapy is not indicated because firstly it can induce resistance and secondly it may increase the risk of colonisation with other organisms such as *P. aeruginosa*. Mearns (1980) has noted that Staphylococcal infection has become less common in the last 30 years as *P. aeruginosa* has increased; this might be due to the increasing use of anti-Staphylococcal agents in the early years. A controlled trial of continuous versus intermittent therapy to delay the onset of chronic Staphylococcal infection (Williams et al 1988b) has demonstrated a reduced colonisation rate of *S. aureus* during the first 2 years of life but there is no evidence as yet of a difference in the rate of colonisation of *P. aeruginosa* according to whether the patient is given continuous antibiotics or only treated during intercurrent infections (controls).

In the young child in particular, viral infections are very common as the infant lacks natural immunity to many of them. Although young CF patients do not seem to be more susceptible than normals to infection with non-bacterial agents, the effects of the colonisation are significantly more damaging to the respiratory tract (Marks 1984). All of the usual respiratory viruses have been implicated in the process but RSV, Parainfluenza and Influenza A appear to be the most common (Wang et al 1984). The mechanism by which the viral agent exacerbates preceding bacterial colonisation in the lung is not understood. It is likely that there is a complex immune-mediated reaction between the virus, the resident bacteria and the host, possibly resulting in altered adherence of the bacterial cell wall to the adjacent tissue such that it has a greater pathogenicity and increased cytotoxic effects. This process will be exacerbated by the altered sputum viscosity which is also part of the basic disorder. Respiratory infections should therefore be treated with an oral anti-Staphylococcal antibiotic. Where *P. aeruginosa* is present consideration should be given to the need for anti-Pseudomonas treatment such as intravenous or inhaled gentamicin.

Whenever a child is seen in the clinic or there is any significant change in respiratory status or symptoms, a cough swab or sputum sample should be obtained for culture. This is then a useful guide to future antibiotic therapy. The agents most commonly used are shown in Table 9.10. When chronic bacterial colonisation is present, any intercurrent respiratory infection should be treated with an appropriate antibiotic. If the patient fails to respond to this then intravenous therapy either in hospital or at home may be necessary. Those whose symptoms deteriorate whenever antibiotics are stopped require continuous oral or inhaled therapy on a long term basis.

Table 9.10 Antibiotic dosage in cystic fibrosis

Type	Route	Individual dose			No of doses/day	Notes
		< 1 yr	Age 1–7	Age 7–14		
Amikacin	IV	←——— 10.0 mg/kg ———→			2	Check levels
Amoxycillin	Oral	125 mg	250 mg	500 mg	3	Better absorption than Ampicillin
Ampicillin	Oral	125 mg	250 mg	500 mg	4	
	IV	←——— 50–100 mg/kg ———→			4	
Augmentin	Oral	62.5 mg	125–250 mg	250–500 mg	3	Amoxycillin + Clavulanic acid. Dose is Amoxycillin
Azlocillin	IV	←——— 100 mg/kg ———→			3	
Carbencillin	IV	←——— 100 mg/kg ———→			4	
Ceftazidime	IV	←——— 50 mg/kg ———→			3	
Cephradine	Oral	125 mg	250 mg	500 mg	4	
Chloramphenicol	Oral	12.5 mg/kg	25 mg/kg	25 mg/kg	4	Check levels
	IV	12.5 mg/kg	25 mg/kg	25 mg/kg	4	Check levels
Ciprofloxacin	Oral	5 mg/kg	125 mg	125–250	2	
	IV	←——— 3–5 mg/kg ———→			2	
Colistin	Nebulised	250 000 units	500 000 units	1 000 000 units	2	

Drug	Route					
Cotrimoxazole	Oral	120 mg	240 mg	480 mg	2	Trimethoprim 1 part Sulphamethoxazole 5 parts
Erythromycin	Oral	125–250 mg	250–500 mg	500 mg	4	
	IV	——————— 12.5 mg/kg ——→			4	
Flucloxacillin	Oral	125 mg	250 mg	500 mg	4	
	IV	——————— 25 mg/kg ——→			4	
Fucidin Sodium Fusidate	Oral	125 mg	250 mg	500 mg	3	
Gentamicin	IV	——————— 2–3 mg/kg ——→			3	Check levels
	Nebulised	40 mg	40 mg	80 mg	2	
Penicillin	Oral	62.5 mg	125–250 mg	250–500 mg	4	
	IV	——————— 50 mg/kg ——→			4	
Tobramycin	IV	——————— 2–3 mg/kg ——→			3	Check levels
	Nebulised	40 mg	40 mg	80 mg	2	
Trimethoprim	Oral	25–50 mg	100 mg	200 mg	2	

Pseudomonas

P. aeruginosa infection is much more difficult to treat. Once colonisation of the lung occurs, it is seldom, if ever, eradicated. This may be because the organism can adhere more efficiently to respiratory mucus in the CF lung than other Gram-negative bacteria (Vishwatah & Ramphal 1984). Once within the CF lung the organism changes from the common non-mucoid to a mucoid form by the production of a mucoid exopolysaccharide (MEP) which is similar to the alginate polysaccharide normally found in seaweed. Micro-colonies of the organism encompassed by this layer of mucus are protected from attack by host defences. It also produces a number of other toxic products such as proteases, elastase and alkaline proteinase which are locally tissue damaging and which increase its pathogenicity. Phospholipase which shows haemolytic activity is also produced, as is exotoxin A which may be toxic for human macrophages, and pyocyanin, a pigment, which inhibits ciliary function (Pitt 1986). The mucoid type of *P. aeruginosa* is found in 60–90% of chronically colonised CF patients but is rare in other conditions apart from bronchiectasis and some types of urinary tract infection. CF patients with chronic *P. aeruginosa* infection have significantly raised antibody levels to MEP although this does not appear to influence colonisation with mucoid or non-mucoid types.

Much of the local tissue damage caused by *P. aeruginosa* infection is immune-mediated; this has been reviewed by Zach (1988). A number of investigators consider that the damage is largely mediated through a type 3 hypersensitivity reaction in which *P. aeruginosa* supplies antigen for an immune complex disease which ultimately leads to the release of lysomsal enzymes and oxygen radicals from stimulated polymorphonuclear leucocytes. Patients with severe disease due to *P. aeruginosa* have high antibody levels against the organism (Doring & Hoiby 1983) and also significant levels of immune complexes present in their serum and sputum (Pitcher-Wilmott et al 1982, Hoiby and Schiotz 1982). There is a correlation between longitudinal variation of these immune complexes as detected in the sputum and alterations in lung function (Schiotz et al 1983). The inflammatory process involves complement activation and the attraction of polymorphonuclear neutrophils (PMNs) into the lung tissue. These cells release proteolytic enzymes which may be locally tissue damaging; normally these proteases are inactivated by local inhibitors but it is thought that in CF this system may be ineffective (Zach 1988). All of these mechanisms ultimately contribute to the development of local airway damage and bronchiectasis, both of which contribute to the abnormal and deteriorating lung function with age which is the cardinal feature of the disease.

In North America another Pseudomonad, *P. cepacia*, has been seen with increasing frequency in recent years (MacLusky et al 1987). This organism has been isolated during intercurrent viral infections such as RSV and Influenza A and it is often resistant to many antibiotics. Its virulence is variable — in some cases it can colonise the lungs for a number of years —

but it is also capable of producing a very rapid deterioration in lung function over a short period.

The majority of patients with established Pseudomonas infection, defined as three sequential positive cultures over a 6-month period, will require intensive intravenous antibiotic therapy from time to time depending on their clinical condition. Indications for treatment include increasing cough and sputum production, breathlessness and a general deterioration in the patient's condition associated with poor appetite and weight loss. A chest X-ray and lung function tests should be performed to assess any change from the patient's previous state and will usually show deterioration. When the organism first appears it is not always necessary to undertake intensive treatment of this kind providing that there is no change in the clinical state. In some cases the Pseudomonas may be present in the lung without evidence of rapid deterioration even for a number of years. Patients with more advanced lung disease will probably require intensive treatment at intervals of 3–4 months at least. Some centres believe that a structured programme of aggressive 3-monthly preventive treatment should be given and that this is associated with a better prognosis (Szaff et al 1983, Hoiby 1984). Other centres utilise monotherapy with agents such as ceftazidime on a 3-monthly basis whether or not there is clinical deterioration in order to control chronic *P. aeruginosa* infection (Phillips & David 1987). Both types of treatment, whether initiated by clinical deterioration or given regularly, are associated with an immediate effect on the patient's general condition. Although the organism is not eradicated from the sputum there is usually significant improvement in lung function, appetite, weight gain, decreased sputum production and a feeling of general well-being. There has not as yet been a controlled trial to demonstrate which approach is more effective, but both have been associated with the improved prognosis which has occurred during the past 20 years (Wilmott et al 1985). Aggressive treatment in Denmark has reduced the annual mortality rate among patients chronically colonised to a level of 1–2% per year but it has also resulted in the emergence of a number of multiply resistant organisms (Pederson et al 1987).

The intravenous treatment is usually given for a period of 10–14 days. It is common practice to give two antibiotics simultaneously and a wide choice of these is available; the most usual combinations are an aminoglycoside such as gentamicin or tobramycin with an acyleurerido penicillin such as azlocillin or a third generation cephalosporin such as ceftazidime. It is useful to admit the patient to hospital for this treatment since a general review of their condition can be undertaken, intensive physiotherapy can also be given and dietary habits and intake with particular reference to total calorie counting (Dinwiddie & Madge 1988) can also be assessed.

Frequent and intensive intravenous therapy does have some disadvantages however, particularly disruption of daily life — especially during school term and among those who are in employment. This has led to an increasing number of patients requesting such therapy at home (Winter et al 1984). Such a treatment regime is entirely practical given suitable support

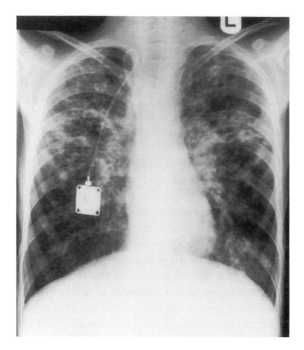

Fig. 9.7   Advanced lung disease in CF: Portacath in situ for frequent parenteral antibiotic therapy.

from the local family practitioner services and hospital back-up for cannula placement (Phillips & David 1987, Williams et al 1988b). This approach allows patients to lead a much more normal life and yet maintain the intensive treatment programme. Another approach to long term therapy is to place a permanent subcutaneous cannula such as a Portacath (Fig. 9.7); this allows repeated access over long periods of time and is associated with a low complication rate if it is properly managed. This type of treatment is probably best supervised by a special nurse liaison sister who is able to visit the patient at home.

Until recently treatment for *P. aeruginosa* could only be given parenterally or by nebuliser. The introduction of ciprofloxacin, an oral anti-Pseudomonal agent, has facilitated the treatment of this organism in CF. Hodson et al (1987) have shown it to be as effective in exacerbations of *P. aeruginosa* infection in CF as standard iv therapy. Although it is important, advance in treatment resistance to this agent has already appeared in a significant number of patients (Scully et al 1986).

An alternative approach to the long term control of chronic *P. aeruginosa* infection is to use nebulised antibiotics. These could also be useful over short periods during intercurrent respiratory tract infections. Hodson et al (1981) showed significant improvement in lung function and a reduction in the need for acute treatment and hospital admissions with regular outpatient treatment using nebulised carbenicillin and gentamicin in combination.

There is also some evidence to show that minimum inhibitory concentration of anti-Pseudomonal antibiotics such as azlocillin may be reduced in the presence of a mucolytic agent (Heaf et al 1983). Some patients benefit from nebulised therapy with a mucolytic agent prior to physiotherapy followed by nebulised antibiotic after treatment. As portable nebulisers are readily available nowadays, this form of treatment is quite suitable for home use. It is important to vent the antibiotic to the outside both in the hospital setting and at home. Examples of antibiotics used in this way are gentamicin, tobramycin, colistin or azlocillin given as monotherapy.

The use of a polyvalent vaccine against *P. aeruginosa* has also been tried in an attempt to prevent infection with the organism, but in a controlled trial no significant difference was found in the numbers colonised or the rate of progress of the disease (Langford & Hiller 1984).

Mucolytic aerosols such as acetylcysteine (Parvolex) or mercaptoethane sulphonate (MESNA) have both been used in CF (Reas 1964, Weller et al 1980). The major mode of action of these compounds is by splitting the glycoprotein disulphide bonds in sputum; this is thought to result in decreased sputum viscosity and improved clearance from the lungs. These compounds are also irritant to the airway and should be used with caution in those who have evidence of bronchospasm; they should not be used if there is any haemoptysis. It is useful to introduce them in a 50% dilution initially and increase to the full concentration if further effect is required. Because of the possible side-effects it is best to reserve this form of treatment for those with particularly thick viscid sputum in whom conventional treatment with physiotherapy, antibiotics and bronchodilators is proving inadequate.

If there is severe bronchiectasis confined largely to a single lobe of the lung, a situation usually seen in younger patients, there is a place for surgical intervention. Lobectomy can be effective and delays the spread of the disease to the other less infected areas of the lungs (Steinkamp et al 1988).

Steroids

The rationale for the use of steroids during exacerbations of lung infection is that the process may be immune-mediated (MacLusky et al 1987, Zach 1988). Those with high immunoglobulin levels appear to have a faster deterioration than those with low or normal immunoglobulin levels. The study of Auerbach et al (1985) using high dose steroids did show a reduction in the rate of progress of lung disease. Steroids obviously have a number of potential long term side-effects including induction of diabetes, hypertension, bone demineralisation, peptic ulceration, poor growth and excess immune suppression; any or all of which may be important to the patient with CF. Oral steroids, however, clearly have a role in the control of severe asthmatic or allergic symptoms and in allergic bronchopulmonary aspergillosis which can accompany Pseudomonas infection. Their role in the treatment of otherwise uncomplicated *P. aeruginosa* infection in CF is currently being investigated further.

Aspergillus

Aspergillus fumigatus is not uncommonly seen in the sputum of patients with CF and many have positive skin tests to it, demonstrating an immediate hypersensitivity reaction to the organism. Despite this, allergic bronchopulmonary aspergillosis (ABPA) is uncommon. It presents with recurrent wheezing in association with deteriorating chest symptoms. Investigations include positive early and late reaction on skin testing, elevated total and specific IgE, the presence of serum precipitins, eosinophilia and a positive culture of the organism from the sputum. The chest X-ray shows fleeting fluffy shadows bilaterally. Patients who show typical symptoms usually respond very well to oral prednisolone, 1 mg/kg/day for a period of 2 weeks with a gradually reducing dosage thereafter. Rarely patients develop invasive bronchopulmonary aspergillosis and require treatment with anti-fungal agents including amphotericin.

Pneumothorax

Pneumothorax (Fig.9.8) is relatively uncommon in young children with CF and is usually a feature of advanced lung disease. Penketh et al (1982) reported an incidence of 19% in 243 adolescent and adult patients. It is

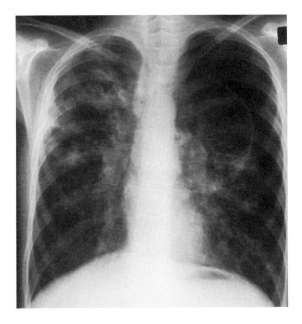

Fig. 9.8 Left pneumothorax in CF: note partial collapse of lung only, due to stiffness of underlying parenchyma.

more common in males than females, affects either side equally and is usually associated with advanced disease and marked airflow obstruction. The majority of patients have an FEV_1 of less than 50% predicted value for height. Recurrences are common and are seen in as many as 50% of cases (Batten & Matthew 1983). The exact cause of the pneumothorax is not clear but in many cases a subpleural bleb is found which may have resulted from previous scarring or localised emphysema. The patient with a pneumothorax usually presents with acute onset pleuric chest pain and increased respiratory difficulty and breathlessness. Any patient who presents in this way should have a chest X-ray to exclude a pneumothorax. The X-ray will often show a small rim of air only since in advanced lung disease the lungs are so stiff that they do not collapse to the same degree as in an otherwise healthy person.

Penketh et al (1982) have reviewed the management of pneumothorax pointing out the high rate of persistent air leak and frequent recurrences either on the same side or the other side. Persistent symptoms and the need for chest drainage are dangerous for the CF patient since they inhibit deep breathing, coughing and bronchial clearance, all of which are likely to worsen the underlying infection.

The management recommended at present is that a small pneumothorax should be observed and treated conservatively with high inspired oxygen, if this can be tolerated, to aid in the reabsorption of air. If the episode does not resolve within 24–48 hours or if there are increasing symptoms intercostal drainage should be instituted along with more intensive treatment for the lung infection. The drain should be placed on suction which will encourage apposition of the pleural surfaces increasing the chance that sufficient adherence will occur obliterating the pneumothorax. If this treatment fails to resolve the problem within 7 days, then chemical pleurodesis or thoracotomy with open pleurodesis or pleurectomy should be performed. Pleurectomy is an absolute contraindication to later heart–lung transplantation in CF so the possibility that this may be necessary in the future must be borne in mind when deciding on the immediate management of an acute pneumothorax.

Haemoptysis

Haemoptysis is another complication more commonly seen in the older CF patient with advanced lung disease. It may occur in as many as 60% of adolescents or adults (Di Sant'Agnese & Davies 1979). Fortunately most patients only have a small amount of bleeding with blood streaking of the sputum and the presence of small clots particularly during severe bouts of coughing. A few have more major episodes of bleeding which are worse in those who have concomitant liver disease with a prolonged prothrombin time. If the haemoptysis is small reassurance and an anxiolytic agent is all that is required. Gentle physiotherapy and antibiotics are continued but nebulised mucolytics are contraindicated as these can exacerbate the bleeding. Correction of anaemia by blood transfusion and clotting abnormalities with vitamin K and fresh plasma should be carried out where necessary. A very small proportion of patients develop a much larger haemoptysis which requires more invasive treatment. The treatment of choice nowadays is bronchial artery occlusion by embolisation. This is a highly specialised procedure and is only available in a few centres. Should embolisation fail to control the bleeding then thoracotomy with ligation of the affected artery or lobectomy is necessary. This is very rare in children but is occasionally required in adults where it is still a high risk procedure.

Cor pulmonale

As the disease progresses and the lungs worsen there is increasing strain on the right heart which results in right ventricular hypertrophy. Pathologically, the blood vessels in the lungs show decreased filling, irregular tapering of peripheral arteries and dilatation of central ones. Arterial pruning and contralateral filling of the bronchial arteries develops. Microscopically, the muscle coat in the small pulmonary arteries is hypertrophied and the muscle extends distally into the arterioles (Tomashefski et al 1983). These changes are exacerbated in the presence of hypoxia and ultimately become irreversible although in the earlier stages oxygen administration will produce some pulmonary vessel dilation and reduction in the pulmonary artery pressure. Unfortunately, many patients at this stage have an elevated carbon dioxide and depend on their hypoxic drive for breathing; this naturally limits the inspired oxygen concentration to less than 28%. Right heart strain may be evident on the ECG and the cardiac ultrasound will show significant right ventricular wall thickening but cardiac enlargement on the chest X-ray is only seen very late in the disease.

Treatment consists of careful attention to daily fluid balance combined with diuretic therapy such as frusemide and spironolactone. Electrolytes should be carefully monitored. Aggressive treatment of the underlying lung infection is vital as part of the aim is to reduce the associated increased pulmonary vascular resistance. The use of continuous home oxygen therapy is helpful in some cases and is currently under investigation (MacLusky et al 1987).

Nasal polyps

Nasal polyps are relatively common in CF — Stern et al (1982) reported a prevalence of 26%. Drake-Lee & Pitcher-Wilmott (1982) were unable to find any association between this complication and allergy which is the usual background in non-CF children. They proposed that polyps were related to chronic sinus infection which is known to be very common in CF. The presence of polyps was also associated with milder clinical disease. It is present practice to remove the polyps when they are causing significant nasal obstruction and interfering with the sense of smell and taste or if they are causing localised discomfort, usually in association with chronic sinusitis and headache.

Heart–lung transplantation

Heart–lung transplantation (Fig. 9.9) offers a new and as yet experimental form of treatment for CF patients with advanced disease (Scott et al 1988). The operation is best reserved at present for those with severe advanced lung disease who have a life expectancy of less than 12–24 months. Based on current mortality rates in the UK it is likely that 50–60 CF patients per year might require assessment for this form of treatment. Careful patient selection is vital if the best results are to be achieved since the number of suitable donor organs is small.

Absolute contraindications to heart–lung transplantation in CF include previous major thoracic surgery such as pleurectomy for pneumothorax (although some patients who have had chemical pleurodeses might be suitable), invasive infection with *Aspergillus fumigatus*, the absence of a positive psychological approach to the illness and a history of poor compliance with treatment in the past, hypoalbuminaemia, HIV antibody or hepatitis B antigen positivity and high dose steroid therapy (greater than 1 mg/kg body weight/day).

Relative contraindications include severe malnutrition, abnormal liver function tests (particularly if associated with cirrhosis), portal hypertension and hypersplenism, although it is technically possible to transplant heart–lung and liver simultaneously (Wallwork et al 1987). Diabetes is not a contraindication.

Patients who are selected for assessment require admission to hospital for approximately one week for detailed review and investigation including lung function tests, exercise tests, blood gases, microbiological assessment, psychological evaluation, liver function tests and measurement of chest size. When donor organs are found arrangements are made for the transplant to take place immediately. The donor organs can survive up to 4 hours and so can be transported a considerable distance in that time if appropriate arrangements are made. The heart from the CF patient can also be used for a heart transplant in another suitable candidate with advanced cardiac disease. Those for whom donor organs have not become available have had a median life expectancy of some 3 months. Heart–lung transplantation should not be undertaken in those with terminal disease since the operative risks are higher.

Postoperatively most patients are usually extubated within 24 hours and are breathing air 48 hours after surgery. Rejection of the organs is a major problem and all patients receive immunosuppression with cyclosporin and azathioprine. Cyclosporin therapy is nephrotoxic and will induce some degree of renal impairment in all patients (Burke et al 1986). Methylprednisolone is used to treat acute rejection episodes. The rejection can affect the lung but not necessarily the heart at the same time — this

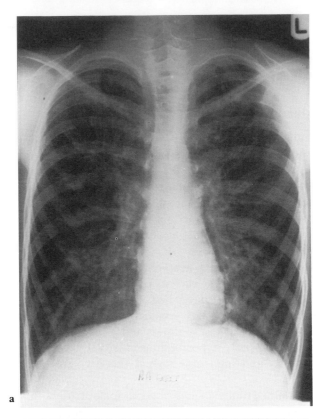

a

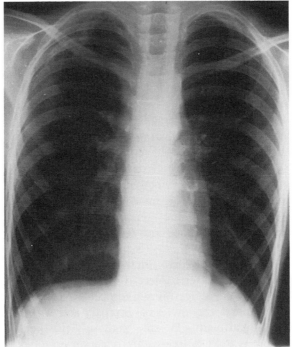

b

Fig. 9.9 Chest X-ray pre and post-heart/lung transplantation in CF.

must be assessed by transbronchial lung biopsy (Higenbottam et al 1988). Bacterial lung infection is another potentially serious postoperative problem because the CF patient still retains many of the pathogenic bacteria in the sinuses, particularly *P. aeruginosa*.

The transplanted patient is able to cough properly because the larynx and trachea are innervated but the airways below the anastomosis are not. Therefore, the cough reflex cannot be initiated from the bronchial tree itself. Mucociliary clearance is also impaired because of the interruption·of the mucociliary escalator at the site of the tracheal anastomosis (Penketh et al 1987a). Most patients show immediate improvement in lung function and a gradual increase in lung volumes towards normal, usually by 4–6 months post-transplantation. In the longer term, however, some patients have developed bronchiolitis obliterans which is a common problem in those who have undergone heart–lung transplantation for other diseases (Burke et al 1986).

At .present there is no evidence that the transplanted organs acquire the abnormality of the disease in the mucus secreting glands. This has been assessed by measurement of the transepithelial potential difference above and below the tracheal anastomotic site up to 2 years after heart–lung transplantation (Wood et al 1988). The abnormality persists in the upper airway but has not been acquired below the site of the anastomosis.

By early. 1989 42 CF patients had received a heart–lung transplant in the UK. The survival rate was 78% in the first year and 66% in the second. One adult with CF is alive and well 3 years post-transplant. The longer term effects of this procedure are not yet known. Heart–lung transplantation thus offers a new approach to those with end stage lung disease but cannot be undertaken as a routine procedure. Further clinical trials confined to nominated transplant centres are required to assess the longer term risks and benefits.

NUTRITION

Almost all patients have some degree of pancreatic insufficiency; this results in malabsorption which leads to a poor nutritional state which can significantly affect growth and development and lower resistance to infection. In addition those who have frequent exacerbations of lung infection become anorexic and catabolic. CF children are also known to have a higher total energy expenditure than normal (Shepherd et al 1988); this too contributes to their increased nutritional requirements. Digestive problems are caused by deficiency of pancreatic enzymes: amylase, trypsin and lipase and also pancreatic bicarbonate. In addition a reduced bile salt pool in the duodenum further impairs the absorption of fat. Young children with CF usually have a large appetite but this is often inhibited during intercurrent infection, and as the pulmonary complications advance anorexia and nausea become common features. These are exacerbated by the swallowing of significant quantities of sputum and frequent bouts of coughing often result in episodes of vomiting during which valuable nutrition is lost. Taking all of these factors together, in addition to the excess loss of undigested fat in the stool, it has been calculated that these children require an intake of 120–150% of the recommended daily allowance to maintain adequate nutrition (Goodchild 1986).

There is a relationship between the nutritional status and the severity of the underlying lung disease, those with the most severe involvement having the greatest difficulty in maintaining weight. There have been a number of studies attempting to improve calorie intake, either by nasogastric feeding, via gastrostomy or by parenteral nutrition, recently reviewed by MacLusky et al (1987). Significant weight gain can frequently be achieved with aggressive nutritional therapy but lung function does not improve at the same time (Lancet 1986); it may however decline at a less rapid rate (Levy et al 1985). Improved nutrition often leads to a better sense of physical well being which can have important psychological benefits for the patient and their compliance with other treatment including for example, physiotherapy and physical exercise. The long term effects of aggressive nutritional support are not yet clear although Corey et al (1988) have shown enhanced survival amongst patients attending a large CF clinic in Toronto where there has always been a policy of high fat, high energy intake. Further studies of this important area are needed.

Children with CF should now have a normal diet which is high in energy with no significant restrictions; where possible a high protein intake should be encouraged with a normal or increased fat content. The advent of enteric coated pancreatic enzymes, such as Creon and Pancrease, has significantly improved the fat absorption when compared to those previously available (Beverley et al 1987). Those who have a poor intake, especially during exacerbations of lung infection, may benefit from intensive calorie counting and education while they are in hospital (Dinwiddie & Madge 1988). Vitamins A, B, C, D and E are routinely given as supplements to all CF children and vitamin K to those who have significant liver disease. For those who have persistent nutritional problems despite these measures antacids such as cimetidine or ranitidine can be used; Durie et al (1980) have reported improved nutrient absorption with the use of these agents. Their use in this situation is associated with increased weight gain in a number of cases but as the long term effects are not yet known, they should only be used in selected cases.

Where the lung disease is very advanced it may not be possible to maintain weight by oral intake alone. Children in this situation benefit from additional feeding particularly at night utilising nasogastric supplementation with a predigested formula but allowing the patient to feed normally during the daytime (Lancet 1986). Some centres have given this nutrition by a gastrostomy tube (MacLusky et al 1987) although in these cases gastro-oesophageal reflux can be a problem. Others have used jejunostomy feeding with a good response in terms of weight gain. The pyschological difficulties in relation to body image which can be associated with these more invasive procedures has meant that they have not gained widespread use in CF clinics.

Newborn babies and infants with CF require special attention to their nutrition particularly if they have had meconium ileus. Whenever possible breast feeding should be encouraged since this provides the best nutritional intake and the presence of lipase in breast milk is likely to encourage satisfactory absorption. The psychological effects of bonding during the period in which a mother is adjusting to the knowledge that her child has CF are also enchanced by breast feeding. A few will gain weight satisfactorily by this method without the addition of pancreatic enzymes but most will in fact require additional enzymes in order to produce optimal weight gain. Nowadays, a normal infant formula is used for those who are unable to establish breast feeding and in all of these cases pancreatic enzymes will be required. Some infants have digestive difficulties following meconium ileus and may need predigested milk such as Pregestimil or Nutramigen with added pancreatic supplements.

Older children with poor nutritional intake can have nutritional supplementation with high calorie drinks such as Build-up, Complan or Fresubin. Carbohydrate containing supplements such as Caloreen, Maxijul or Hical can be added to food or drinks increasing their calorie content without altering the taste. Medium chain triglycerides (MCT) can also be used for cooking, particularly if there is persistent intolerance to other types of dietary fat. CF children can also suffer from other gastrointestinal problems such as coeliac disease or lactose intolerance. The appropriate investigations and management should be undertaken for these conditions if there is persistent failure to respond to normal dietary measures. Pancreatic dysfunction and the nutritional care of the CF patient have recently been reviewed by Durie & Forstner (1989) and Durie & Penchary (1989).

Another important abdominal complication of CF is meconium ileus equivalent (MIE) more correctly termed distal intestinal obstruction syndrome (DIOS). This presents with signs of acute or subacute intestinal obstruction due to the accumulation of a thick sticky 'meconium-like' faecal mass in the lower bowel, usually in the caecal area.

Clinical features include colicky abdominal pain, vomiting, abdominal distension and constipation; in severe cases complete intestinal obstruction develops. The typical X-ray features are shown in Fig. 9.10. This complication occurs in approximately 10% of CF patients but has become much less common since the introduction of enteric coated enzymes. The differential diagnosis includes acute appendicitis, obstruction from stricture formation or adhesions following previous abdominal surgery for neonatal meconium ileus and intussusception.

Treatment depends on the severity; in mild cases there is usually a good response to increased pancreatic enzyme intake, oral lactulose and acetylcysteine (Fabrol). Gastrografin is often effective orally if the initial measures are unsuccessful. If acute obstruction occurs nasogastric suction and intravenous fluids are required; oral gastrografin is continued initially fol-

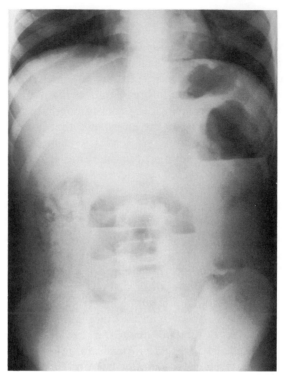

Fig. 9.10   Distal intestinal obstruction syndrome (meconium ileus equivalent in CF).

lowed by a gastrografin enema. The use of a non-absorbable solution of propylene glycol (Golytley) has proved very useful in this condition (Cleghorn et al 1986), providing complete obstruction has not occurred.

Significant liver disease occurs in 5–10% of paediatric patients and biliary cirrhosis in 10% of adolescents and adults (MacLusky et al 1987). There may or may not be biochemical evidence of hepatic disease but eventually complications such as portal hypertension, hypersplenism, and oesophageal varices come to light; these can result in massive haematemesis. Children with significant varices require sclerotherapy for these on a number of occasions; they frequently also have significant pulmonary disease at this stage and the risk of anaesthesia is significant (Stamatakis et al 1982, Price 1986).

Approximately 8% of adults develop diabetes mellitus as a significant complication (Batten 1983, Finkelstein et al 1988). Many CF children have impaired glucose tolerance but only 2–3% develop overt diabetes. When this does occur it makes the nutritional management more difficult. Diabetes can be precipitated at any age by the use of steroid therapy for the underlying lung disease, so this potential complication should always be borne in mind. Routine urine testing for glucose should always be performed on any patient who is losing weight as other signs such as polyuria and polydipsia may not be particularly obvious in the early phase of the illness. Most patients with diabetes require treatment with insulin which should be monitored in the usual way including the measurement of glycosylated haemoglobin values — HbA1c. Finkelstein et al (1988) reported a significantly reduced survival for CF patients with diabetes than for those without this complication. Fewer than 25% of those with diabetes mellitus survived to 30 years whereas nearly 60% of the non-diabetic CF population reached this age. Close hospital supervision and dietary support is needed for these patients.

Arthropathy

A number of patients complain of pains and reduced mobility in their joints. This may occur for three major reasons (Phillips & David 1986):

1. Cystic fibrosis arthropathy (CFA), specifically related to CF.
2. Hypertrophic pulmonary osteoarthropathy (HPOA), a condition related to those with chronic pulmonary disease.
3. Incidental juvenile rheumatoid arthritis.

The overall incidence is 1–2% of CF children.

CFA usually presents with acute pain, swelling, limited joint movement and low grade fever. It is not specifically associated with the severity of the underlying lung disease. Large joints such as knees and ankles are usually affected. X-ray of the joint is normal, a few patients develop an erythematous rash which may occasionally be purpuric. This condition is thought to be related to an immune-mediated mechanism associated with chronic lung infection and inflammation. It usually settles spontaneously after symptomatic treatment with non-steroid anti-inflammatory agents.

HPOA is seen in patients with advanced lung disease and consists of an arthritis and periostitis; periosteal changes are seen in the long bones on X-ray or by radioisotope scans. Joint effusions are a frequent complication. Treatment consists of anti-inflammatory agents avoiding aspirin which can cause gastrointestinal bleeding and checking that liver function is satisfactory if agents metabolised by this route, such as paracetamol, are used.

Psychosocial problems

The psychological and social aspects of this disease form a very significant part in its morbidity. The knowledge that the child has a life long and life threatening illness naturally comes as a great shock to any family and much time has to be spent in the early period after diagnosis in counselling the parents with regard to the long term effects, not only on the patient but on the family and indeed on future generations. As the disease advances, and particularly as chronic lung infection sets in, a number of serious psychological effects begin to appear in relation to the chronic nature of the disease and its physical limitations. Frustration develops which comes from being unable to lead a normal life. As patients become older they also have an increasing insight into the long term prognosis, particularly if the disease is progressing and frequent admission to hospital is required. These problems are exacerbated when other friends with CF die.

The incidence of psychological disturbance in the parents is also high; Bywater (1981) found that 44% of the mothers of CF children were depressed and that marital breakdown was a major factor in 18% of the families studied. Pinkerton et al (1985) found that some adult patients, despite comparable degrees of physical disability, coped more successfully than others with daily life. Those who coped less well had twice as many hospital admissions even though their lung function was better. They also compared unfavourably in terms of jobs, family and sexual relationships, and knowledge and understanding of their disease.

The social aspects involve the patient and family in frequent visits to the hospital for outpatient review and admission at regular intervals for intensive intravenous treatment if it is not practical to give this at home. These stresses have significant effects on the family in terms of time involved both in travelling and staying at the hospital and also in relation to absence from full time education and employment. There are considerable financial complications for the family, as the parents or the patient may not be able to earn in the normal way during periods of illness and may or may not be eligible for financial help such as the Attendance or Mobility Allowance which can alleviate some of these problems. Although children in the UK receive prescriptions free of charge, this does not apply to adults with CF at the present time nor indeed to children in some EC countries and in North America.

Prognosis

The prognosis for CF patients has improved dramatically over the last 30 years. There used to be an excess mortality among those who presented with meconium ileus but this has now virtually disappeared (Dodge et al 1988). Chronic Pseudomonas infection does however significantly worsen the prognosis (Wilmott et al 1985). The survival rate to 16 years for those attending large CF centres is 70–75% (Wilmott et al 1983, Schiotz et al 1983). Dodge et al (1988) have reported a 50% survival to 21 years for males and 17 years for females in the UK between 1980 and 1985. The annual increase in surviving CF adults in the UK is estimated at 100 per year. Increasing numbers of adults are seen in their 30s and 40s leading a reasonable quality of life (Penketh et al 1987b). MacLusky et al (1987) have however suggested that although the median life expectancy for adult CF patients in North America is now close to 30 years there is evidence of plateauing of this with little change in the figures for the last 7–10 years. It is likely that new treatments will be developed when the gene is isolated and the underlying biochemical abnormality is more clearly understood both of which should occur in the near future. Not all CF patients suffer from severe disease and some adults have now reached the pensionable age of 65.

Note: Much useful help and information on CF can be obtained from The Cystic Fibrosis Research Trust, 5 Blyth Road Bromley, Kent, BRI 3RS, UK.

REFERENCES

Abman S H, Ogle H W, Butler-Simon N, Rumack C M, Accurso F J 1988 Role of respiratory syncytial virus in early hospitalisations for respiratory distress of young infants with cystic fibrosis. Journal of Pediatrics 113: 826–830

Anderson D H 1938 Cystic fibrosis of the pancreas and its relation to celiac disease, a clinical and pathological study. American Journal of Disease in Childhood 56: 344–399

Anderson C M, Goodchild M C (eds) 1976 Cystic fibrosis manual of diagnosis and management. Blackwell Scientific, Oxford pp 9–23

Auerbach H S, Williams M, Kirkpatrick J A et al 1985 Alternate day prednisolone reduces morbidity and improves pulmonary function in cystic fibrosis. Lancet II: 686–688.

Batten J C 1983 The adolescent and adult. In: Hodson M E, Norman A P, Batten J C (eds) Cystic fibrosis. Ballière-Tindall, London, pp 209–218

Batten J 1988 Cystic fibrosis in adolescents and adults. 10th International Cystic Fibrosis Congress. Excerpta Medica Asia Pacific Congress Series 74: 187–194

Batten J C, Matthew D J 1983 The respiratory system. In: Hodson M E, Norman A P, Batten J C (eds) Cystic fibrosis. Balliere-Tindall, London, pp 105–131

Beaudet A, Bowcock A, Buchwald M et al 1986 Linkage of cystic fibrosis to two tightly linked DNA markers: joint report from a collaborative study. American Journal of Human Genetics 39: 681–693

Beverley D W, Kelleher J, MacDonald A, Littlewood J M, Robinson T, Walters M P 1987 Comparison of four pancreatic extracts in cystic fibrosis. Archives of Disease in Childhood 62: 564–568

Bishop H C, Koop C E 1957 Management of meconium ileus: resection, Roux-en-Y anastomosis and ileostomy irrigation with pancreatic enzymes. Annals of Surgery 145: 410–414

Brock D H J 1983 Amniotic fluid alkaline phosphatase isoenzymes in early prenatal diagnosis of cystic fibrosis. Lancet II: 941–943

Brock D H J 1988 Prenatal diagnosis of cystic fibrosis. Archives of Disease in Childhood 63: 701–704

Brock D H J, Barron L, Bedgood D, Haywood C 1985 Prospective prenatal diagnosis of cystic fibrosis. Lancet I: 1175–1178

Brock D H J, Curtis A, Holloway S, Burn J, Nelson R 1986 DNA typing to avoid need for prenatal diagnosis of cystic fibrosis. Lancet II: 393

Buchwald M, Tusi L-C, Riordan J R 1988 The genetics of cystic fibrosis. Mid 1987. 10th International Cystic Fibrosis Congress. Excerpta Medica, Asia Pacific Congress Series 74: 3–9

Burke C M, Theodore J, Baldwin C et al 1986 Twenty-eight cases of human heart–lung transplantation. Lancet I: 517–519

Bywater M 1981 Adolescents with cystic fibrosis: psychosocial adjustment. Archives of Disease in Childhood 56: 538–543

Carter E P, Barrett A D, Heeley A F, Kuzemko J A 1984 Improved sweat test method for the diagnosis of cystic fibrosis. Archives of Disease in Childhood 59: 919–922

Cerney F J, Pullano T O, Cropp G J A 1982 Cardiorespiratory adaptations to exercise in CF. American Review of Respiratory Disease 126: 217–222

Chrispin A R, Norman A P 1974 The systematic evaluation of the chest radiograph in cystic fibrosis. Pediatric Radiology 2: 101–106

Cleghorn G J, Stringer D A, Forstner G G, Durie P R 1986 Treatment of distal intestinal obstruction syndrome in cystic fibrosis with a balanced intestinal lavage solution. Lancet 1: 8–11

Corey M, McLaughlin F J, Williams M, Levison H 1988 A comparison of survival, growth and pulmonary function in patients with cystic fibrosis in Boston and Toronto. Journal of Clinical Epidemiology 41: 583–591

Cropp G J, Pullano T P, Cerney F J, Nathanson T J 1982 Exercise tolerance and cardiorespiratory adjustments at peak work capacity in CF. American Review of Respiratory Disease 126: 121–126

Crossley J R, Elliot R B, Smith P A 1979 Dried blood spot screening for cystic fibrosis in the newborn. Lancet I: 472–474

David T J 1986 Nasal polyposis, opaque paranasal sinuses and usually normal hearing: the otorhinolaryngological features of cystic fibrosis. Journal of the Royal Society of Medicine 79 (Suppl 12): 23–26

Devlin J, Beckett N J, David T J 1989 Elevated sweat potassium, hyperaldosteronism and pseudo-Bartter's syndrome: a spectrum of disorders associated with cystic fibrosis. Journal of Royal Society of Medicine 82 (Suppl 16): 38–43

Dinwiddie R 1986 Management of the chest in cystic fibrosis. Journal of the Royal Society of Medicine 79 (Suppl 12): 6–9

Dinwiddie R 1987 Cystic fibrosis. In: Evans J N G (ed) Scott-Brown's Otolaryngology, Vol 6. Butterworths, London, pp 527–533

Dinwiddie R, Madge S 1988 Intensive calorie counting in C F: an effective way of achieving weight gain? 10th International Cystic Fibrosis Congress. Excerpta Medica Asia Pacific Congress Series 74: 165

Di Sant' Agnese P A, Davis P B 1979 Cystic fibrosis in adults, 75 cases and a review of 232 cases in the literature. American Journal of Medicine 66: 121–132

Dodge J A, Goodall J, Geddes D et al 1985 The BPA cystic fibrosis survey. Archives of Disease in Childhood 60: 1098

Dodge J A, Goodall J, Geddes D et al 1988 Cystic fibrosis in the United Kingdom 1977–85: an improving picture. British Paediatric Association Working Party on Cystic Fibrosis. British Medical Journal 297: 1599–1602

Donnison A B, Schwachman H, Gross R E 1966 A review of 164 children with meconium ileus seen at the Children's Medical Centre, Boston. Pediatrics 37: 833–837

Doring G, Hoiby N 1983 Longitudinal study of immune response to *Pseudomonas aeruginosa* antigens in cystic fibrosis. Infection and Immunology 42: 197–201

Drake-Lee A B, Pitcher-Wilmott R W 1982 The clinical and laboratory correlates of nasal polyps in cystic fibrosis. International Journal of Pediatric Otorhinolaryngology 4: 209–214

Durie P R, Bell L, Linton W, Corey M L, Forstner G G 1980 Effect of cimetidine and sodium bicarbonate on pancreatic replacement therapy in cystic fibrosis. Gut 21: 778–786

Durie P R, Forstner G G 1989 Pathophysiology of the exocrine pancreas in cystic fibrosis. Journal of the Royal Society of Medicine 82, (Suppl 16): 2–10

Durie P R, Pencharz P B 1989 A rational approach to the nutritional care of patients with cystic fibrosis. Journal of the Royal Society of Medicine 82, (Suppl 16): 11–20

Edlund L P, French R W, Herbst J J et al 1986 Effects of swimming programme on children with cystic fibrosis. American Journal of Disease in Childhood 140: 80–83

Farrell M, Rodeck C H, Law H-Y et al 1986 First trimester prenatal diagnosis of cystic fibrosis with linked DNA probes. Lancet I: 1402–1405

Feldman G L, Williamson R, Beaudet A L, O'Brien W E 1988 Prenatal diagnosis of cystic fibrosis by DNA amplification for detection of KM19 polymorphism. Lancet ii: 102

Finkelstein S M, Wielinski C L, Elliot G R et al 1988 Diabetes mellitus associated with cystic fibrosis. Journal of Pediatrics 112: 373–377

Frates R C, Kaizu T T, Last J A 1983 Mucus glycoproteins secreted by respiratory epithelial tissue from cystic fibrosis patients. Pediatric Research 17: 30–34

Geddes D M 1984 Physical exercise in cystic fibrosis. In: Lawson D (ed) Cystic fibrosis: horizons. Wiley, Chichester, pp 114–133

Gibson L E, Cooke R E 1959 A test for the concentration of electrolytes in sweat in cystic fibrosis of the pancreas utilising pilocarpine by iontophoresis. Pediatrics 23: 545–549

Goodchild M 1986 Practical management of nutrition and gastrointestinal tract in cystic fibrosis. Journal of the Royal Society of Medicine 79 (suppl 12): 32–35

Goodchild M, Dodge J A (eds) 1985a Clinical and diagnostic features in cystic fibrosis. Cystic Fibrosis. Manual of diagnosis and management, 2nd edition. Ballière Tindall, London, pp 27–46

Goodchild M C, Dodge J A (eds) 1985b Management of respiratory disease. In: Cystic

Fibrosis. Manual of diagnosis and management 2nd edition. Ballière-Tindall, London, pp 53–85

Green A, Dobbs P, Pennock C 1985 A study of sweat sodium and chloride: criteria for the diagnosis of cystic fibrosis. Annals of Clinical Biochemistry 22: 171–176

Hadorn B, Zopi G, Shmerling D, Prader A, McIntyre I, Anderson C M 1968 Quantitive assessment of exocrine pancreatic function in infants and children. Journal of Pediatrics 73: 39–50

Hay J C, Geddes D M 1985 Transepithelial potential difference in cystic fibrosis. Thorax 40: 493–496

Heaf D P, Webb G J, Matthew D J 1983 In vitro assessment of combined antibiotic and mucolytic therapy for *Pseudomonas aeruginosa* in cystic fibrosis. Archives of Disease in Childhood 58: 824–826

Heeley A F, Heeley M E 1987 Biochemical screening of the neonatal population for the early detection of cystic fibrosis in East Anglia 1980–86. In: Insights into Paediatrics. Glaxo Laboratories, Greenford, pp 49–58

Higenbottam T W, Stewart S, Wallwork J 1988 Transbronchial lung biopsy to diagnose lung rejection and infection in heart–lung transplant. Transplant Proceedings 20: 767–769

Hjelm M, Brown P, Briddon A 1986 Sweat sodium related to amount of sweat after sweat test in children with and without cystic fibrosis. Acta Paediatrica Scandinavica 75: 652–656

Hodson M E, Gaskell D V 1983 Physiotherapy. In: Hodson M E, Norman A P, Batten J C (eds) Cystic fibrosis. Ballière-Tindall, London, pp 219–241

Hodson M E, Penketh A R L, Batten J C 1981 Aerosol carbenicillin and gentamicin treatment for *Pseudomonas aeruginosa* infection in cystic fibrosis. Lancet II: 1137–1139

Hodson M E, Beldon I, Power R et al 1983 Sweat test to diagnose cystic fibrosis in adults. British Medical Journal 281: 1381–1383

Hodson M E, Butland R J A, Roberts C M, Smith J, Batten J C 1987 Oral ciprofloxacin compared with conventional intravenous treatment for *Pseudomonas aeruginosa* infection in patients with cystic fibrosis. Lancet I: 235–237

Hoggs W A, Schonberg S A, Golbus M S 1985 Prenatal diagnosis by chorionic villous sampling: lessons of the first 600 cases. Prenatal Diagnosis 5: 393–400

Hoiby N 1984 The management of Pseudomonas chest infection — the way forward. In: Lawson D (ed) Cystic fibrosis: horizons. Wiley, Chichester, pp 87–95

Hoiby N, Schiotz P O 1982 Immune complex mediated tissue damage in the lungs of cystic fibrosis patients with chronic *Pseudomonas aeruginosa* infection. Acta Paediatricia Scandinavica 301 (Suppl): 63–73

Holtz F J, Olinsky A, Phelan P D 1981 Variability of airways hyper-reactivity and allergy in cystic fibrosis. Archives of Disease in Childhood 56: 495–499

Kerem B, Rommens J M, Buchanan J A et al 1989 Identification of the cystic fibrosis gene: Genetic analysis. Science 245: 1073–1080

Kessler W R, Anderson D H 1951 Heat prostration in fibrocystic disease of the pancreas and other conditions. Pediatrics 8: 648–656

Khun P, Landau L, Phelan P D 1984 Nebulised gentamicin in children with cystic fibrosis. Australian Paediatric Journal 20: 43–45

Knowles M, Gatzy J, Boucher R 1981 Increased bioelective potential difference across respiratory epithelia in cystic fibrosis. New England Journal of Medicine 305: 1489–1495

Knowles M, Gatzy J, Boucher R 1983 Relative ion permeability of normal and cystic fibrosis nasal epithelium. Journal of Clinical Investigation 71: 1407–1410

Kramm E R, Crane M M, Sirkin M G, Brown M L 1962 A cystic fibrosis pilot survey in three New England States. American Journal of Public Health 52: 2041–2057

Kuzemko J A, Heeley A F 1983 Diagnostic methods and screening. In: Hodson M E, Norman A P, Batten J C (eds) Cystic fibrosis. Ballière-Tindall, London, pp 21–30

Kuzemko J A 1986 Screening: early neonatal diagnosis and prenatal diagnosis. Journal of the Royal Society of Medicine 79 (suppl 12): 2–5

Kylzycki L L, Shauf V 1974 Cystic fibrosis in blacks in Washington D C. American Journal of Disease in Childhood 127: 64–67

Lancet 1986 Supplementary nutrition in cystic fibrosis. Lancet I: 249

Langford D T, Hiller J 1984 Prospective controlled study of polyvalent Pseudomonas vaccine in cystic fibrosis — three year results. Archives of Disease in Childhood. 59: 1131–1134

Levin S 1963 Fibrocystic disease of the pancreas. In: Goldschmidt E (ed) Genetics of migrant and isolate populations. Williams and Wilkins, Baltimore, p 293

Levy L D, Durie P R, Pencharz P B, Corey M L 1985 Effect of long term nutritional rehabilitation on body composition and nutritional status in malnourished children and adolescents with cystic fibrosis. Journal of Pediatrics 107: 225–230

Littlewood J 1986 The sweat test. Archives of Disease in Childhood 61: 1041–1043

MacLusky I B, Canny G J, Levison H 1987 Cystic fibrosis. Pediatric Reviews and Communications 1: 343–389

Mabogunje O A, Wang Chun I, Mahour G H 1982 Improved survival of neonates with meconium ileus. Archives of Surgery 117: 37–40

Marcotte J E, Grisdale R K, Levison M, Coates A L, Canny G J 1986 Multiple factors limit exercise capacity in cystic fibrosis. Paediatric Pulmonology 2: 274–281

Marks M 1984 Respiratory viruses in cystic fibrosis. New England Journal of Medicine 311: 1695–1696

Matthew D J, Warner J O, Chrispin A R, Norman A P 1977 The relationship between chest radiographic scores and respiratory function tests in children with cystic fibrosis. Pediatric Radiology 5: 198–201

Mearns M B 1980 Natural history of pulmonary infection in cystic fibrosis. In: Sturgess J M (ed) Perspectives in Cystic Fibrosis. Proceedings of the 8th International Cystic Fibrosis Conference, Toronto. Canadian Cystic Fibrosis Association, Toronto, pp 325–334

Meindl R S 1978 Hypothesis: a selective advantage for cystic fibrosis heterozygotes. American Journal of Physical Anthropology 74: 39–45

Mornet E, Simon-Bohy B, Serre J L et al 1988 Genetic differences between cystic fibrosis with and without meconium ileus. Lancet I: 376–378

Muller F, Aubrey M C, Gasser B, Duchatel F, Boue J, Boue A 1985 Prenatal diagnosis of cystic fibrosis II. Meconium ileus in affected fetuses. Prenatal Diagnosis 5: 104–117

Nielson O H, Larsen B F 1982 The incidence of anaemia, hypoproteinaemia and oedema in infants as presenting symptoms of cystic fibrosis. Journal of Pediatric Gastroenterology and Nutrition 1: 355–359

Nielson O H, Thomsen B L, Green A, Anderson P K, Hauge M, Schiotz P O 1988 Cystic fibrosis in Denmark 1945–1985. An analysis of incidence, mortality and influence of centralised treatment on survival. Acta Paediatrica Scandinavica 77: 836–841

Orenstein D M, Franklin B A, Doershuk C F et al 1981 Exercise conditions and cardiopulmonary fitness in cystic fibrosis. The effect of a three month supervised running program. Chest 80: 329–398

Papp Z, Toth Z, Szako M, Szeifort G T 1985 Early prenatal diagnosis of cystic fibrosis by ultrasound. Clinical Genetics 28: 356–358

Pederson S S, Jensen T, Hoiby N, Koch C, Flensborg E W 1987 Management of *Pseudomonas aeruginosa* lung infection in Danish cystic fibrosis patients. Acta Paediatrica Scandinavica 76: 955–961

Penketh A R L, Knight R K, Hodson M E, Batten J C 1982 Management of pneumothorax in adults with cystic fibrosis. Thorax 37: 850–853

Penketh A R L, Higenbottam T, Hakim M, Wallwork J 1987a Heart and lung transplantation in patients with end stage lung disease. British Medical Journal 295: 311–314

Penketh A R L, Wise A, Mearns M B, Hodson M E, Batten J C 1987b Cystic fibrosis in adolescents and adults. Thorax 42: 526–532

Peterson N T, Hoiby N, Mordhurst C M, Lind K, Flensborg E W, Bruun B 1981 Respiratory infections in cystic fibrosis patients caused by virus, chlamydia and mycoplasma — possible synergism with *Pseudomonas aeruginosa*. Acta Paediatricia Scandinavica 70: 623–628

Phelan P D, Gracey M, Williams H E, Anderson C A 1969 Ventilatory function in infants with cystic fibrosis. Physiological assessment of inhalation therapy. Archives of Disease in Childhood 44: 393–396

Phillips B M, David T J 1986 Pathogenesis and management of arthropathy in cystic fibrosis. Journal of the Royal Society of Medicine 79 (Suppl 12): 44–50

Phillips B M, David T J 1987 Management of the chest in cystic fibrosis. Journal of the Royal Society of Medicine 80 (Suppl 18): 30–37

Pinkerton P, Trauer T, Duncan F, Hodson M E, Batten J C 1985 Cystic fibrosis in adult life: a study of coping patterns. Lancet II: 761–763

Pitcher-Wilmott R W, Levinsky R J, Matthew D J 1982 Circulating immune complexes containing Pseudomonas antigens in cystic fibrosis. Archives of Disease in Childhood 57: 577–581

Pitt T 1986 Biology of *Pseudomonas aeruginosa* in relation to pulmonary infection in cystic fibrosis. Journal of the Royal Society of Medicine 79 (suppl 12): 13–18

Price J 1986 The need to avoid general anaesthesia in cystic fibrosis. Journal of the Royal Society of Medicine 79 (Suppl 12): 10–12

Prior J A, Webber B A, Hodson M E, Batten J C 1979 Evaluation of the forced expiratory technique as an adjunct to postural drainage in treatment of cystic fibrosis. British Medical Journal 2: 417–418

Quinton P M 1983 Chloride impermeability in cystic fibrosis. Nature 301: 421–422

Raeburn J A 1983 Genetics and genetic counselling. In: Hodson M E, Batten J C, Norman A (eds) Cystic fibrosis. Ballière-Tindall, London, pp 1–12

Reas H W 1964 The use of N-acetylcysteine in the treatment of cystic fibrosis. Journal of Pediatrics 65: 542–557

Reid L, de Haller R 1964 Lung changes in cystic fibrosis. In: Hubble D (ed) Cystic fibrosis. Chest and Heart Association, London, p 21

Rickham P P, Boeckman C R 1965 Neonatal meconium obstruction in the absence of mucoviscidosis. American Journal of Surgery 109: 173–177

Righetti A B B, Mighavacca M, Prampolini L, Guinta A 1976 Extensive neonatal screening of CF. Proceedings of VII International Cystic Fibrosis Conference. p 153

Riordan J R, Rommens J M, Kerem B et al 1989 Identification of the cystic fibrosis gene: Cloning and characterisation of complementary DNA. Science 245: 1066–1078

Roberts G, Stanfield M, Black A, Redmond A 1988 Screening for cystic fibrosis: a four year regional experience. Archives of Disease in Childhood 63: 1438–1443

Rommens M J, Iannuzzi M C, Kerem B et al 1989 Identification of the cystic fibrosis gene: Chromosome walking and jumping. Science 245: 1059–1065

Sauder R A, Chesrown S E, Loughlin G M 1987 Clinical application of transepthelial potential difference measurements in cystic fibrosis. The Journal of Pediatrics 111: 353–358

Schiotz P O, Jorgensen M, Flensborg E W et al 1983 Chronic *Pseudomonas aeruginosa* lung infection in cystic fibrosis. Acta Paediatrica Scandinavica 72: 283–287

Schwachman H, Mahmoodian A, Neff R K 1981 The sweat sodium and chloride levels. Journal of Pediatrics 98: 576–578

Scott R C, Higenbottam T, Hutter J et al 1988 Heart lung transplantation for cystic fibrosis. Lancet II: 192–194

Scully B E, Neu H C, Parry M F, Mandell W 1986 Oral ciprofloxacin therapy of infections due to *Pseudomonas aeruginosa*. Lancet I: 819–822

Selander P 1962 The frequency of cystic fibrosis of the pancreas in Sweden. Acta Paediatricia Scandinavica 51: 65–67

Sharples P M, Hope P L, Wilkinson A R 1988 False positive in prenatal diagnosis of cystic fibrosis. Lancet I: 558

Shepherd R W, Holt T L, Vasques-Velasquez L, Coward W A, Prentice A, Lucas A 1988 Increased energy expenditure in young children with cystic fibrosis. Lancet I: 1300–1303

Stamatakis J D, Howard E R, Psacharopoulos H T, Mowat A P 1982 Injection sclerotherapy for oesophageal varices in children. British Journal of Surgery 69: 74–75

Steinkamp G, Hardt H, Zimmerman H J 1988 Pulmonary resection for localised bronchiectasis in cystic fibrosis. Acta Paediatrica Scandinavica 77: 569–575

Stern R C, Boat T F, Wood R E, Matthews L W, Doershuk C F 1982 Treatment and prognosis of nasal polyps in cystic fibrosis. American Journal of Diseases of Children 136: 1067–1070

Stroobant J 1986 Viral infections in cystic fibrosis. Journal of the Royal Society of Medicine 79 (suppl 12): 19–22

Super M, Ivison A, Schwartz M, Giles L, Elles R G, Read A P 1987 Clinical experience of prenatal diagnosis of cystic fibrosis by use of linked DNA probes. Lancet II: 782–784

Szaff M, Hoiby N, Flensborg E W 1983 Pulmonary pathology. In: Hodson M E, Norman A P, Batten J C (eds) Cystic fibrosis. Baillière-Tindall, London, pp 31–51

Tomashefski J F, Vawter G F, Reid L 1983 Pulmonary pathology. In: Hodson M E, Norman A P, Batten J C (eds) Cystic fibrosis. Baillière-Tindall, London, pp 31–35

Tyrell J C, Weller P H, Martin J 1986 Face mask physiotherapy in cystic fibrosis. Archives of Disease in Children 61: 598–601

Vishwantah S, Ramphal R 1984 Adherence of *Pseudomonas aeruginosa* to human tracheobronchial mucin. Infection and Immunology 45: 177–202

Wagget J, Johnson D G, Borns P, Bishop H C 1970 The non-operative treatment of meconium ileus by gastrografin enema. Journal of Pediatrics 77: 407–411

Wainwright R J, Scrambler P J, Schmidtke T et al 1985 Localisation of cystic fibrosis locus to human chromosome 7 cen-q 22. Nature 318: 384–385

Wallwork J, Williams R, Caine R 1987 Transplantation of liver, heart and lungs for primary biliary cirrhosis and primary pulmonary hypertension. Lancet II: 1882–1884

Wang L T K, Turtle S, Davidson A G F 1982 Secretin-pancreoyymin stimulation test and confirmation of the diagnosis of cystic fibrosis. Gut 23: 749–750

Wang E E L, Prober C G, Manson B, Corey M, Levison M 1984 Association of respiratory viral infections with pulmonary deterioration in patients with cystic fibrosis. New England Journal of Medicine 311: 1653–1658

Warner J O, Taylor B W, Norman A P, Soothill J F 1976 Association of cystic fibrosis with allergy. Archives of Disease in Childhood 51: 507–511

Warwick W J 1982 Prognosis for survival with cystic fibrosis: the effects of early diagnosis and cystic fibrosis centre care. Acta Paediatrica Scandinavica (Suppl 301): 27–31

Webber B A 1988 Is postural drainage necessary? 10th International Cystic Fibrosis Congress. Excerpta Medica Asia Pacific Congress Series 74: 29–35

Weller P H, Ingram D, Preece M A, Matthew D J 1980 Controlled trial of intermittent aerosol therapy with sodium-2-mercaptoethane sulphonate in cystic fibrosis. Thorax 35: 42–46

White R, Woodward S, Leippert M et al 1985 A closely linked genetic marker for cystic fibrosis. Nature 318: 382–384

Wilcken B, Chalmers G 1985 Reduced morbidity in patients with cystic fibrosis detected by neonatal screening. Lancet II: 1319–1321

Wilcken B, Brown A R D, Urwin R, Brown D A 1983 Cystic fibrosis screening by dried blood spot trypsin assay: results in 75 000 newborn infants. Journal of Pediatrics 102: 383–387

Williams C, Williamson R, Loutelle C, Loeffler R, Smith J, Ivinson A 1988a Same day, first trimester antenatal diagnosis for cystic fibrosis by gene amplification. Lancet ii: 102–103

Williams J, Alfaham M, Ryley H C, Goodchild M C, Weller P H, Dodge J A 1988b Screening for cystic fibrosis in Wales and the West Midlands. 10th International Cystic Fibrosis Congress. Excerpta Medica Asia Pacific Congress Series 74: 20–21

Williams J, Smith H L, Woods C G, Weller P H 1988c Silastic catheters for antibiotics in cystic fibrosis. Archives of Disease in Childhood 63: 658–659

Williamson R, Crampton J M, Clarke B E 1983 Research perspectives: the basic defect in cystic fibrosis. In: Hodson M E, Norman A P, Batten J C (eds) Cystic fibrosis. Baillière-Tindall, London, pp 260–272

Wilmott R W, Tyson S L, Dinwiddie R, Matthew D J 1983 Survival rates in cystic fibrosis. Archives of Disease in Childhood 58: 835–838

Wilmott R W 1985 Allergy and infection in cystic fibrosis. In: Milner A D, Martin R J (eds) Neonatal and Pediatric Respiratory Medicine. Butterworths, London, pp 190–210

Wilmott R W, Tyson S L, Matthew D J 1985 Cystic fibrosis survival rates. The influence of allergy and Pseudomonas aeruginosa. American Journal of Disease in Childhood 139: 669–673

Winter R J D, George R J D, Deacock S J et al 1984 Self administered home intravenous antibiotic therapy in bronchiectasis and adult cystic fibrosis. Lancet I: 1338–1339

Wood A M, Jackson M, Miller M, Higenbottam T, Wallwork J 1988 Transepithelial potential difference in the transplanted lung of patients with and without cystic fibrosis. American Review of Respiratory Diseases 137: 220

Wright S W, Norton N E 1966 Genetic studies in cystic fibrosis in Hawaii. American Journal of Human Genetics 20: 157–169

Zach M, Oberwaldner B, Hausler F 1982 Cystic fibrosis, physical exercise versus chest physiotherapy. Archives of Disease in Childhood 57: 587–589

Zach M 1988 Lung disease in cystic fibrosis — current concepts. 10th International Cystic Fibrosis Congress. Excerpta Medica Asia Pacific Congress Series 74: 72–79

10. Aspiration syndromes

A number of conditions are seen following the inhalation of foreign material into the tracheobronchial tree. The symptoms and signs may be acute or chronic depending on the type of inhalation and the time during which the foreign material has been present in the respiratory tract. This is best considered under the headings of acute inhalation, mainly in regard to foreign bodies, and chronic or recurrent inhalation, most commonly seen in patients who have feeding or swallowing difficulties.

ACUTE ASPIRATION

Acute syndromes usually occur as the result of the aspiration of a foreign body into the lower respiratory tree. Sometimes, there is a clear history of a sudden episode of choking while eating or playing with food or small toys. This form of aspiration is most common in the 1–3 year old child (Evans 1987), particularly in late infancy and in the toddler age group when the child has become mobile and therefore has access to materials which can be inhaled. There may be a sudden onset of coughing, gagging, wretching and vomiting and difficulty in breathing. This can be followed by more chronic symptoms with respiratory indrawing and persistent wheezing and cough. The offending agent often causes partial airway obstruction leading to overinflation of one lung and retained secretions within it which will contribute to the wheeziness. Parents should be particularly suspicious where a child who has never had a previous history of wheeze has an episode without obvious evidence of respiratory infection where wheezing is a prominent feature. Boys are twice as likely to inhale a foreign body as girls.

The most common foreign bodies are foodstuffs, especially peanuts, pieces of apple, carrot, beans and pips or seeds. Small plastic and metal toys are becoming increasingly common causes of this problem and, like most foodstuffs, plastic objects are not radio-opaque so will not be seen on plain chest films (Rothmann & Boeckmann 1980).

The most common site for impaction is the right main stem bronchus followed by the left main stem bronchus and the trachea. Less commonly, the objects may be inhaled into the right middle or lower lobe bronchus and occasionally into the left lower lobe bronchus. Aspiration into the upper

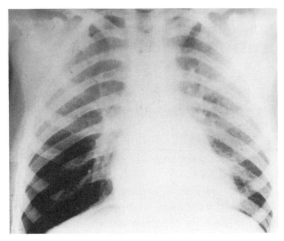

Fig. 10.1   Foreign body inhalation: expiratory film showing hyperlucent right lower lobe indicating air trapping.

lobe bronchi is uncommon. Occasionally, foreign bodies may pass from one major bronchus to the other during fits of coughing and some objects, such as plastic beads, have a hole in the middle through which air can pass even though the object is largely obstructing the airway (Kosloshe 1980).

Physical examination will often reveal poor air entry over the affected lung which is hyper-resonant to percussion. Wheezing may also be heard and there is respiratory distress of a greater or lesser degree.

Chest X-ray should be taken on inspiration and expiration (Fig. 10.1). The classical features on the expiratory film are overinflation of the lung with decreased lung markings on the affected side secondary to airway obstruction. Screening of the chest can also be helpful in demonstrating poor air entry into the affected zone and mediastinal shift away from this area during expiration. The diaphragm on the affected side will also be pushed downwards and shows reduced movement.

Unrecognised acute aspiration

If the aspiration episode is not noted by any other person because the child was alone at the time, or it is thought to be due to the onset of respiratory infection, a different series of mechanisms comes into play. Increasing oedema of the bronchial mucosa, especially if the inhaled object is vegetable matter, will produce obstruction of the bronchus over a period of hours and certainly within the first day or two of the aspiration episode. The lung distal to the obstructed bronchus collapses and almost inevitably develops secondary pneumonic changes. This will be demonstrated as consolidation on the chest X-ray with loss of lung volume on the film. The previously noted overinflation will have disappeared by this stage. It is not uncommon for the child's symptoms to become much less acute by this period and for there only to be a persistent cough and the wheezing to be much less prominent. This diagnosis should always be considered in a child who presents with apparent pneumonia which does not clear with the usual treatment and who shows persistent changes on the chest X-ray. In Cohen's series (Cohen et al 1980) 26% of foreign body inhalations were only recognised 10 days to one month after the event. When an episode is unrecognised more damage occurs distal to the aspirated foreign body and this is likely to leave residual changes for a very long period. Ultimately, this area of lung will become bronchiectatic if the foreign body or the obstruction is not relieved.

The use of ventilation/perfusion lung scans (Fig. 10.2) has recently been helpful in delineating a number of these problems. It may be useful in children who have a history of wheezing with no obvious foreign body present or where there is uncertainty that it has all been removed. Longitudinal studies of ventilation/perfusion lung scan have also shown persisting residual damage in the lungs of children who have inhaled a foreign body. These show non-ventilation and poor perfusion of the affected lung area, even though this may appear aerated on the chest X-ray. This occurs because the ventilatory turnover of gas in this area of the lung is very slow and considerably longer than the half life of the Krypton isotope used in the scan (12 seconds). The degree of this relates to the time for which the foreign body has been present in the lower respiratory tract before removal. Such changes may persist for a number of years in the more severe cases (Gordon et al 1987) (Figs 10.2a and 10.2b).

Treatment

Treatment of children who have aspirated a foreign body into the airway is by urgent bronchoscopy and removal. This is usually effective in relieving the airway obstruction and in ensuring that there is no other abnormality in the lower respiratory tract. Most children tolerate the procedure without complication but pneumothorax can occur postoperatively and a postoperative chest X-ray is mandatory. It is usual practice to treat these patients with physiotherapy and antibiotics because of the associated bacterial contamination of the lower respiratory tract and the inflammatory/pneumonic process which so commonly occurs distal to the site of foreign body obstruction. Steroids such as dexamethasone may be used where there is significant generalised oedema of the airway or where the bronchoscopy has been particularly difficult.

A small percentage of cases show persisting signs after initial bronchoscopy and may require a repeat examination to ensure the foreign body has been completely removed. In a few it may prove impossible to remove the foreign body by bronchoscopy and thoracotomy and bronchotomy is required in order to remove it if it has lodged in a more distal part of the

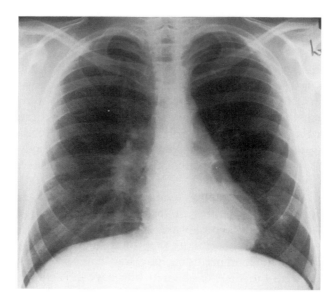

Fig. 10.2a Chest X-ray after recovery from peanut inhalation 4 weeks in left lower lobe before removal.

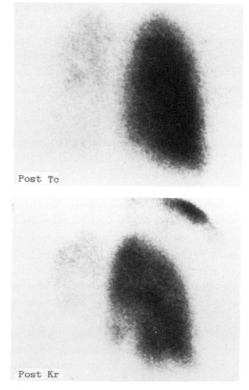

Fig. 10.2b Posterior V/Q lung scan post peanut inhalation. Non-functioning left lower lobe, severely reduced function left upper lobe. Peanut removed 4 weeks post inhalation.

tracheobronchial tree (Evans 1987). All these patients will require physiotherapy on a regular basis to aid clearance of lung secretions and resolution of any associated infection.

CHRONIC ASPIRATION

Chronic aspiration of saliva and foodstuffs, usually liquid or semi-solid, is a common cause of lower respiratory tract disease in children. It is often under-recognised and many children with these conditions are considered to have either recurrent lower respiratory tract infection or asthma (Spitz 1987). Unless there is an obvious underlying congenital abnormality or physiological defect, such as swallowing inco-ordination, which is evident clinically, these syndromes can be difficult to diagnose. This is especially the case where the aspiration is intermittent and where a single investigation such as a barium swallow which only looks at cross-sectional information might not reveal the problem.

The condition is most commonly seen in infants and young children who have a variety of structural or functional abnormalities of the upper airway, oesophagus or gastro-oesophageal junction. They classically present with recurrent episodes of wheezing and lower respiratory tract infection with significant overinflation of the lungs. In some cases, more acute symptoms are seen such as apnoeic attacks, which can be life threatening, or episodes in which there is the rapid onset of dyspnoea, cough, wheeze and respiratory difficulty, particularly during feeding. A proportion of patients also develop upper gastrointestinal bleeding. If the reflux is severe then chronic oesophagitis can develop which in some cases results in stricture formation — this is more likely in children who are mentally handicapped. Apart from saliva, milk is the substance most commonly inhaled into the lower respiratory tree.

The major conditions which underlie children with this problem are as follows:

1. Poor oesophageal function and gastro-oesophageal sphincter tone resulting in frequent reflux of milk into the lower oesophagus up to the pharynx. This condition may be seen with or without an associated hiatus hernia. It is particularly common in children who have other congenital abnormalities such as cerebral palsy or evidence of abnormal neurological development (Spitz 1982). There is also an increased incidence of these problems in infants who have pyloric stenosis.

2. Inco-ordination of sucking or swallowing. This may be seen in children who are entirely normal in every other way and can be transient, tending to improve as the nervous system and general neuromuscular co-ordination matures. It is, however, also more common in children who have other neurological or physical abnormalities.

3. An extra communication between the larynx, trachea or bronchus and the oesophagus or stomach. Examples of this include tracheo-oesophageal fistula and cleft larynx.

Presenting features

The presenting features of these syndromes will depend on the cause, frequency and severity of the inhalation episodes. Some infants will present from birth with recurrent wheeze, cough and overinflation. They most commonly have either tracheo-oesophageal fistula, with or without oesophageal atresia, or major swallowing inco-ordination, such as occurs in bulbar palsy. Those who have significant reflux, with or without hiatus hernia, often have obvious episodes of vomiting and difficulty in retaining feeds. The constant exposure of the lower respiratory tract to foreign material, most commonly milk protein, produces an acute inflammatory response which causes a pneumonitis leading to oedema of the airways, airway obstruction and often an associated broncho-constriction secondary to the coughing episodes. Those who have more major episodes of aspiration present with recurrent pneumonia evident on the chest X-ray, most commonly seen in the upper zones in infants who tend to be supine most of the time. This is particularly likely in those who are left lying flat with a bottle for comfort. Those who are fed in the more erect position tend to aspirate into the right middle and lower lobes and this is the more common site of disease in the older patient. In the worst cases, the recurrent aspiration episodes may lead to severe parenchymal lung disease and ultimately bronchiectasis, although this is much less common nowadays because of the frequent use of antibiotics to treat lower respiratory tract infections.

Investigation

Investigation of the child who is suspected of recurrent aspiration follows lines designed to exclude the most common pathological processes already mentioned. History and physical examination will reveal a pattern of feeding difficulties or may be suggestive of swallowing inco-ordination, particularly if symptoms such as cough and wheeze are associated with feeds. Examination may reveal tachypnoea at rest, overinflation of the lungs, intercostal indrawing and bilateral wheezing on auscultation. It is important to evaluate the child neurologically since the underlying problem is often secondary to neurological disturbance of the swallowing mechanism or some other generalised process including rare conditions such as Werdnig Hoffman disease or familial dysautonomia (Riley-Day Syndrome).

Further investigation will include PA and lateral chest X-ray to demonstrate overinflation, increased bronchial line shadowing and possibly patchy consolidation. The lateral view is particularly helpful in demonstrating generalised air trapping. A barium swallow should be performed by an experienced radiologist and the specific features seen in recurrent aspiration should be considered. These will include difficulty in sucking and swallowing, nasal escape and particularly spillover of contrast medium from the oesophagus into the trachea during swallowing, reflux from the stomach with or without a hiatus hernia present, and possibly abnormal gastric function, such as delayed gastric emptying or pyloric narrowing (Gordon et al 1987).

Any degree of reflux will be exacerbated by the presence of narrowing in the stomach or beyond. Particular observation should be made on the X-ray for evidence of pyloric stenosis and for malrotation of the upper small bowel at the duodenal flexure. Tracheo-oesophageal fistula cannot adequately be excluded by barium swallow alone. This requires a tube oesophagram in which radio-opaque medium is injected under pressure into a nasogastric tube placed in the upper oesophagus. Other techniques such as radioisotope milk scan can be helpful in demonstrating reflux but have not proven useful in making the diagnosis of milk aspiration into the lungs. The most accurate method for assessing reflux into the lower oesophagus is by direct pH measurement using a catheter tip electrode. This allows continuous measurement over several hours with the child in all positions while performing normal activities. This technique allows a quantitative demonstration of frequent or prolonged episodes of reflux in excess of the minor and intermittent ones which occur in normal infants and young children (Spitz 1987). A small number require oesophagoscopy to exclude oesophagitis as further evidence of significant gastro-oesophageal reflux and to exclude stricture formation.

Treatment

This will naturally depend on the nature of the underlying lesion. Where an anatomical abnormality such as a tracheo-oesophageal fistula is found, this should be repaired surgically. Children who have significant reflux and aspiration without a hiatus hernia should receive medical treatment in the first instance (Carre 1985). This includes thickening of the feeds with Nestargel, antacids such as alginic acid (Gaviscon) (Cucchiara et al 1984), and propping up during and after feeds at an angle of no greater than 30 degrees in order to diminish mechanical regurgitation from the stomach (Ovenstein & Whittington 1983). If theophylline has been given for wheezing it should be withdrawn, if possible, as this relaxes the gastro-oesophageal sphincter. Other agents such as domperidone may improve oesophageal motility. Those who have a hiatus hernia and reflux who do not respond to this conservative medical approach, or who are having major aspiration episodes even in the absence of a hernia, require surgical treatment. This would include repair of the hiatus hernia if present and Nissen's fundoplication to prevent further regurgitation. Spitz & Kirtane (1985) have reported on the results and complications of this procedure. Thirty-nine per cent of 106 children presenting for surgery had mental retardation and 27% had reflux strictures. The eventual success rate was 92% but 19% required a second operation: prolapse of the fundoplication through the oesophageal hiatus was the commonest complication occurring in 7% of patients.

It is important to remember that when this operation has been done, the child can no longer vomit. If in a subsequent illness acute intestinal obstruction develops then the physical sign of vomiting is no longer present. Overall however this procedure has been extremely helpful in cases with severe reflux and aspiration.

Children who have major swallowing difficulties due to neurological inco-ordination in addition to reflux may not respond to these measures. In a small proportion of cases other feeding methods may be required. These would include continuous nasogastric feeding, nasojejunal feeding or a gastrostomy placed at the time of a fundoplication. This allows feeding and growth to occur and prevents milk in particular from passing through the pharyngeal area. Unfortunately these children also tend to inhale saliva thus, although the problem may be significantly improved, it may not be completely alleviated.

Fortunately most children with recurrent reflux and aspiration, in the absence of hiatus hernia, outgrow this problem as the nervous system matures and the gastro-oesophageal sphincter tone improves, usually after the age of one year.

Lipoid inhalation pneumonia

Some children develop a chronic inhalation pneumonitis from repeated exposure to oily substances such as petroleum products sucked into the mouth or from medication including certain nose drops or vitamin preparations prepared in an oily base. If there is any coughing or struggling during the administration of these substances direct inhalation can result. Figure 10.3 shows the X-ray changes which can occur as a result of chronic exposure over a period of time.

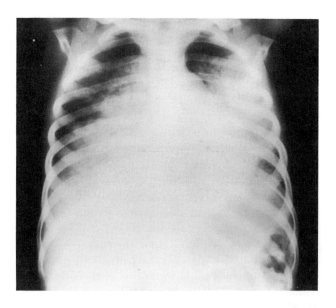

Fig. 10.3   Lipoid inhalation pneumonia: acute lung changes secondary to use of oily nasal drops. Courtesy of Dr G Fischer.

The pathological changes usually constitute an inflammatory response with or without secondary infection. If the changes are acute or have developed over a short period of time they are usually reversible. If they are chronic there is a significant risk that permanent damage including airway obstruction and pulmonary fibrosis will occur.

DROWNING

Aspiration of water into the lungs occurs in drowning or near-drowning incidents. There are more than 2000 child deaths per annum from drowning in the United States. This occurs at any age in childhood and is more common in those who have not learnt to swim (Webster 1967). Many instances, however, occur even in quite shallow water — especially with infants and very young children. The upper airway can become submerged even in quite shallow water such as a garden pond or the bathtub.

The pathology of drowning depends on the nature of the asphyxial event. So called 'dry drowning' occurs when water is not aspirated into the lungs but where there is severe laryngospasm or breath holding sufficient to result in profound hypoxia and often secondary cerebral damage. Those who do actually aspirate water will undergo different changes depending on whether this is fresh or salt water and on whether or not it contains large numbers of potentially pathogenic micro-organisms. Two-thirds of near drowning incidents in the UK occur in fresh water (Harries 1985). The final common pathway of damage is via hypoxia which occurs quite rapidly once the airway is obstructed, either by laryngospasm or by water. The changes produced by different types of drowning will be considered under separate headings.

Dry drowning

About 10–15% of patients with drowning incidents do not aspirate water into the lungs (Modell 1977). The main damage in these cases occurs due to asphyxia. If they can be removed from the water without gasping and subsequent aspiration and immediately resuscitated, the respiratory component of their illness is relatively easily to reverse. Their main treatment will consist of correction of acid–base imbalance and general supportive measures including maintenance of circulation, blood pressure and cerebral perfusion pressure.

Fresh water

Fresh water aspiration (Fig. 10.4) results in marked ventilation/perfusion imbalance. The fresh water is not hypertonic so is absorbed into the circulation across the alveolar wall. As a result of this there is reduced alveolar volume with loss of surfactant and the lungs collapse. This worsens the underlying pulmonary disease and leads to increasing hypoxia, hypercarbia

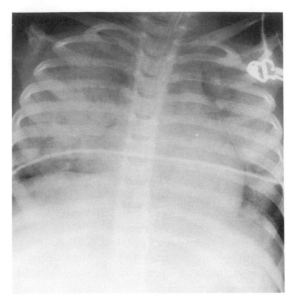

Fig. 10.4   Fresh water drowning.

and acidosis. Large amounts can also be swallowed and when this, plus the water in the lungs, is absorbed systemically there is haemodilution and hypokalaemia. Red cell haemolysis also occurs — this releases potassium into the circulation but despite this hypokalaemia is more common than hyperkalaemia after near drowning in fresh water.

Salt water

Those who aspirate sea water undergo a different sequence of events. The alveoli are filled with a hypertonic solution which draws fluid from the circulation into the alveolar space. These alveoli remain perfused initially but as they are not ventilated large intrapulmonary shunts occur with consequent hypoxia and hypercarbia. Hypernatraemia is a constant feature of salt water immersion.

Hypothermia is a common feature among those who are submerged under water. Breathing stops when the head is submerged but the heart continues to beat. Heat is lost very quickly because the thermal conductivity of water is much greater than air. If the water aspirated into the lungs is cold and it is absorbed into the circulation this will contribute to central cooling of the body generally including the brain where it produces cerebral hypothermia. This sequence of events is similar to that used for preservation of brain function during hypothermia induced prior to open heart surgery and it may partly explain why some cases of near drowning can survive intact after many minutes of immersion (Harries 1985).

Another contributory factor to pulmonary damage is the aspiration of gastric contents either during the acute episode or while the patient is being resuscitated. This is likely to contain gastric acid and probably bacteria and vegetable matter from the water; this is estimated to occur in as many as 25% of cases (Conn 1987).

Treatment

The treatment of all cases of drowning or near drowning is to correct hypoxia, hypercarbia and acidosis, to avoid circulatory collapse or overload and to maintain cerebral perfusion pressure with appropriate control of cerebral oedema if this is present. Those with severe changes in acid–base status and prolonged hypoxia are most at risk. Artificial ventilation and the application of positive end expiratory pressure is particularly helpful in those who have inhaled water directly into the lungs. Monitoring of blood pressure and central venous pressure will allow the correct adjustments to be made in overall fluid balance and ventilation. There is no place for routine steroid therapy in these patients. Antibiotics and chest physiotherapy are useful, particularly in those who require ventilation.

The overall mortality is about 20%. In the series of 140 cases reported by Conn (1987) the long term neurological outcome for those who were concious or semiconcious by the time they arrived in hospital was excellent with only a 5% mortality and 95% of cases showing complete recovery. Those who were unconcious on arrival at hospital had a mortality of 38.5% but even in these circumstances almost 50% made a complete recovery. Those who have raised intracranial pressure after any form of near drowning have a uniformly poor outcome (Dean & McComb 1981).

SMOKE INHALATION

The pulmonary complications of smoke inhalation are a common problem among children rescued from house fires. The type and severity of the injury depends not only on the duration and severity of the inhalation period but also on the presence of toxic substances and carbon monoxide which is inevitably present in the smoke itself. There may be acute heat injury to the upper airway but inhalation into the lungs more commonly products an acute toxin-induced inflammatory response at epithelial level. Inhalation into the smaller airways stimulates bronchospasm and subsequently results in an obliterative bronchiolitis. Alveoli respond to the stress by the production of interstitial and alveolar wall oedema and haemorrhage in some cases.

Treatment

Treatment of the child with smoke inhalation consists of acute respiratory support based on review of the chest X-ray (Fig. 10.5), analysis of blood gases and acid–base status and an assessment of the carbon monoxide level. High concentration oxygen may help to displace carbon monoxide from haemoglobin, to which it binds tightly. Tracheal intubation and mechanical

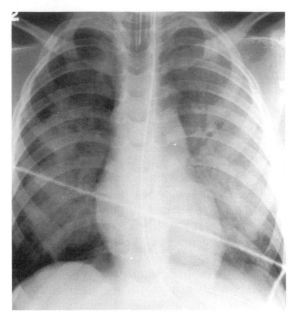

Fig. 10.5   Smoke inhalation.

ventilation will be necessary for those with significant respiratory failure. Careful assessment of fluid balance is necessary since pulmonary oedema is common. If this is a problem, increased end expiratory pressure on the ventilator is helpful. Bronchospasm should be relieved by the use of bronchodilators such as salbutamol or terbutaline and theophylline if necessary. Antibiotics are given to cover any associated infection. There is no proven place for steroids except when there is severe bronchoconstriction. Children who are unconcious have usually suffered more prolonged stress from inhalation of toxins, hypoxia or both. They require continuous monitoring of blood pressure, central venous pressure and possibly intracranial pressure (Dinwiddie & Stroobant 1985) in order to ensure that an adequate cerebral circulation is maintained until recovery occurs.

REFERENCES

Carre I J 1985 Management of gastro-oesophageal reflux. Archives of Disease in Childhood 60: 71–75
Cohen S R, Herbert W I, Lewis G B Jr, Geller K A 1980 Foreign bodies in the airway. Five year retrospective study with special reference to management. Annals of Otology, Rhinology and Laryngology 89: 437–442
Conn A W 1987 Drowning and near drowning. In: Behrman R E, Vaughan V C (eds) Nelson Textbook of Pediatrics, Saunders, Philadelphia, pp 220–223
Cucchiara S, Staiano A, Romaniello G, Capobianco S, Auricchio S 1984 Antacids for cimetidine for gastro-oesophageal reflux and peptic oesophagitis. Archives of Disease in Childhood 59: 842–847
Dean M J, McComb J G 1981 Intracranial pressure monitoring in severe pediatric near drowning. Neurosurgery 9: 627–630

Dinwiddie R, Stroobant J 1985 Monitoring and treatment of raised intracranial pressure in children. Journal of the Royal Society of Medicine 78: 185–186

Evans J N G (ed) 1987 Foreign bodies in the larynx and trachea. In:Scott Brown's otolaryngology 5th edn. Paediatric Otolaryngology, Butterworths, London, pp 438–448

Gordon I, Dinwiddie R, Matthew D J 1987 Respiratory System. In: Gordon I (ed) Diagnostic Imaging in Paediatrics. Chapman and Hall, London, pp 27–57

Kosloshe A M 1980 Tracheobronchial foreign bodies in children. Pediatrics 66: 321–323

Harries M 1985 Near drowning and its management. Respiratory Disease in Practice 2: 14–15

Modell J H 1977 Drowning and near drowning. In: Kendig E L, Chernick V (eds) Disorders of the respiratory tract in children. Saunders, Philadelphia, pp 498–510

Ovenstein S R, Whittington P E 1983 Positioning for prevention of infant gastroesophageal reflux. Journal of Pediatrics 103: 534–537

Rothmann B F, Boeckmann C R 1980 Foreign bodies in the larynx and tracheobronchial tree in children. A review of 225 cases. Annals of Otology, Rhinology and Laryngology 89: 434–436

Spitz L 1982 Surgical treatment of gastroesophaeal reflux in severely mentally retarded children. Journal of the Royal Society of Medicine 75: 525–529

Spitz L, Kirtane J 1985 Results and complications of surgery for gastro-oesphageal reflux. Archives of Disease in Childhood 60: 743–747

Spitz L 1987 Diseases of the oesophagus. In: Evans J N G (ed) Scott-Brown's otolaryngology, 5th edn. Paediatric Otolaryngology. Butterworths, London, pp 534–553

Webster D P 1967 Pool drownings and their prevention. Public Health Report 82: 587–600

11. Pulmonary tuberculosis

Tuberculosis (TB) is a disease which has been prevalent all through the history of mankind. Evidence of its spread throughout the body has been found as long ago as Palaeolithic times (Guthrie 1958). The organism itself is usually of low grade virulence but it can cause significant chronic disease resulting in serious symptoms which develop over a period of time. The organism was first observed by Koch in 1882 to be an acid fast bacillus — *Mycobacterium tuberculosis*. This illness is one of the best examples of a disease in which chronic infection is a balance between the numbers and virulence of the organism present against the general and specific ability of the host to resist it. This results in a wide variety of presentation of the illness, especially in children.

EPIDEMIOLOGY

Although the incidence of the disease in the UK has been falling over the past 20 years (Table 11.1) cases are still seen among those who have lived or travelled abroad to areas of the world where there continues to be a higher prevalence. A number of children also acquire the infection in this country from relatives or other contacts, often in the home, who have come from endemic areas. The notification rate for white children under the age of 15 years in the UK was 2.4/100 000 in 1983. The rate for Indian children was 32/100 000 and for Pakistani and Bangladeshi children 52/100 000 (MRC Report 1988). The disease is also more prevalent in lower socioeconomic groups and in the malnourished. The incidence increases with age and although it affects males and females equally in early childhood it is more common in females in later childhood. There is a higher incidence where housing conditions are poor, especially if there is overcrowding. It is also seen more frequently in other ethnic groups such as Eskimos and North American Indians. This is not necessarily due to genetic or racial differences in susceptibility but is probably related to poorer socioeconomic circumstances.

Those who are immunocompromised either due to a primary defect of the immune system or secondary to chemotherapy for malignant disease are also at increased risk. This is particularly likely if the abnormality affects cell-mediated immunity. Enquiry should always be made of parents as to

Table 11.1 Notifications of pulmonary tuberculosis in children (<15 years) in England and Wales 1966–1986

| Year | Age | | | Total |
	0–4	5–9	10–14	
1966	473	423	295	1191
1967	480	372	306	1158
1968	484	351	323	1158
1969	364	334	292	990
1970	336	304	284	924
1971	363	333	298	994
1972	305	325	289	919
1973	307	313	274	894
1974	272	275	315	862
1975	235	244	319	798
1976	214	268	291	773
1977	217	247	277	741
1978	227	208	223	658
1979	184	242	280	706
1980	211	235	265	711
1981	178	160	204	542
1982	144	153	181	478
1983	156	118	155	429
1984	173	113	123	409
1985	128	92	103	323
1986	119	111	127	357

Courtesy of Communicable Disease Surveillance Centre, Colindale, London

whether they are consanguinious since this will increase the chance of the child having an inherited defect of the immune system.

PATHOGENESIS

The major mode of spread of infection is airborne, usually adult to child. Infection can also be acquired via the gut or cervical lymph nodes (with atypical mycobacteria) although this is less common. Fetal infection through haematogenous spread from the maternal bloodstream or inhalation of infected amniotic fluid at birth has occurred but is extremely rare in clinical practice.

The most common route of infection is directly through the upper respiratory tract. Once in the lower respiratory system it migrates to the periphery of the lung where it establishes itself just beneath the pleural surface. This primary infection occurs more frequently in the lower lobes than the upper in young children and in the apical area in the older child and adolescent. The organism then multiplies and elicits an inflammatory response from the host; this lesion then constitutes the primary focus. The local immune response initially involves acute inflammatory cells such as neutrophils and mononuclears but this is soon followed by a much more chronic, mainly lymphocytic, response resulting in the typical caseation and granuloma formation which is classical of TB. This lesion often calcifies over a period of 1–2 years and is called a Ghon focus. Shortly after initial

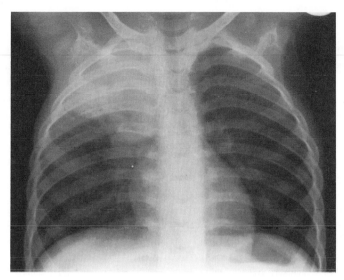

Fig. 11.1   Pulmonary tuberculosis showing consolidation of right upper lobe with hilar adenopathy.

invasion there is spread to the regional lymph nodes resulting in hilar adenopathy which may be visible on the chest X-ray (Fig. 11.1). This is more likely to occur if the child's nutritional state is poor. The combination of the primary focus plus regional lymph node enlargement forms the primary complex.

Children with pulmonary TB demonstrate a wide variety of signs and symptoms. These will vary from no systemic upset to severe weight loss and wasting in those with generalised miliary spread. Most children undergoing primary infection have few if any symptoms but occasionally complain of lassitude and anorexia in combination with poor weight gain. Low grade fever is also seen. Cough is usually a feature of more advanced disease such as post-primary spread and is rarely associated with sputum production except where there is rupture of a primary focus into the adjacent bronchus. Culture of the organism is important if possible and sputum or early morning gastric washings are the best samples to examine. Positive cultures for tubercle bacilli are obtainable in 19–20% of paediatric cases (MRC 1988).

Sensitivity to tuberculoprotein

Any patient with an intact cell-mediated immune system who is infected with *Mycobacterium tuberculosis* will develop sensitivity to tuberculoprotein about 6 weeks after initial infection. This is a form of delayed hypersensitivity reaction and may be used as a specific test for previous infection with the organism. The two most commonly used are the Mantoux and Heaf tests.

The Mantoux test is the more accurate and involves intradermal injection of 0.1 ml of purified protein derivative (PPD). This comes in various strengths and if a positive reaction occurs there is an area of induration at the site of injection which is recorded in millimetres diameter at 48 hours. The standard solutions of PPD are 1 in 10 000 containing 10 tuberculin units per ml or 1 in 1000 dilution containing 100 tuberculin units per ml. In practice 0.1 ml of 1 in 1000 solution (10 units) is injected intradermally and a positive reaction is counted as induration of 5 mm or more at 48 hours. If significant infection is suspected then the 1 in 10 000 solution should be used since a strongly positive response can cause a severe localised skin reaction which may ulcerate. Sensitivity to tuberculoprotein appears between 4 and 8 weeks after initial contact with the organism. The reaction may be reduced or absent in the following situations: advanced TB, the malnourished, those with suppressed cell-mediated immunity (including HIV), steroid therapy and transiently following measles.

The Heaf test is commonly used for population screening. It involves the use of a multipuncture skin test technique utilising a spring loaded gun with six needles previously primed with tuberculoprotein of known strength. The result is quantified in terms of induration at the puncture sites which will vary from small individual lesions at each site to complete coalescence in the more reactive case. Recent surveys in the UK indicate that only 1 in 1000 school children tested at the age of 13 has a positive reaction.

CLINICAL PATTERNS OF INFECTION

Clinical TB in children is seen in four major forms:

1. Primary infection with little or no systemic symptoms, primary complex disease.
   Diagnosis is made by a positive Mantoux or Heaf reaction. The chest X-ray is normal or only shows minimal change.
2. Local spread to regional lymph nodes.
   Diagnosis is made by a positive skin test and by the chest X-ray which shows definite changes including hilar adenopathy.
3. Post-primary spread.
   Positive skin test with evidence of consolidation on chest X-ray and hilar adenopathy.
4. Generalised spread.
   Immediate — miliary TB with generalised tuberculous broncho-pneumonia (Fig. 11.2).
   Late — involvement of other organs including meninges, kidneys, skin, bones and joints 1–7 years after primary infection.

Primary complex disease

Most children with a primary complex are asymptomatic. They may be found when there is other evidence of possible TB such as erythema nodosum or spontaneous Mantoux conversion; this may be discovered

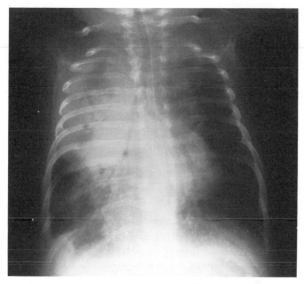

Fig. 11.2   Tuberculous bronchopneumonia: bilateral hilar adenopathy, consolidation of the right upper zone and generalised overinflation due to airway narrowing.

during contact testing of a known case. Evidence of a previous primary complex may also be found by a positive screening test at school prior to BCG immunisation.

It is important to perform a chest X-ray on all of those who have any systemic upset and in any case where active disease is suspected. If a discrete lesion is found then a full course of antituberculous chemotherapy is indicated as this will localise the primary focus and greatly reduce the risk of later haematogenous spread to other organs. A few children go on to develop a small pleural effusion in relation to their primary focus and they too require full treatment. Those who are immune-suppressed may go on to develop more florid miliary spread especially in the lungs. This requires aggressive treatment and elucidation of the immune defect if this has not already been undertaken.

Regional lymph node disease

Regional lymph node involvement is virtually universal in any case of primary TB. The degree to which they are involved varies from minor enlargement to a much greater increase in size with abscess formation due to caseation. In the lung the nodes involved are at the hilum and these may be visible as hilar adenopathy on the chest X-ray. Similar changes are sometimes seen in the axillary lymph nodes following BCG. Enlarged hilar nodes can lead to partial or complete obstruction of the adjacent bronchus; this initially causes air trapping with lobar overinflation and subsequently collapse behind the obstruction. In these cases there is usually also lobar consolidation from the primary disease. A full course of chemotherapy is indicated; the inflammatory response in glands obstructing the airway can be reduced by a short course of oral steroid therapy providing antituberculous chemotherapy is already established. Occasionally surgical resection of the enlarged glands is required. A few children develop persistent airway obstruction which can lead to tuberculous bronchiectasis but this is rare in the UK if the child is otherwise healthy.

EXTRATHORACIC TUBERCULOSIS

Primary tuberculous lesions in the lung usually heal leaving a small calcified scar or minor hilar adenopathy. The more serious infections however disseminate throughout the bloodstream to other parts of the body. In the extremely malnourished or the severely immune deficient child this may be relatively rapid and can be fatal within a short space of time. This is miliary TB and in this situation the chest X-ray will also show widespread mottled shadowing throughout both lung fields — fortunately this presentation is rare. A similar pattern is occasionally seen following the administration of BCG to immune deficient infants in the neonatal period. Haematogenous spread most commonly appears within 3–5 years of the primary complex. The organs most likely to be affected include the central nervous system, bones, joints and kidneys (Fig. 11.3).

Tuberculous meningitis

TB meningitis is a major cause of death in children following untreated primary infection. It may be the presenting feature although there will usually have been a previous unrecognised primary lung lesion. Presentation

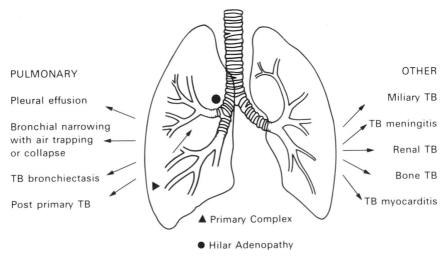

PULMONARY

Pleural effusion

Bronchial narrowing
with air trapping
or collapse

TB bronchiectasis

Post primary TB

OTHER

Miliary TB

TB meningitis

Renal TB

Bone TB

TB myocarditis

▲ Primary Complex

● Hilar Adenopathy

Fig. 11.3   Complications of pulmonary tuberculosis in children.

is with irritability, neck stiffness and meningism. Headache, restlessness and anorexia are common but fever is not usually a prominent feature at this stage. Localised spread within the brain can lead to the formation of a tuberculous cerebral abscess. As the disease progresses hydrocephalus and increased intracranial pressure occur leading to the onset of coma, further cerebral depression and death if not treated.

Fundal examination may reveal tubercles in the choroid. Cerebrospinal fluid examination typically shows an increase in white cells, mainly lymphocytes, with an elevated protein and decreased sugar level and no organisms on initial microscopy. A proteinaceous fibrinous web forms in the CSF if it is left to stand and acid-fast bacilli may be seen on careful microscopy of a centrifuged specimen examined by direct immunofluorescence. A latex particle agglutination test is now available for rapid detection of TB antigen in CSF (Krambovitis et al 1984).

Intensive treatment with antituberculous chemotherapy is required and it may be necessary to monitor and treat the patient for raised intracranial pressure. Appropriate drainage procedures for hydrocephalus are sometimes required. Mortality is of the order of 30–40% and morbidity among survivors is common although complete recovery is possible.

Renal tuberculosis

A sterile pyuria is not uncommon in children with active pulmonary TB and indicates renal colonisation — in most cases this disappears as appropriate treatment is given for the lung disease. More generalised renal disease is a late feature and usually occurs some 5–7 years after the primary infection. At this stage there are obvious lesions within the renal tract and there is caseation in the renal parenchyma. This complication is again more common in the malnourished. Diagnosis is by discovery of the primary complex or by the detection of typical acid-fast bacilli in early morning urine specimens. Treatment is with intensive chemotherapy and surgical treatment is occasionally required.

Tuberculosis of bones and joints

This is also a late manifestation following primary lung infection which may or may not be obvious. Bony involvement is seen from a few months to several years after primary infection. The spread to the bones is haematogenous and those most frequently involved are the spine and either of the hip joints. The small bones of the hands or feet can also be infected resulting in tuberculous dactylitis. TB of the spine (Pott's disease) most commonly affects the lower thoracic or upper lumbar region and occasionally the cervical spine. Presentation is with intermittent pain and irritability and the onset of kyphosis. The absence of major toxicity distinguishes it from other acute infective lesions. Treatment is with antituberculous chemotherapy, orthopaedic support and surgical drainage of the abscess where necessary. TB of the hip presents with a limp and sometimes pain in the joint. Progression of the disease can lead to destruction of the femoral head. The absence of toxic features again distinguishes it from acute pyogenic osteomyelitis and arthritis. Treatment is with appropriate antituberculous chemotherapy.

Other manifestations

TB can also present with other manifestations such as phlyctenular conjunctivitis, chorioretinitis or erythema nodosum. Occasionally skin lesions are seen (lupus vulgaris). These are clues to the diagnosis and a search should be made for the primary site of infection. Abdominal TB is due to infection acquired through the gut and used to be seen following the ingestion of infected milk before bovine tuberculin testing was routine. Mesenteric lymph nodes were commonly involved and occasionally there was a TB peritonitis. Cervical lymph node TB is still seen as a manifestation of primary infection via the tonsils. Nowadays this is usually caused by infection with atypical mycobacteria. Other causes of lymphadenopathy must be excluded such as Hodgkin's disease and non-Hodgkin's lymphoma. Treatment is with appropriate antituberculous chemotherapy although abscess drainage is sometimes necessary both for diagnostic and treatment purposes.

CONTACT TRACING

The most important factor in preventing the spread of TB is to establish the source of infection. This will involve screening other family members and anyone with whom the patient has been in contact during the appropriate time. This applies particularly to other members of the household, especially those who have come from other areas of the world with a continuing high prevalence of TB. The Community Health Service or the local Chest Clinic will usually organise the necessary contact tracing in the UK.

BCG IMMUNISATION (BACILLE CALMETTE GUERIN)

This is one of the most important measures which has reduced the incidence of TB worldwide. Improved public health, hygiene and general nutrition of the population are also important factors. The vaccine used is of bovine origin and consists of a live bacillus which has been passaged by repeated culture to attenuate its virulence. Immunisation is offered to school children in the UK after routine screening using the Heaf test. The paediatric dose is 0.1 ml BCG given intradermally. Various sites are used but the lower part of the outer aspect of the upper arm is recommended as it is easy for others to check for evidence of previous immunisation and it leaves less of a scar (Sanders & Dickson 1982). The injection results in a slowly developing red indurated lesion at the site which is initially open and then gradually crusts over during the next 6 weeks. Some children develop regional lymph node enlargement in the axilla and very occasionally these ulcerate, in which case oral isoniazid should be given for 6 weeks.

Neonates should be immunised in the first week (0.05 ml dose) if there is a higher risk of family or communal exposure to the organism (Curtis et al 1984, Packe & Innes 1988). This would include those whose parents or relatives who come from or travel to countries with a high incidence of the disease. Children who themselves will travel frequently to Africa, the Middle East, Asia and South America or who have family history of a close living relative with TB. The protective effect of neonatal BCG is estimated to vary between 64% and 75% (Curtis et al 1984, Packe & Innes 1988).

TREATMENT

All children with active TB require treatment; this includes those who have shown Mantoux conversion, particularly in the younger age groups. Treatment is designed to deal effectively with the primary lesion and to prevent the later complications in other organs which arise as a result of haematogenous spread. Chemotherapy is the basis of modern treatment but must be combined with measures to improve general health and nutrition. Other contributory factors such as immune deficiency must be elucidated and treated appropriately if possible.

Until recently the duration of chemotherapy for TB was 9 months. A number of different regimes were in use all utilising a combination of two or three antituberculous drugs given simultaneously (British Thoracic Association 1980). New recommendations have suggested the possibility of successful treatment with a regime lasting 6 months in some cases (American Thoracic Society 1986, Drug and Therapeutics Bulletin 1988). Treatment is maintained for the entire period with rifampicin and isoniazid. This is supplemented with pyrazinamide during the first 2 months. Others have further supplemented this regime with ethambutol or streptomycin during the first 2 months if drug resistance is likely to be a problem. Ethambutol has potential ophthalmic side effects which are difficult to monitor in children so should probably be avoided. Appropriate dosage for these agents is given in Table 11.2.

Table 11.2 Drugs used to treat pulmonary tuberculosis

Drug	Single daily dose	Maximum daily dose
Isoniazid	10–20 mg/kg oral	300 mg
Pyrazinamide	15–30 mg/kg oral	2 g
Rifampicin	10–20 mg/kg oral	600 mg
Streptomycin	20–40 mg/kg im	1 g
Ethambutol	25 mg/kg oral, 1st 60 days 15 mg/kg after 60 days	2.5 g

A baby whose mother has active TB should receive isoniazid for the first 3 months or until his or her mother is known to be sputum negative. If after this time the baby is tuberculin test negative and has a normal chest X-ray isoniazid is stopped but the infant is then given isoniazid resistant BCG. If the baby has become tuberculin test positive, and especially if the chest X-ray is abnormal, then he must be given a further course of isoniazid in combination with rifampicin (American Thoracic Society 1986). It is not necessary to separate mother and infant in the neonatal period if both are known to be receiving adequate medication.

REFERENCES

American Thoracic Society 1986 Treatment of tuberculosis and tuberculosis infection in adults and children. American Review of Respiratory Disease 134: 355–363
British Thoracic Association 1980 Lancet 1: 1182–1183
Curtis H M, Leck I, Bamford F N 1984 Incidence of childhood tuberculosis after neonatal BCG vaccination. Lancet 1: 145–148
Drug and Therapeutics Bulletin 1988 Chemotherapy for pulmonary tuberculosis in Britain. 26: 1–4
Guthrie D (ed) 1958 A History of Medicine. Nelson, London, p 2
Krambovitis E, McIllmurray M B, Lock P E et al 1984 Rapid diagnosis of tuberculous meningitis by latex particle agglutination. Lancet 2: 1229–1231
Medical Research Council Tuberculosis and Chest Diseases Unit 1988 Tuberculosis in children: a national survey of notifications in England and Wales in 1983. Archives of Disease in Childhood 63: 266–276
Packe, G E, Innes J A 1988 Protective effect of BCG vaccination in infant Asians: a case-control study. Archives of Disease in Childhood 63: 277–281
Sanders R, Dickson M G 1982 BCG vaccination scars: an avoidable problem? British Medical Journal 285: 1679–1680

12. Rare diseases of the lung

There are a number of unusual lung conditions whose aetiology is obscure and which cross the boundaries between many areas already discussed such as congenital malformation, infection and abnormal reactions to environmental factors. Some of those which are seen from time to time in clinical practice are discussed in this chapter.

INTERSTITIAL PNEUMONITIS (Idiopathic) — FIBROSING ALVEOLITIS

These terms describe a group of uncommon conditions in which there is an inflammatory process mainly affecting the interstitium, the alveolar space or both of these. The aetiology is unclear but it is probably multifactorial and may represent the end stage of a number of different processes (Nash 1982).

The condition may present at birth, in infancy or later in childhood — most paediatric cases begin below the age of 5 years. There is a gradual onset of breathlessness without major respiratory difficulty, at least in the beginning, and there is usually a dry irritating cough. As the illness progresses the blood begins to desaturate and cyanosis appears. Physical examination reveals tachypnoea even at rest and showers of fine crepitations throughout both lungs on deep inspiration. Chest X-ray (Fig. 12.1) shows a diffuse haziness with a granular appearance throughout both sides and low volume lungs on inspiration. Blood gases show a typical alveolar block pattern with hypoxia and hypocapnia in the initial stages leading to hypercapnia in more advanced cases.

Investigations should be undertaken to rule out major immune deficiency infection by organisms such as bacteria, viruses or fungi or reaction to extrinsic allergens. The diagnosis can only be made by open lung biopsy. When this is done the tissue should be carefully subdivided and cultured for the usual organisms and histologically examined for evidence of *Pneumocystis carinii*. In true fibrosing alveolitis a variety of histological changes are seen. These vary from a pure interstitial inflammatory infiltrate with an increase in alveolar macrophages to a much more proliferative fibrotic or desquamative picture, occasionally with giant cell formation, and with large amounts of cellular debris in the alveoli obstructing them. This represents

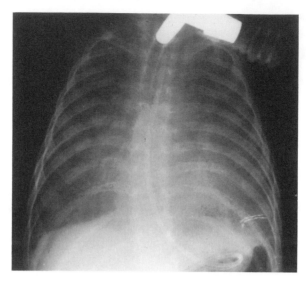

Fig. 12.1   Congenital desquamative interstitial pneumonitis.

the full blown picture of desquamative interstitial pneumonitis (DIP). In pure DIP the histological changes principally affect the type II pneumocytes which can be seen in degenerative forms actually separating from the alveolar wall.

The disease probably represents an abnormal host reaction as immune complexes and a number of cytotoxic immune-mediated enzymes have been found in the alveolar wash from these patients (Roberton 1985). There may also be a genetic predisposition as cases have been seen in siblings (Farrell et al 1986) and there is a higher than expected incidence of HLA antigen DR2 in affected cases (Libby et al 1983).

The rate of progress is very variable. Some patients show a relentless downhill course and die within a few months. Others progress more slowly and the disease process waxes and wanes over several years. The disease can burn out spontaneously after a period of several months without any specific treatment. These children are usually left with a degree of pulmonary fibrosis and at this stage the granularity on the X-ray is much more coarse and honeycomb-like in its appearance; they usually have a good prognosis. Treatment is otherwise unsatisfactory; a few children respond to oral steroid therapy but many do not. Immunosuppressive agents such as azathioprine are sometimes helpful and more recently chloroquine has also been used (Springer et al 1987). Unless there is a response to these agents the prognosis is poor.

SHWACHMAN'S SYNDROME

This rare condition involving pancreatic hypoplasia with bone marrow dysfunction is characterised by exocrine pancreatic deficiency, short stature and neutropenia. Other signs of bone marrow dysfunction such as hypoplastic anaemia and thrombocytopenia are also often seen (Aggett et al 1980). Over 50% of children with this syndrome have metaphyseal dysplasia with a characteristic X-ray appearance. Almost all children under the age of three have abnormally short ribs with flared ends which leads to reduced lung volumes at all ages. There is a neutrophil mobility defect and although lung disease is not a major feature most patients do suffer from recurrent respiratory infection thus making the condition resemble cystic fibrosis in many ways, particularly in the early years. This syndrome can be differentiated from cystic fibrosis by the normal sweat electrolytes, the presence of bony abnormalities of the ribs and pelvis and the neutropenia. Its cause and inheritance pattern are not known precisely although it is thought probably to be an autosomal recessive condition in the few families in which more than one case has occurred. The prognosis is variable; 15–25% die from intercurrent infection but if they survive the early years of life some spontaneous improvement with age is to be expected (Walker-Smith et al 1983).

ALVEOLAR PROTEINOSIS

This is another extremely rare form of interstitial pneumonitis. In this condition the type II pneumocytes become lipid laden and subsequently desquamate into the alveolar spaces. The onset is gradual and the physical signs and X-ray changes are similar to those seen in idiopathic interstitial pneumonitis. The patient becomes increasingly cyanosed and oxygen dependent. A number of these patients also have thymic alymphoplasia. Specific diagnosis is made only at open lung biopsy. There is no effective treatment although bronchial lavage may temporarily slow down the relentless progression of the disease. Most cases in children are fatal within a matter of months from the diagnosis.

AUTOIMMUNE LUNG DISEASE

Inflammatory processes affecting the lung are seen in some patients with chronic multisystem disease which is immune-mediated and non-infective in origin. These include rheumatoid arthritis, systemic lupus erythematosus, dermatomyositis, Goodpasture's syndrome (with associated glomerular disease) and polyarteritis nodosa.

Changes of varying severity are seen. The most common pattern is one of interstitial pneumonitis leading on to pulmonary fibrosis (Roberton 1985). The X-ray changes are similar to those described in idiopathic interstitial pneumonitis and the lung function tests show a restrictive pattern with impairment of diffusion. There may be some airflow obstruction due to peribronchial inflammation (Begin et al 1982). Unilateral or bilateral pleural effusions can also occur.

Treatment if required is usually with immunosuppressive agents such as oral prednisolone or azathioprine used to suppress the more generalised disease process. If it is not rapidly progressive this approach will often control the pulmonary manifestations very effectively. There is however a significant risk of secondary infection in the lungs with opportunistic agents such as *Pneumocystis carinii* or *Aspergillus fumigatus* because of the immune suppression. Some of these patients also develop an associated weakness of the respiratory muscles and those of deglutition; there is then an added risk of lung infection secondary to aspiration (Walport 1987). Over the longer term many of these autoimmune conditions burn out. If the lungs have been involved they are often left fibrotic with coarse streaky honeycomb shadows on the chest X-ray. If this does happen without too much restriction of lung function then the long term prognosis is good.

SARCOIDOSIS

Sarcoidosis of the lung is an uncommon disease in childhood and is more often see in adolescents and young adults. The condition is due to a multisystem granulomatous disorder of unknown cause. It typically presents with a dry irritant cough and breathlessness. There is hilar lymphadenopathy with or without patchy infiltrates on the chest X-ray. There may be evidence of involvement of other organs such as the eyes with uveitis or iritis or the skin with erythema nodosum. Immunological investigation typically reveals hyperimmunoglobulinaemia and impaired cell-mediated immune response. There is a marked increase in local immunoglobulin production within the lung (Rankin et al 1983).

Diagnosis is by biopsy of an affected superficial lymph node if one is available — this will show non-caseating epithelioid cell granulomata. The Kveim test is also used to make the diagnosis. Antigenic material is obtained from affected human sarcoid tissue and is injected intradermally. If a nodule appears at the site of injection it is biopsied at 4–6 weeks and shows typical sarcoid follicles. In practice however it is often difficult to obtain suitable antigen for the test.

Patients with mild disease may show spontaneous resolution. Treatment with steroids is indicated for ophthalmic complications. As recurrence is common these may have to be continued for some time so should only be given to patients with serious manifestations of the illness. Steroids are not indicated for the pulmonary manifestations which are usually self limiting in children.

HISTIOCYTOSIS

Histiocytosis is a term used to describe a number of non-malignant conditions typified by abnormalities of the mononuclear phagocytes (histiocytes). The major type affecting the lungs was previously known as Histiocytosis X but this has now been reclassified as Class I: Langerhans-cell histiocytosis on the basis of specific ultrastructural and enzymatic features (Chu et al 1987). This can affect various organs throughout the body including the lungs.

There is usually widespread infiltration of histiocytic and other inflammatory cells in the interlobular, alveolar, peribronchial and perivascular areas of the lung. This leads to obstruction of the terminal bronchioles with secondary microcyst formation which gives a fibrotic honeycomb appearance on the chest X-ray (Fig. 12.2). These cysts may rupture causing air leak including pneumothorax, pneumomediastinum and interstitial emphysema. Pneumothorax may be persistent or recurrent requiring intercostal drainage and occasionally pleurectomy to control it. Treatment of the underlying disorder may require steroids and cytotoxic agents such as vincristine.

The long term prognosis is variable and depends on the activity of the basic disease process. This may cease spontaneously after a period of time leaving the lungs fibrotic and prone to secondary infection. Other cases show a steady deterioration despite drug therapy and have a fatal outcome after a period of several years.

PULMONARY HAEMOSIDEROSIS

This is a rare condition of the lungs characterised by repeated episodes of intra-alveolar haemorrhage, production of bloodstained sputum containing haemosiderin laden macrophages and acute anaemia. It is usually first seen in early childhood and waxes and wanes in severity over a number of years. The most common pattern is of acute episodes of intrapulmonary haemorrhage with asymptomatic periods between. Despite this, microscopic haemorrhages continue and can lead to chronic anaemia. Most cases in childhood are idiopathic but some are secondary to other problems. A number of children have been described in whom there are features of cow's milk protein intolerance with associated antibodies present in the blood. These patients respond to withdrawal of cow's milk from the diet. Another condition in which there is a similar clinical picture is Goodpasture's syndrome where there is pulmonary haemosiderosis in combination with progressive proliferative or membranous glomerulonephritis. This disease is also thought to have an immunological basis. It is usually seen in young adult males. The renal disease can lead to chronic renal failure and death; some patients show an improvement in their lung condition following bilateral nephrectomy. Pulmonary haemosiderosis can also occur secondary to heart disease such as mitral stenosis and in collagen vascular disease such as polyarteritis or as a manifestation of rheumatoid arthritis.

In any type of pulmonary haemosiderosis the same symptoms occur during periods of acute haemorrhage. The patient may be febrile and usually complains of being short of breath and wheezy. There is a moist cough and mild to moderate haemoptysis. The sputum may be frankly bloodstained or rust coloured depending on the timing and severity of the bleeding. If it is swallowed there may be melaena as well. Auscultation of the chest does not reveal any characteristic added sounds although coarse crepitations may be heard if there has been recent significant bleeding. Anaemia develops secondary to the haemorrhage which is severe can

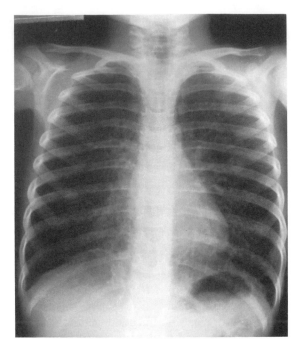

Fig. 12.2   Histiocytosis: generalised honeycomb appearance of the lung.

induce shock. Manv patients become iron deficient as a result of the bleeding although in spite of this there is excessive iron deposition in the lung itself. The chest X-ray (Fig. 12.3) shows widespread mottled shadows in both lung fields which become more confluent during periods of acute bleeding.

Treatment of acute episodes is with blood transfusion and intravenous hydrocortisone. Some cases are controlled by low dose, alternate day, oral steroid therapy or agents such as azathioprine, and others are able to discontinue therapy completely between acute episodes. Oral iron should be given to correct the anaemia. The long term prognosis is very variable and depends on the frequency and severity of bleeding episodes. Acute massive haemorrhage can occur without warning and may be fatal. Some patients develop an associated myocarditis which itself significantly increases the morbidity of the disease.

CENTRAL HYPOVENTILATION SYNDROME (ONDINE'S CURSE)

This term applies to any condition where there is loss of central control of breathing in the absence of an obvious structural lesion in the central nervous system itself. It was termed 'Ondine's curse' by Severinghaus & Mitchell in 1962 because of a curse which the water nymph Ondine placed upon her lover Hans who had jilted her. This made him take control of all his autonomic functions only by a conscious act. This went well until he

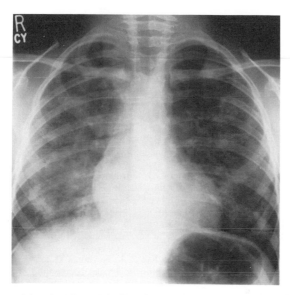

Fig. 12.3   Haemosiderosis: bilateral fluffy infiltrates due to intraparenchymal haemorrhage.

fell asleep. 'A single moment of inattention and I forget to breathe'. 'He died they will say because it was a nuisance to breathe'. Nowadays the term is applied to anyone who has failure of central respiratory drive whether awake or asleep. By definition central apnoea occurs when there is no detectable airflow at the nose or mouth and there is cessation or severe reduction in the amplitude of respiratory movements (Apps 1985).

The condition can present at birth and in this form may occasionally be familial. It can also present later if there is loss of functional control of breathing at brainstem level. Precipitating factors include viral encephalitis (including RSV), meningitis, congenital hypogammaglobulinaemia, neurodegenerative disease, microscopic infiltration by tumour, metabolic disease and hypoxic brain insult. A number are idiopathic.

Affected patients demonstrate hypoventilation to varying degrees. This may occur only while asleep or throughout the day and night. Some have true apnoea lasting more than 20 seconds which may or may not be associated with bradycardia. Others merely have a blunted response to CO_2 stimulation. All become hypoxic at times and this may lead to pulmonary hypertension and cor pulmonale.

Treatment consists of respiratory support which may involve tracheostomy and long term ventilation at home. Central stimulation of breathing can sometimes be achieved with the use of drugs including theophylline, acetazolamide or medroxyprogesterone. Pacing of the diaphragm has also been used successfully. The long term prognosis depends on the underlying cause, some infants improve spontaneously as the nervous system matures. If the primary cause such as infection or hypogammaglobulinaemia can be eliminated then the prognosis may be excellent (Price & Dinwiddie 1989).

REFERENCES

Aggett P J, Cavanagh N, Matthew D J, Pincott J R, Sutcliffe J, Harries J T 1980
Shwachman's syndrome. Archives of Disease in Childhood 55: 331–347
Apps M C 1985 Sleep apnoea: the dangers. Respiratory Disease in Practice 2: 6–12
Begin R, Masse S, Contin M, Menard H A, Bureau H A 1982 Airway disease, in a subset of
nonsmoking rheumatoid patients. Characterisation of the disease and evidence for an
autoimmune pathogenesis. American Journal of Medicine 72: 743–750
Chu T, D'Angio G J, Favara B, Ladisch S, Nesbit M, Pritchard J 1987 Histiocytosis
syndromes in children. Lancet 1: 208–209
Farrell P M, Gilbert E F, Zimmerman J J et al 1986 Familial lung disease associated with
proliferation and desquamation of type II pneumocytes. American Journal of Disease in
Childhood 140: 262–266
Libby D M, Gibofsky A, Fotimo M, Waters S J, Smith J P 1983 Immunogenetic and
clinical findings in idiopathic pulmonary fibrosis: association with B-cell alloantigen
HLA-DR2. American Review of Respiratory Disease 127: 618–622
Nash G 1982 Pathological features of the lung in the immunocompromised host. Human
Pathology 13: 841–858
Price H, Dinwiddie R 1989 Ondine's curse: a new association. Journal of the Royal Society
of Medicine 82: 366–367
Rankin J A, Naegel G P, Schrader C E, Mathay R A, Reynolds H Y 1983 Air-space
immunoglobulin production and levels in bronchoalveolar lavage fluid of normal subjects
and patients with sarcoidosis. American Review of Respiratory Disease 127: 442–448
Roberton D 1985 The lung in immunological disease. In: Milner A D, Martin R J (eds)
Neonatal and pediatric respiratory medicine. Butterworths, London, pp 126–160
Severinghaus J, Mitchell R A 1962 Ondine's curse. Failure of respiratory center
automaticity while awake. Clinical Research 10: 122
Springer C, Maayan C, Katzir Z, Ariel I, Godfrey S 1987 Chloroquine treatment in
desquamative interstitial pneumonia. Archives of Disease in Childhood 62: 76–77
Walker-Smith J A, Hamilton J R, Walker WA (eds) 1983. Disorders of the exocrine
pancreas. In: Practical paediatric gastroenterology. Butterworths, London, pp 316–317
Walport M J 1987 Respiration and connective tissue disease. British Medical Journal
294: 392–393

13. Radiology and pulmonary disease

Modern methods of imaging the respiratory system are among the most valuable techniques available for elucidating the complex pathology which often affects it. These procedures, especially those involving exposure to radiation, must only be used after careful consideration of the most appropriate tests in any individual case. Imaging of the respiratory system is used for various purposes including establishment of the diagnosis, assessment of extent and severity of disease and to follow the natural history of specific conditions over a period of time.

A number of imaging techniques are available including plain X-rays, dynamic studies such as screening, and contrast procedures such as barium swallow, radioisotope lung scan, ultrasound, computed tomography of the chest, digital subtraction angiography and pulmonary angiography. Magnetic resonance imaging and associated techniques will also contribute increasingly in the future (O'Callaghan et al 1988). Many procedures involve exposure to radiation to a greater or lesser degree and the potential information gained must always be weighed against the cumulative hazards of repeated X-rays. Radiological investigation should always be seen in the context of the overall assessment of the patient; most children will simultaneously be undergoing a number of other tests many of which will yield complementary information.

Before deciding on a particular imaging technique a careful history and physical examination should be undertaken in order to assess the overall clinical picture and to decide on the most appropriate investigations. It is usual to begin with the more simple examinations such as plain X-ray and to move to the more dynamic or invasive procedures should the intial

Table 13.1 Paediatric imaging techniques

Plain chest X-ray (PA, AP, lateral)	Fluoroscopy of the chest
Postnasal space	Ventilation/perfusion lung scan
Sinuses	Digital vascular imaging
Lateral neck	Thoracic CT scan
Filter view of large airways	Magnetic resonance imaging
Ultrasound of the chest	Pulmonary angiography
Barium swallow	Bronchography
Tube oesophagram	

evaluation prove inconclusive. Table 13.1 shows the investigations available in the paediatric age group.

UPPER RESPIRATORY TRACT

X-rays of the sinuses, postnasal space (PNS) and lateral neck are useful in the investigation of the upper respiratory tract. Sinus and PNS films are usually performed at the same time. Frontal views of the sinuses are combined with lateral views of the post nasal space. The maxillary sinuses are variable in the time of their appearance (Kovatch et al 1984) but are usually visible after the age of 2 years (Gordon et al 1987) and the ethmoid and frontal sinuses are seen in older children. The nasal septum and the turbinates should also be visible on the film. Mucosal thickening and the presence of fluid in the antra may be seen on the X-ray. These indicate the presence of an acute, or more commonly chronic, process within the sinuses which may be infective or allergic in origin with failure to clear accumulated mucus or mucopurulent material, particularly in the antra. The PNS X-ray is useful for assessing airway obstruction secondary to adenoid hypertrophy and the degree of tonsillar enlargement. This picture also includes the posterior pharyngeal space. Lesions which may occlude this include a retropharyngeal abscess or tumour and structural abnormalities such as hypoglossia with posterior displacement of the tongue as in Pierre Robin syndrome.

The lateral neck X-ray is useful in assessing the posterior pharyngeal area, epiglottis and the extrathoracic trachea. It is important to ensure that the film is taken in the true lateral position and that the neck is extended (Phelps 1987). The soft tissues of the posterior pharyngeal space between the cervical spine and trachea should not be greater in thickness than the width of the vertebral body adjacent to them. The lateral neck X-ray is also valuable in investigation of the child with stridor. It is however dangerous to perform this procedure in any child who is suspected of having acute epiglottitis since extension of the neck can precipitate complete respiratory obstruction. It is useful to assess other pathology after acute epiglottitis has been excluded in theatre through direct visualisation. Narrowing of the trachea below the larynx may be seen due to acute infection, allergy or exacerbation of an underlying congenital narrowing. The possibility of a laryngeal foreign body should also be considered although not all of these are radio-opaque. External tracheal narrowing or compression may be seen although a barium swallow is often more helpful in delineating the exact site of such a lesion.

LOWER RESPIRATORY TRACT

Frontal chest X-ray

This is usually taken in the postero-anterior (PA) direction on deep inspiration. The antero-posterior (AP) position is preferred for the neonate and young infant. It is again important to ensure that the film is straight. Rotation can produce apparent signs of pathology even when none is present. During a full inspiration the diaphragm should lie between the fifth and sixth anterior rib ends. Note should be made as to whether the picture was taken in the erect or supine position, and this should be marked on the film. There is usually a fluid level present in the stomach in the erect position if air has been swallowed. The picture should be inspected for evenness of aeration in both lung fields as overinflation may indicate air trapping and areas with decreased air entry will appear more radio-dense and thus obscure the edges of adjacent structures such as the cardiac border, the diaphragm or the vertebral bodies. Apparent 'expiratory' films may be seen in some children who cannot take a full inspiration because of underlying intrinsic lung pathology such as interstitial pneumonitis or pneumonia. Generalised shadowing in both lung fields may indicate other problems such as pulmonary oedema secondary to cardiac failure or fluid overload and conditions such as hyaline membrane disease or group B streptococcal pneumonia in the neonate.

Careful examination should also be made for air leak such as interstitial emphysema, pneumothorax, subcutaneous (surgical) emphysema, pneumomediastinum or pneumopericardium. The neonate in the supine position may not always demonstrate these clearly and a horizontal lateral beam X-ray may be necessary to demonstrate air behind the sternum. Fluid accumulation in the chest is not easily seen in the supine film and may only appear as a haziness throughout the lung fields or as loss of clarity over the apices of the lungs rather than the bases as seen in the erect view.

Apart from areas of obvious consolidation within the lung it is important to assess the vascular appearance as this may show congestion where there is a high blood flow; this appearance can be unilateral or bilateral. It occurs for example in unilateral pulmonary artery atresia when the entire cardiac output goes through the other normal lung. There may be segmental or more generalised areas of significantly reduced blood flow leading to a hyperlucent appearance on the X-ray as for example after obliterative bronchiolitis following adenovirus infection. This appearance can be unilateral and, when combined with evidence of reduced lung volume on the more affected side, comprises the condition known as McLeod's or Swyer-James syndrome (Cumming et al 1971). Foreign bodies may be visualised in the plain film but they are not always radio-opaque.

Lateral chest X-ray

This is performed where it is important to have a two-dimensional view of the lungs. It is particularly helpful when there is thought to be significant hyperinflation or airway obstruction not easily seen on the PA film or where it is important to visualise the posterior surface of the diaphragm or the vertebral bodies. It should not be performed routinely but only when specifically indicated. The lateral aspect of the thoracic trachea is well seen on this view and it should be inspected for evidence of AP indentation or compression. Areas of lung collapse are more clearly localised with a simultaneous lateral film, as are zones of bronchial wall thickening such as occur in bronchiectasis, for example, in cystic fibrosis. The vertebal bodies normally become more translucent over the lower thoracic spine. Posterior consolidation or a mass lesion in this position obscures or blunts this appearance; this is known as the 'disappearing vertebra sign'.

Filter view

This is a very useful technique for visualising the major airways (Fig. 13.1). It consists of a coned AP mediastinal view using a high voltage (130–140 kV) magnification technique with a copper/tin/aluminium filter close to the tube (Gordon et al 1987). This reduces the bone density and highlights the soft tissues and air-filled structures. It is particularly helpful in elucidating airway narrowing or compression including obstructive lesions and those caused by foreign body inhalation. In congenital malformation of the lungs the major bronchial anatomy is outlined. It can also be utilised by the cardiologist in the assessment of cardiac situs, especially in the neonate (Deanfield & Chrispin 1981).

Oblique view

The oblique view is occasionally used to visualise unilateral lung disease although it is usually performed in conjunction with fluoroscopy. It is a

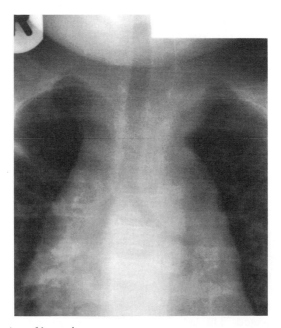

Fig. 13.1   Filter view of large airways.

standard view taken during radioisotope lung scans where it highlights the functional aspects of the lung brought nearer to the gamma camera.

Fluoroscopy

This is useful for children with air trapping such as occurs in foreign body inhalation, congenital lobar emphysema or secondary to narrowing caused by enlarged mediastinal glands. It also visualises dynamic changes in tracheal calibre such as occur during different phases of breathing in tracheomalacia, where marked compression on expiration may be seen. Diaphragmatic movement can easily be assessed by this technique.

Barium swallow

Barium swallow is one of the most useful investigations available for the investigation of children with chest disease. It allows visualisation of mediastinal structures, evaluation of compressive lesions such as aberrant blood vessels lying between the oesophagus and trachea, and functional abnormalities such as gastro-oesophageal reflux with or without associated hiatus hernia. The presence of a tracheo-oesophageal fistula cannot be excluded on a barium swallow and this requires a pressure injected tube oesophagram for proper evaluation. The barium swallow can also be used to assess swallowing incoordination and to attempt to exclude recurrent aspiration into the tracheobronchial tree. These dynamic images should be stored on video for later review and teaching.

Radioisotope lung scan (V/Q scan)

Radioisotope scans (Fig. 13.2) have proved a major advance in the investigation of lung disease in children (Gordon et al 1981). Their particular

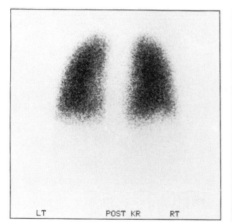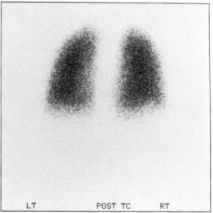

Fig. 13.2   Normal posterior view Krypton ventilation and Technetium perfusion radioisotope lung scan.

advantage is that they can be performed at any age, especially in infancy and early childhood when patient coordination with other lung function tests is not possible. Regional ventilation (V) is assessed using Krypton-81 (^{81}Kr), an inert isotope, with a half life of 13 seconds. This has a rapid turnover in the lung and therefore only reaches areas of effective ventilation which are actively contributing to gas exchange (Fazio & Jones 1975). The radiation dose is less than one chest X-ray. Perfusion (Q) is assessed by injection of macroaggregates labelled with Technetium-99 (^{99}Tc) which has a half life of 6 hours. These are trapped within the pulmonary capillary bed temporarily occluding approximately 1% of them and giving an image of dynamic pulmonary perfusion. They do not enter the systemic circulation unless there is a significant right to left shunt when the macroaggregates are also seen in the kidneys. The radiation dose of a Technetium perfusion scan is equivalent to 1.5 minutes of screening (Gordon et al 1987). It is usual to perform both ventilation and perfusion scans consecutively in order to assess matched V/Q defects (Fig. 13.3).

Analysis of the lung scan should include evaluation of underventilation secondary to lung damage as may occur after acute or chronic infection or congenital malformation including a sequestrated segment. Matched perfusion-ventilation abnormality will be seen in pulmonary hypoplasia, congenital lobar emphysema and secondary to lung damage following infective lesions such as obliterative bronchiolitis and McLeod's syndrome (Fig. 13.4). Ventilation with no perfusion is seen in conditions such as sequestration and congenital absence or segmental atresia of the pulmonary artery. If such an atretic vessel can be reconstructed the scan is useful in assessing the patency of the vessel.

Lung scans can also be used to assess the progress and natural history of disease over a period of years. This is important in those with uncommon

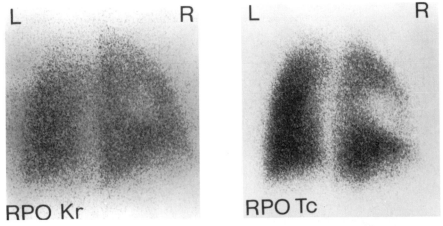

L   R   L   R

RPO Kr   RPO Tc

Fig. 13.3 Imaging techniques demonstrating severely reduced ventilation and perfusion posterior oblique position (RPO) showing segmental ventilation/perfusion abnormality 18 months after lung abscess in right middle lobe.

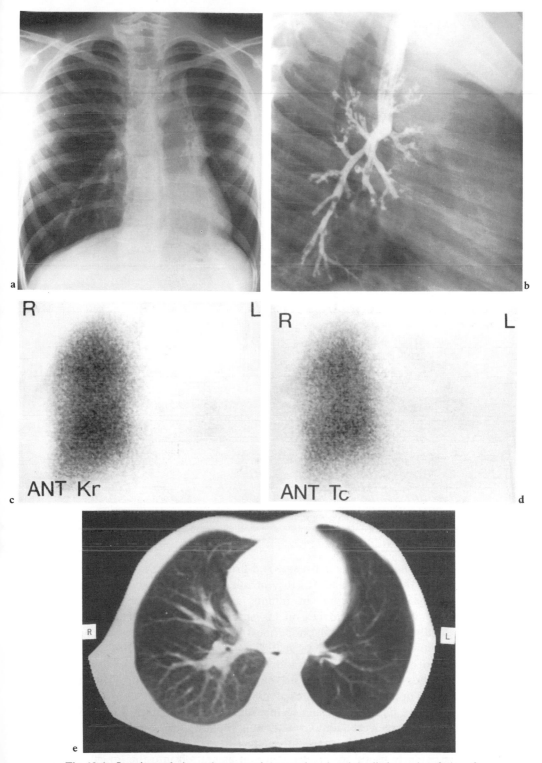

Fig. 13.4 Imaging techniques demonstrating severely reduced ventilation and perfusion of left lung following adenovirus obliterative bronchiolitis – – McLeod or Swyer-James Syndrome: (a) shows left hyperlucent lung; (b) demonstrates 'pruning' of distal bronchi; (c) and (d) show absent ventilation and perfusion on the lung scan and (e) shows marked underperfusion on thoracic CT scan.

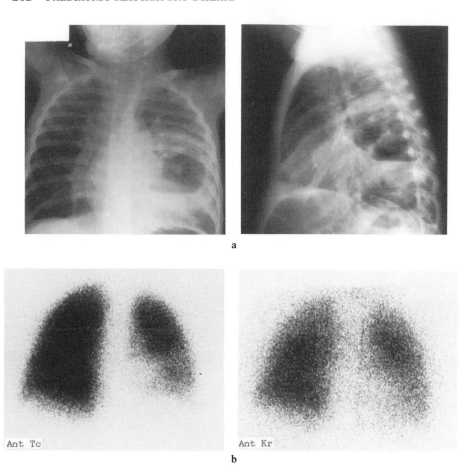

Fig. 13.5 (a) Infected pneumatoceles left lower lobe. (b) Anterior Technetium perfusion/Krypton ventilation scan showing virtually absent perfusion and impaired ventilation of left lower lobe. Infected cysts in a case of lobar sequestration.

conditions such as immune deficiency and bronchiectasis or in the long term follow up of those who have a history of inhaled foreign body or diaphragmatic hernia. These studies in infants and young children have also shown that when the child lies on his side ventilation and perfusion are preferentially distributed to the uppermost lung regardless of its appearance on the plain chest X-ray (Heaf et al 1983). This is the opposite of the adult pattern and has important implications for treatment as it suggests that in unilateral lung disease the infant or young child should be nursed with the normal lung uppermost (Davies et al 1985).

Radioisotope milk scans using technetium-99 may be helpful in evaluating gastro-oesophageal reflux, although continuous oesophageal pH monitoring gives a more quantitative measurement. Milk scans have not been particularly useful in the evaluation of aspiration into the lungs themselves.

Bronchography

Bronchography is a potentially dangerous procedure and requires general anaesthesia in a patient whose lung function is already compromised. It should therefore only be performed after careful consideration and full investigation using other less invasive techniques. It is useful in delineating the exact extent of lung disease such as in bronchiectasis when subsequent surgery is planned. Care must be taken to ensure that the radio-opaque medium is instilled unilaterally and careful observation of the patient after the procedure is necessary.

Digital subtraction angiography

This is a computerised technique involving peripheral venous injection of a radio-opaque medium and the production of images by computerised analysis. It demonstrates vascular lesions well and is useful for the study of children who have haemangiomatous malformations of the lung or abnormal vascular anatomy (Fig. 13.6) such as lobar sequestration or anomalous pulmonary venous drainage. As it is less invasive and involves a lower radiation dose than direct pulmonary angiography this investigation is likely to gain in popularity in the future.

Computerised tomography (CT) of the chest

This procedure requires higher doses of radiation than other X-ray techniques but with modern equipment this is decreasing and the imaging time is much shorter than previously. This is particularly important for young children who may be unable to lie still for any time and who therefore require general anaesthesia. Present scanners can visualise lesions down to 2 mm in diameter. It is helpful where there may be a mass lesion around the airway or in the mediastinum which cannot easily be visualised by other means. Such lesions include duplication cysts or enlarged glands such as occur in tuberculosis or other chronic infections. It is also valuable in those with malignant disease in the chest as it not only delineates the size and position of the lesion but, with use of special filters on the computer analysis, it is possible to assess the density of the tissue involved to show if it is likely to be solid or liquid. Sequential cuts of the major airways can also be taken and this is helpful in determining the exact position of a lesion in relation to the surrounding structures such as large airways or blood vessels.

Ultrasound

Ultrasound of the chest is useful in assessing fluid accumulation or a solid mass. It is used in cases of pleural effusion including chylothorax, malignant pleural effusion or empyema although if the tissue is intensely

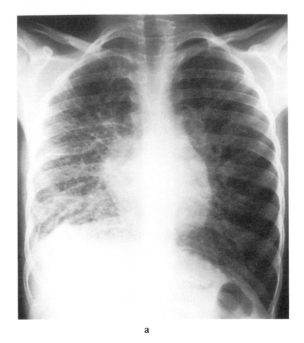

a

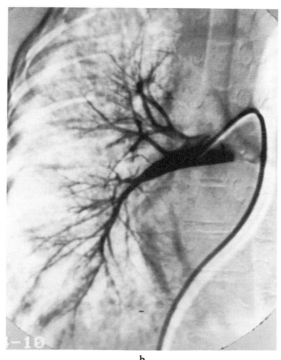

b

Fig. 13.6 (a) Severe parenchymal lung damage secondary to chronic infection in an immune deficient child; (b) digital subtraction angiography showing destruction of peripheral pulmonary vasculature in same patient with resultant severe pulmonary hypertension.

inflammatory, such as in a dense pleural effusion, this delineation may not be so easy. Ultrasound is widely used for the assessment of cardiac lesions including the precise anatomy of the pulmonary arterial and venous systems. It is also valuable in determining the volume and position of mediastinal or pericardial fluid collections. Unfortunately ultrasound does not pass through air-filled cavities so it is not helpful in examination of pathology in aerated areas of the lung. It is however useful where fluid is to be aspirated from the pleural cavity in determining the depth and direction of the needle or drain to be used in this procedure. The diaphragm is well visualised by ultrasound, especially on the right side. Ultrasound can therefore be used to assess diaphragm movement and whether or not the muscle is intact or unusually thin, such as in eventration or diaphragmatic hernia.

Pulmonary angiography

Direct pulmonary angiography is still an extremely useful investigation. It is the most invasive and involves the largest exposure to radiation. It is of greatest value where there is complex vascular anatomy involving the pulmonary arteries or veins or within the lung itself such as sequestration or arteriovenous malformation. It is most frequently performed prior to surgery in order to outline the vascular anatomy precisely.

REFERENCES

Cumming G R, MacPherson R I, Chernick V 1971 Unilateral hyperlucent lung syndrome in children. Journal of Pediatrics 78: 250–260
Davies H, Kitchman R, Gordon G, Helms P 1985 Regional ventilation in infancy. Reversal of the adult pattern. New England Journal of Medicine 313: 1626–1628
Deanfield J E, Chrispin A R 1981 The investigation of chest disease in children by high kilovoltage filter beam radiography. British Journal of Radiology 54: 856–860
Fazio F, Jones T 1975 Assessment of regional ventilation by continuous inhalation of radioactive krypton 81 m. British Medical Journal 3: 673–676
Gordon I, Helms P, Fazio F 1981 Clinical applications of radionuclide lung scanning in infants and children. British Journal of Radiology 54: 576–585
Gordon I, Matthew D J, Dinwiddie R 1987 Respiratory system. In: Gordon I (ed) Diagnostic imaging in paediatrics. Chapman and Hall, London, pp 27–57
Heaf D P, Helms P, Gordon I, Turner H M 1983 Postural effects of gas exchange in infants. New England Journal of Medicine 308: 1505–1508
Kovatch A L, Wald E R, Ledesma Medina J et al 1984 Maxillary sinus radiographs in children with non-respiratory complaints. Pediatrics 73: 306–309
O'Callaghan C O, Chapman B, Coxon R et al 1988 Evaluation of infants by echo planar imaging after repair of diaphragmatic hernia. Archives of Disease in Childhood 63: 186–189
Phelps P D 1987 Radiology of the ear, nose and throat. In: Evans J N G (ed) Scott-Brown's otolaryngology, 5th edn. Butterworths, London, pp 4–25

14. Artificial ventilation of children

Edward Sumner

Nowadays, mechanical ventilation is standard practice in all paediatric and neonatal intensive care units. Mechanical ventilation first became widely used for anaesthesia after its introduction by Kirari in 1946, but it was not until after the 1952 outbreak of poliomyelitis in Denmark that initial scepticism of its use in paediatrics was overcome. The lower respiratory reserve of infants and young children means that increasing numbers require respiratory support during acute illness and this is now available with greatly reduced morbidity, even for patients with a very low birth weight (Fig. 14.1).

Donald & Lord (1953) were the first to describe the use of mechanical ventilation for infants with neonatal respiratory distress. During the early years this treatment carried a very high mortality and morbidity. Subsequently, however, following the introduction of continuous distending pressure by Gregory et al (1971), and the refinement of ventilator settings, described by Reynolds (1974), the manufacturers of mechanical ventilators produced machines specifically for use in infants. The subsequent development of neonatal and infant ventilators has greatly increased the safety and flexibility of respiratory support for patients in the paediatric age group. The basic purpose of mechanical ventilation is to reduce or replace the work of breathing and its associated energy requirement and added oxygen con-

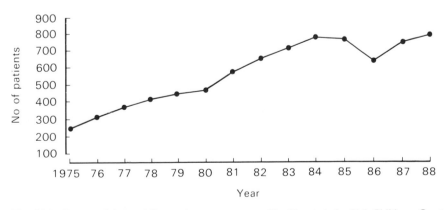

Fig. 14.1 Increased demand for respiratory support at The Hospitals for Sick Children, Great Ormond Street, from 1975 to 1988.

sumption, and to maintain a stable clinical state with physiological gas exchange and normal pH.

Modern ventilators are highly sophisticated and their function is closely monitored using inbuilt alarm systems. The patient is monitored by frequent arterial blood gas measurements and continuous analysis of oxygen levels by the use of an oxygen saturation monitor or a transcutaneous probe to measure $TcPo_2$. The carbon dioxide level can also be measured continuously by transcutaneous probe or via an end tidal CO_2 monitor attached to the ventilator circuit at the endotracheal tube connector. Despite these aids the management of the patient requiring artificial ventilation requires a high level of clinical experience from nurses, paediatricians and anaesthetists working together in specialised units.

RESUSCITATION

Apart from at the time of birth and in patients with primary cardiac disease, the need for acute resuscitative techniques in paediatrics is mainly confined to those who have acute respiratory problems. The lower respiratory reserve of infancy makes respiratory failure a common sequel to pathology in other systems. Equipment for artificial ventilation must be instantly available in all clinical areas and initial resuscitation is usually undertaken by trained members of the nursing staff using bag and mask for artificial ventilation for which the Ambu, Laerdal or Cardiff type is satisfactory.

Diagnosis of cardiopulmonary arrest may be made from the ECG, but it is commonly diagnosed clinically by observation of the usual signs of deep cyanosis, gasping respiration or apnoea and absent arterial pulsation. These signs are seen in conjunction with loss of consciousness and dilated pupils.

The establishment of an oral airway by intubation is an essential part of initial resuscitation – this protects the lungs from aspiration of regurgitated gastric contents and allows the patient to be ventilated efficiently with 100% oxygen. A full range of laryngoscopes and endotracheal tubes suitable for all age groups should be readily available, as well as an ECG monitor, defibrillator, appropriate drugs and intravenous equipment. It is especially important to have uncut endotracheal tubes of adequate length available for those patients whose airway may be narrowed, for example by oedema (Fig. 14.2).

External cardiac massage, at its most effective, achieves a cardiac output 50% of normal and may be performed by rhythmic compression of the ventricles between the centre of the sternum and the vertebral column (Phillips and Zideman 1986). For neonates, the chest may be encircled by the hand and pressure applied with the thumb over the sternum. ECG monitoring is vital for the diagnosis and assessment of response to treatment in patients with cardiac arrest. Commonly, manual ventilation with 100% oxygen will reverse hypoxia and acidosis and lead to restoration of the circulation without recourse to other methods of support. Intravenous access

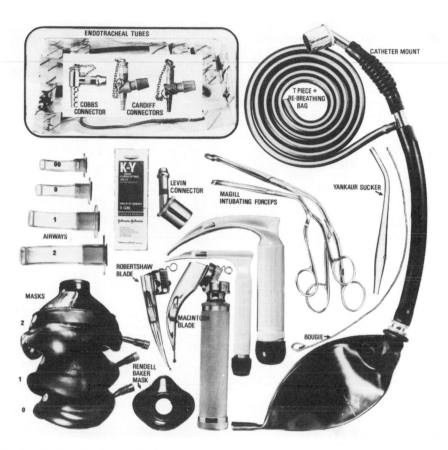

Fig. 14.2   Standard paediatric resuscitation equipment.

is, however, mandatory and a central line, for example via the internal jugular vein, is preferable. Drugs such as adrenaline, calcium chloride and sodium bicarbonate may all be necessary and are best given centrally whenever possible. Severe tissue damage may ensue if calcium or adrenaline are given into a peripheral vein and extravasate into the surrounding tissues. Adrenaline may be effective when administered via the endotracheal tube (Greenberg et al 1981). Adrenaline and calcium increase the myocardial tone and are used with the aim of converting asystole to ventricular fibrillation. Optimal action of these drugs requires a normal pH so it is important to attempt correction of underlying metabolic acidosis at the same time as their administration. Frequent blood gas measurement will facilitate this aspect of resuscitation. Ventricular fibrillation is treated with the use of external DC shock starting at a level of 2 Watt seconds/kg on the first attempt increasing by 2–4 Watt seconds/kg to a maximum of 8 Watt seconds/kg in subsequent attempts. A list of useful drugs and suitable dosages is shown in Table 14.1.

Table 14.1   Drugs used in cardiopulmonary resuscitation

Drug	Dose	Administration
Adrenaline (1/10000)	0.1 ml/kg	IV, ET tube or intracardiac
Atropine (0.5 mg/ml)	0.03 mg/kg	IV
Calcium chloride (10%)	Bolus of 0.25 ml/kg	IV slowly or intracardiac
Diazepam (5 mg/ml)	0.2 mg/kg	IV
Dopamine (40 mg/ml)	5–10 μg/kg/min	IV infusion 5–10 ml/hr of 6 mg/kg in 100 ml 5% Dextrose
Hydrocortisone (50 mg/ml)	10 mg/kg	IV
Isoprenaline		
100 μg/ml	Bolus of 0.5 ml	IV
1 mg/ml for dilution	1 μg/kg bolus	IV infusion of 0.4 mg in 100 ml 5% Dextrose
	0.02–0.2 μg/kg/min infusion	= 4 μg/ml
Lignocaine (1%)	0.1 ml/kg	IV
Naloxone	0.01 mg/kg	IV
neonatal 0.02 mg/kg		
adult 0.4 mg/kg		
Sodium bicarbonate (8.4%)	To correct Base excess $\times \dfrac{\text{kg wt}}{5}$ mmol. HCO_3 (= ml 8.4%)	IV

After a successful resuscitation, continued respiratory support is often necessary and it is at this stage that oral endotracheal intubation is exchanged for the preferred nasal type.

INTUBATION

Prolonged nasotracheal intubation for respiratory support is known to be safe and is now standard practice. The technique became established during the 1970s with the availability of suitable tissue tested plastic for endotracheal tubes and following the work of the Australians McDonald & Stocks (1965) who proved that prolonged intubation has a very low morbidity. Patients at The Hospitals for Sick Children have been maintained under exceptional circumstances by this route of intubation for periods of up to 8 months. Mechanical ventilation is possible by other methods, including a nasal prong (Moretti et al 1981) and it is also technically possible using a face mask, but this technique is not recommended. Nasal intubation allows for better fixation in the long term, makes mouth care easier and permits the infant to suck as this reflex increasingly develops with age. When ventilation is needed for more than 4–6 weeks a tracheostomy is usually required. For routine endotracheal intubation inert PVC or silastic endotracheal tubes are used, uncuffed for patients under the age of 12 years. It is important to allow a small air leak around the tube when a pressure of 30 cmH_2O is applied to the airway. This leak should be tested for on a daily basis; its presence greatly reduces a risk of tube-induced subglottic stenosis (Dinwiddie 1988). The tube should be radio opaque so that it can easily be seen on X-ray. Shouldered tubes are no longer used as they have a significantly greater resistance to airflow and may be associated with a higher incidence of laryngeal trauma.

The infant larynx is high and anterior so that intubation is easier with a straight bladed laryngoscope. At The Hospitals for Sick Children, the Tunstall Oxford pattern of endotracheal tube connector for nasotracheal intubation is favoured (Reid & Tunstall 1966). The infant is initially intubated orally and hand ventilated by an assistant. The patient is usually paralysed with suxamethonium during this period. The length of the nasal tube is determined by passing the uncut tube under direct vision to the level of the larynx. It is then cut to the estimated length allowing its tip to lie some 2 cm above the carina. The tracheal length is approximately the distance between the thyroid cartilage (larynx) and sternal manubrium. The oral tube is then removed and the larynx quickly intubated using the nasal tube introduced with the aid of Magill intubating forceps if necessary. After intubation, the position of the tube is checked by auscultation and confirmed by chest radiography at the earliest opportunity. A note is made of the size and length of the tube so that when a routine change occurs after 1–2 weeks, the correct size and length may be selected. The maximum time a tube is left in one nostril is a period of 14 days as ulceration may occur after this period. Earlier change to the other nostril may be necessary, especially in patients with persistent cyanosis or those with low cardiac output. The nostrils should be inspected daily at the same time as the air leak around the tube is checked (Figure 14.3).

Complications of intubation include accidental dislodgement of the tube, blockage by inspissated secretions and subglottic stenosis, all of which are

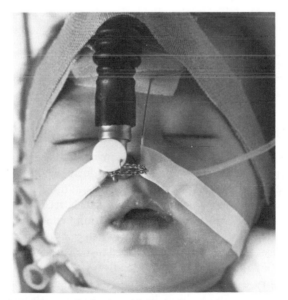

Fig. 14.3   Fixation of nasotracheal tube with Tunstall connector.

preventable. Accidental dislodgement of the tube is prevented by using the correct size and length and by careful fixation. A nasal tube should be fixed both at the nose and to the forehead so that traction on the ventilator tubing is not directly transmitted to the tube. Firm fixation is central to the management of respiratory support. Blockage by inspissated secretions is avoided by full humidification of inspired gases (35–44 mg of water vapour per litre gas flow at 37°C equivalent to 80–100% relative humidity) from the heated water bath type of humidifier such as the Bennett Cascade or Fisher Paykell (Tarnow-Mordi et al 1986). In addition, 0.5–1.0 ml normal saline is instilled down the tube for suction every 30–60 minutes depending on the patient's condition. The smaller the tube, the more care is necessary to prevent it from becoming blocked.

The most serious long term hazard of intubation is subglottic stenosis. This is avoidable by ensuring that the tube is never too tight in the sub-glottic cricoid ring of cartilage. This can be achieved by making certain that there is always a demonstrable air leak between the tube and the mucosa when the patient is hand ventilated up to pressures of 30 cmH$_2$O. When the trachea is intubated for infective lesions, such as laryn-gotracheobronchitis or acute epiglottitis, exactly the same criteria are used for estimating the size of the endotracheal tube, although usually the tube bore is considerably smaller than normal in order to achieve the necessary leak. During the past 10 years at The Hospitals for Sick Children, London, there have been very few complications from endotracheal tube intubation and subglottic stenosis has been extremely rare.

Other complications from tracheal intubation include loss of cilia and their activity within the airway (Gau et al 1987), particularly in the presence of high oxygen requirements and when humidity is less than ideal. The tube itself has an irritant action on the mucosal surface, increases the production of secretions and contributes to the onset of bronchopulmonary dysplasia and secondary lung infection. After extubation there is a period of at least 12–24 hours during which the glottis remains incompetent with increased risk of aspiration. Right upper lobe collapse is also a frequent post-extuba-tion complication (Spitzer & Fox 1982).

CARE OF THE ENDOTRACHEAL TUBE

During prolonged intubation, particularly in the paralysed patient, the in-stillation of normal saline and suction of the endotracheal tube take the place of natural expulsion of lung secretions by coughing. The suction pro-cedure is not without risk and episodes of cardiac arrest from hypoxaemia have been reported. The degree of desaturation which occurs is directly proportional to the length of time during which suctioning takes place and the negative pressure which is used. The disturbance caused is greater than an equal length of time of apnoea, especially in those with underlying car-diac or respiratory disease (Fox et al 1978). The negative pressure applied causes airway collapse and reduces lung compliance with increased right to left shunting in proportion to the amount of atelectasis. The collapsed areas of lung may persist after the suction is finished and some alveoli require pressure of up to 25 cmH$_2$O to reopen.

Suction may also contribute to mucosal damage with loss of ciliated epithelium and its replacement with squamous cells which are much less efficient in terms of mucociliary clearance. The squamous areas are seen more commonly in the right main bronchus than the left main bronchus and higher in the respiratory tract rather than lower (Sackner et al 1973). Suction catheters with whistle tips are particularly damaging. Suction pressure should be limited to 100–150 mmHg and suction time to 15 seconds or less with suction taking place only on withdrawal of a sterile soft catheter. Negative pressure appears in the airway when a catheter diameter exceeds 70% of the narrowest part of the ET tube. Devices do exist whereby IPPV or distending pressure can continue during suction, but these are not in common use.

Hyperventilation with 100% oxygen for 30 seconds before suction will prevent associated hypoxaemia and bradycardia unless the underlying disease itself demands a high inspired oxygen concentration. Manual ventilation with oxygen after suction with a few sustained breaths of up to 25 cmH$_2$O pressure will re-expand alveoli collapse by suction. Regular hyperventilation and physiotherapy, including percussion, vibration and postural drainage, is thus a vital part of respiratory care and should take place at frequent intervals in intubated patients. The effect of these procedures on Pao$_2$ should also be monitored.

EXTUBATION

Before extubation, the contents of the stomach should be aspirated and the trachea and nasal passages suctioned for the last time. The endotracheal tube is removed with positive pressure so that secretions are immediately expelled by coughing. Nasojejunal feeds are withheld for 4 hours post-extubation and nasogastric feeding for 12–16 hours as glottic closure is inhibited after extubation. It is important for the patient to receive adequate humidity and, if necessary, increased oxygen via a face mask or loose fitting acrylic headbox in order to maintain adequate Pao$_2$. Blood gases should be checked at regular intervals until the patient is stable. The inspired gases should be warmed and humidified and cold gases should not be administered over the trigeminal area of the face in neonates because of their response by cold receptors in this area which may lead to increase in oxygen consumption, irrespective of the environmental temperature (Adamson et al 1965).

Patients who are dependent on CPAP may have this continued after extubation using a nasal prong. This technique helps to maintain the functional residual capacity in patients with non-compliant lungs. Limited reintubation for physiotherapy and suction is sometimes necessary as lobar collapse or consolidation, especially in the right upper lobe, is very common after extubation (Roper & Fisk 1976, Spitzer & Fox 1982). Bronchoscopy is seldom necessary for routine lung toilet in young children.

Stridor after extubation is not unusual, particularly if the endotracheal tube has been too large or if the original air leak has disappeared. The incidence of this complication is higher when extubation takes place after 24 hours of intubation and in patients with hypotonia, such as those with Down's syndrome. Oedema of the larynx is treated by humidity and the administration of dexamethasone, 0.25 mg/kg iv single dose (maximum 8 mg) 0.1 mg/kg iv 6-hourly for 24 hours. Should reintubation be necessary a smaller endotracheal tube is used, again allowing for a small air leak. Post-extubation oedema may also be treated with nebulised adrenaline (2.25% solution).

TRACHEOSTOMY

Tracheostomy, the complications of which are always more severe than in-tubation, may be indicated for infants requiring prolonged management of chronic respiratory failure. This alternative airway is considered if, after 4–6 weeks of intubation, the weaning from respiratory support has failed. It may be considered earlier if there has been persistent loss of air leak around the smallest suitable endotracheal tube, or if there are underlying abnorma-lities of the airway. Tracheostomy has advantages from the social point of view because handling, nursing and stimulation of the patient are easier and it also shortens the dead space. In addition the tracheostomy tube has a low-er resistance to gas flow than the appropriate endotracheal tube for the same size of patient. Infant tracheostomy is an operation requiring great skill; cartilage should not be excised if possible and the use of stay sutures to the tracheal edge allows reinsertion of the tube should accidental dislodgement occur before the tract has epithelialised (see pages 87–90).

MECHANICAL VENTILATORS

Many ventilators are now manufactured which are suitable for use throughout the paediatric age group. It is important that the inspiratory flow rates are low enough to provide the small tidal volumes needed for paediatric patients (Mushin et al 1980). Mechanical ventilators may be clas-sified into two basic groups: the volume pre-set flow generating type, for example the Elema-Servo 900 range, and the pressure limited time cycled flow generating type, such as the Bourns BP 200 (Fig. 14.4).

Flow generator volume pre-set ventilators cope with changes in lung compliance but not with large leaks in the delivery system including the tubing, humidifier and endotracheal tube. They are more effective in de-livering constant tidal volumes. Peak inspiratory pressure becomes a func-tion of the inspiratory flow rate, pre-set tidal volume and total pulmonary compliance. This pressure is the variable and changes in it reflect changing compliance. Ventilator wave form tends to be of the sine wave type. These

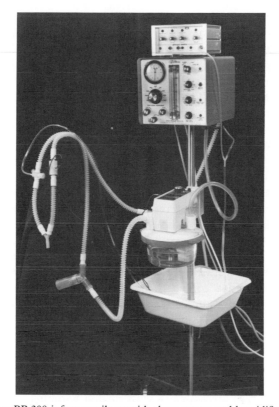

Fig. 14.4   Bourns BP 200 infant ventilator with alarm system and humidifier.

machines are usually larger and with more working parts but have useful inbuilt metering of inspired and expired gas volumes (Fig. 14.6).

Pressure limited, timed cycled, flow generating machines do cope with leaks in the delivery system but not with changes in lung compliance. Tidal volume becomes a function of the pre-set peak inspiratory pressure and the lung compliance. Thus the tidal volume is the variable though it is not usually directly monitored because of the difficulty and expense of metering small gas volumes. It is indirectly assessed by frequent arterial Pa_{CO_2} estimations or by continuous transcutaneous measurement. Peak airway pressure is, however, easy to control and square wave ventilation simple to produce.

The lungs of small babies are at risk of developing bronchopulmonary dysplasia (BPD) during intubation and mechanical ventilation (Milner 1980). The condition is suspected when there is a need for increased ventilator pressures and inspired oxygen concentrations to maintain adequate blood gases after the age of 3–4 weeks. It is confirmed by typical X-ray changes or often histologically at post mortem (Bancalari 1985). There is no exact agreement as to the causes but they include endotracheal intubation, high peak airway pressures over 30 cmH_2O, high inspired oxygen concentrations (over 60%), poor mucociliary function causing retained secretions and chronic lower respiratory tract infection, persistent patent ductus arteriosus or other cause of high pulmonary blood flow with left to right shunt (Taghizadeh & Reynolds 1976), and high fluid intake resulting in pulmonary oedema (O'Brodovich & Mellins 1985). This condition may lead to long term ventilation and subsequently oxygen dependence for many months. Death or chronic respiratory failure may result, particularly during the first 2 years of life when intercurrent respiratory tract infections are particularly common. Those who survive may have persistent failure to thrive and poor weight gain despite adequate supportive therapy (Yu et al 1983). BPD is fully discussed in Chapter 3.

It is important that all ventilators should be robust, reliable and simple to use. All parts of the patient circuit, including those within the machine, should be autoclavable and sets of tubing available to change every 48 hours. Bacteriological evidence suggests that this interval is optimal for reduction of infection (Craven et al 1982). Infected patients will require isolation depending on the type of organism which has been cultured. Most modern ventilators require piped compressed air and oxygen to allow free adjustment of FiO_2 between 0.21 and 1.00. Adequate humidity should be provided with a heated water bath humidifier capable of delivering 100% saturated gas to the patient at temperatures of up to 37°C. Humidifiers such as the Bennett Cascade and Fisher Paykell are suitable. In practice, a lower temperature of 35 to 36°C is set as excessive condensation within the tubing can become a problem at higher temperatures. Some ventilator circuits, for example the Sechrist, are supplied with heated patient tubing which minimises the temperature drop from humidifier to patient but these systems are relatively more expensive.

RATE

Alveolar ventilation is optimal when patients are ventilated close to their spontaneous breathing rate. Ventilators must have the facility for wide rate variation, preferably from 1 to 150 breaths/min. The rate chosen will depend on the patient's underlying condition and most patients will start at a fairly low rate of 20–40 breaths/min and their rate thereafter will be varied according to the response and the blood gas measurement. More rapid rates of 60–120 breaths/min have been investigated, particularly in the neonate (Field et al 1984).

HIGH FREQUENCY VENTILATION

Conventional mechanical ventilation (CMV) may be unsuccessful in the control of respiratory failure in patients with very poor lung compliance or areas with widely differing compliance, those with severe bronchopulmonary dysplasia, large bronchopleural fistula or severe interstitial emphysema. High frequency ventilation has been introduced with the hope that it would have a less inhibiting effect on cardiac output and a lower incidence of BPD. Various forms of high frequency ventilation are described (Frantz 1985): high frequency positive pressure ventilation (HFPPV) using rates of 60–150 breaths/min on presently available ventilators; high frequency jet ventilation (HFJV) utilising rates of 180–600/min (3–10 Hz) — jet pulses are injected through a cannula into the endotracheal tube along with humidification; and high frequency oscillation utilising rates of 180–3000/min (3–50 Hz). Oscillations are delivered through the endotracheal tube into the airway by a high frequency pump oscillator or airflow interruptor.

High frequency ventilation may produce adequate gas exchange at lower mean airway pressure in pre-term infants (Frantz et al 1983) although it has not yet been shown to be superior to conventional ventilation in respiratory distress syndrome. High frequency jet ventilation has been used successfully in patients with bronchopleural fistula and in viral pneumonia and larger studies of its use have been undertaken by Rouby et al (1983) and Carlon et al (1983) but this did not show any significant advantage over conventional ventilation. High frequency jet ventilation is particularly likely to cause tracheal mucosal damage, increased lung secretions and blockage of the endotracheal tube. High frequency oscillation differs from the other techniques in that much faster rates are used. At these rates tidal volume is less than dead space volume and gas exchange is thought to occur by three different mechanisms including bulk flow by convection, convective mixing between lung units and augmented diffusion (Frantz 1985). Infants suffering from respiratory distress syndrome or pulmonary interstitial emphysema have been shown to maintain adequate gas exchange at lower pressure swings than with conventional ventilation and those with interstitial emphysema showed some clinical improvement (Frantz et al 1983). The exact place of these new methods of ventilation in paediatric intensive care is not yet clear and further studies are required before this question can be clearly answered.

MEAN AIRWAY PRESSURE

Mean airway pressure (MAP) is the mean pressure transmitted to the airway over a series of respiratory cycles and is represented by the area under the curve of inspiratory and expiratory pressure. Boros et al (1977) demonstrated that increasing MAP causes improved oxygenation in babies with hyaline membrane disease by decreasing atelectasis within the lung and consequently improving right to left shunting of blood (Fig. 14.5). MAP may be increased on the ventilator by four techniques: increasing inspiratory flow rate to give a square wave pattern, increasing peak inspiratory pressure, prolonging inspiratory time during each respiratory cycle and, finally, increasing positive end expiratory pressure (PEEP).

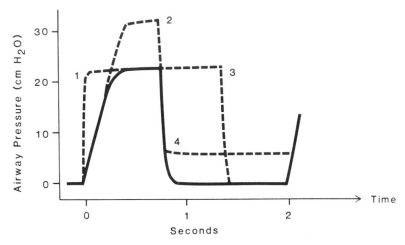

Fig. 14.5   Mean airway pressure may be increased by:
1. Increased flow rate giving square wave pattern.
2. Increased peak inspiratory pressure.
3. Reversed inspiratory:expiratory time ratio.
4. Increased positive end expiratory pressure.

WAVE FORM

The wave form used in mechanical ventilation may be varied according to the clinical situation. A sine wave form is produced by flow generating machines utilised in volume cycled ventilation and approximates most closely to physiological breathing. It is particularly advantageous for patients with maldistribution of ventilation. Square waves are more commonly used in small babies, especially those with hyaline membrane disease, who have uniformally abnormal time constants within the lung — this produces improved oxygenation, especially if used in conjunction with reversed inspiratory to expiratory ratios.

INSPIRATORY:EXPIRATORY (I:E) RATIO

Reynolds (1974) showed that reversal of I:E from the usual 1:1 or 1:2 to 2:1 or greater was useful in increasing oxygenation when the lungs were stiff secondary to surfactant deficiency. The response to change in I:E ratio is, however, unpredictable and, in certain cases, may lead to a fall in Pa_{O_2} and cardiac output due to a decreased venous return. For each individual patient the optimum level of ventilator settings has to be found by trial and error and frequent blood gas monitoring. High I:E ratios should be reduced or reversed during weaning in order to avoid air trapping and to allow for improved lung compliance. More recently, shorter inspiratory time has gained favour as respiratory rates have increased (Field et al 1985).

CONSTANT DISTENDING PRESSURE (CDP)

All modern mechanical ventilators for paediatric use have the facility for the application of constant distending pressure (CDP) during IPPV (PEEP) or during spontaneous breathing (CPAP). CDP has two major effects, firstly it results in recruitment of collapsed alveoli, thus increasing the alveolar area available for gas exchange and preventing atelectasis at end expiration. This maintains the FRC and results in improved lung compliance and reduces intrapulmonary right to left shunt. The second effect is to distend the small airways so that resistance to gas flow is minimised and the work of spontaneous breathing is reduced (Cogswell et al 1975). Excessive CDP increases dead space to tidal volume ratio and may result in increased Pa_{CO_2}. PEEP of up to 10 cm H_2O is used routinely after cardiopulmonary bypass, in patients with pulmonary oedema, or in any child with increased pulmonary interstitial oedema; this promotes gas exchange and allows the Fi_{O_2} to be reduced to a lower, possibly less damaging, level.

Fox & Shutack (1981) have usefully reviewed the various ventilator settings that may be used for infants with different forms of lung disease. Over-distension of the lung by the use of CDP may result in a fall of cardiac output because of reduction in venous return with an effect which will be most marked in those who are hypovolaemic or in cardiac failure. Over-distension of areas of the lung already fully inflated will increase pulmonary vascular resistance by compression of the vascular bed. This will result in secondary right to left shunting of blood and further hypoxaemia.

The level of CDP is usually maintained until it is possible to reduce Fi_{O_2} to less than 0.6. The pressure is then reduced in a stepwise manner with a blood gas check at each level. When a pressure of 4–5 cmH$_2$O is reached, weaning from the ventilator may begin. Extubation should occur at a level of 2–3 cm of CPAP as this is equivalent to the resistance of the upper airway (Fox et al 1977).

INTERMITTENT MANDATORY VENTILATION (IMV)

All modern ventilators have the facility for spontaneous breathing through the same patient circuit as used during ventilation; this results in intermittent mandatory ventilation (IMV) which is particularly useful during weaning as it allows the patient to breath spontaneously with a constant distending pressure. This method of weaning is a great advance as it allows a gradual transition from mechanical ventilation to spontaneous breathing, although it may not decrease the actual time of weaning itself (Downs et al 1973). An IMV system ideally has a continuous fresh gas flow so that no extra work of breathing is involved for the patient. The long response time of the ventilator and tubing and the large inspired volume necessary make the demand flow type of IMV (Siemans Servo series) suitable only for older children and adults. It is possible to convert such a system into a continuous flow type by producing a parallel fresh gas flow into the inspiratory circuit using a one way valve and reservoir bag (Fig. 14.6) (Bingham et al 1986).

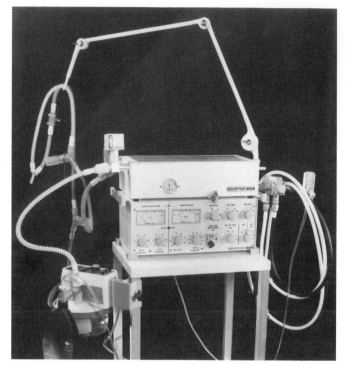

Fig. 14.6   Servo 900B ventilator with parallel circuit for continuous flow intermittent mandatory ventilation (IMV).

ALARM

Alarm systems which warn of disconnection, excess airway pressure or apnoea are mandatory, but those which signal electrical power failure, drop in gas supply pressure or inadvertent change in inspired oxygen concentration are also useful. However, alarms should not be irritatingly oversensitive or they will be disregarded by the nursing staff. The increasing use of muscle relaxants for patients during mechanical ventilation makes such systems absolutely vital.

APPLICATION OF MECHANICAL VENTILATION

There is no standard technique for applying mechanical ventilation to children and no wide agreement as to which method is the most effective or physiological. Formulae exist for ventilator settings based on weight or body surface area of the patient for use in children with volume cycled machines. These are, however, of little practical help because they take no account of the reduced pulmonary compliance nor of the internal compliance of the tubing and humidifier unit. The decision to start mechanical ventilation will depend on the patient's underlying condition. Most patients will be in respiratory failure and ventilation is usually required when inspired oxygen concentration is in excess of 60% to maintain an adequate Pao_2 of 8 kPa (60 mmHg) or the $Paco_2$ is greater than 9 kPa (68 mmHg).

A pre-set tidal volume of 8–10 ml/kg at a frequency of 20–25 per minute and a peak inspiratory pressure not initially exceeding 25 cmH_2O are useful starting figures. Inspiratory time may be set between 0.5 and 1 second and PEEP at 4–5 cmH_2O with the inspired oxygen concentration at 60%, unless the patient is severely hypoxic when higher initial concentrations are needed. With pressure generating machines, the peak pressure is set at 15 cmH_2O if the lung compliance is normal but a higher level of up to 25 cmH_2O is useful for patients with stiff lungs. Observation of chest movement and auscultation of the lung fields give some guide to the adequacy of ventilation but direct and frequent blood gas measurements are essential for the maintenance of patients on mechanical ventilation. Most patients in the intensive care unit will require placement of an arterial line for repeated sampling. Oxygen and carbon dioxide levels may also be monitored using transcutaneous electrodes throughout childhood (Marsden et al 1985, Cheriyan et al 1986). End tidal CO_2 measurement is also useful in those who have radiologically normal lungs (Helms 1986).

Inspired oxygen concentration is maintained at a level which gives a Pao_2 of 10–12 kPa (75–90 mmHg) saturation 90–95% and the initial setting is usually related to the Fio_2 requirement before IPPV was instituted. Particular care should be taken with pre-term babies who are at risk of the development of retinopathy of prematurity.

Most clinicians aim for a $Paco_2$ of 3.5–5 kPa (34–48 mmHg) if this is easily achieved with reasonable peak inflation pressures. Greater hyperventilation is used only to overcome transitional circulation in the neonate (Peckham & Fox 1978), or as part of therapy to reduce intracranial hypertension. Prolonged hyperventilation is not desirable as this will reduce cerebral blood flow and may result in alkalosis with associated potassium loss and a shift of the oxygen dissociation curve from the left to the right.

Ventilator settings of rate, wave form, inspiratory pause, expiratory type and distending pressure are adjusted to achieve optimal alveolar ventilation and gas exchange at minimal mean airway pressure and inspired oxygen concentration. There are very few basic rules:

1. Square wave ventilation with a prolonged inspiratory time is effective in increasing Pao_2 in those with uniformly stiff lungs.
2. Sine wave ventilation is more appropriate for patients with maldistribution of alveolar ventilation.
3. Minute ventilation is determined basically by rate and peak inflation pressures and by patient size.
4. Excessive pressures may damage the lungs and increase the risk of air leak and bronchopulmonary dysplasia, especially in the neonate.
5. Excess distending pressure reduces cardiac output, increases $Paco_2$, pulmonary artery pressure and right to left shunt.

6. Selection of I:E ratio must allow full expiration to avoid air trapping, for example in asthma. These patients benefit from an I:E ratio of at least 1:2.

SEDATION

Most babies and children can be ventilated using basic sedatives if the blood gases and pH are normal and the patient is otherwise comfortable. Suitable drugs for use in intubated children include:

1. Morphine, 0.2 mg/kg iv as necessary, or infusion 2 ml/h iv of 0.5 mg/kg in 50 ml of 5% dextrose.
2. Diazepam, 0.2 mg/kg iv as necessary.
3. Chloral hydrate, 30 mg/kg by nasogastric tube 4-hourly.

Mild hyperventilation to maintain the $Paco_2$ between 3.5 and 5 kPa (34–38 mmHg) helps to reduce the drive to spontaneous ventilation in many patients in addition to the administration of small doses of sedative drugs. It is, however, increasingly necessary to use muscle relaxants, such as pancuronium (0.1 mg/kg iv as necessary), to paralyse patients with severe respiratory disease who need limitation of peak airway pressure (deliberate hypoventilation with raised $Paco_2$) and changes in I:E ratio who would otherwise not be controlled and in whom the risk of higher pressures would be more likely to produce lung damage. Such patients include those with severe RDS, meconium aspiration syndrome, transitional circulation, those with a low cardiac output and patients ventilated for asthma. Paralysed patients must also be sedated appropriately with morphine, diazepam or chloral hydrate as described above. There is evidence that gas exchange is improved and bronchopulmonary dysplasia may be reduced by paralysis (Pollitzer et al 1981) and that there may also be an associated reduction in pneumothorax and intraventricular haemorrhage in the neonate (Greenough et al 1984).

Each ventilated patient should have a chart where the ventilator settings are plotted at frequent intervals and on which the prescription for new settings is written and signed by the medical staff. Changes in ventilator variables, such as tidal volume, expired minute volume or peak expiratory pressure, should be recorded by the nursing staff so that trends in pressure and volume may be observed as lung compliance changes during the course of the illness. A circuit for manual ventilation with a supply of pure oxygen must also be provided for every patient on mechanical ventilation. This is useful for giving manual breaths during suction and physiotherapy periods and should there be ventilator mechanical or electrical failure.

WEANING

As the patient improves and the ventilator settings are decreased, weaning may begin. This can generally be achieved when peak inflation pressures are less than 25 cmH$_2$O, $Paco_2$ less than 6 kPa (45 mmHg) and Pao_2

greater than 10 kPa (75 mmHg) in less than 50% oxygen. Cardiovascular stability must also be maintained but the use of inotropic support such as dopamine, 2–10 μg/kg/min, is not a contraindication to weaning and may indeed be helpful. pH should be within the normal range. Sedation should not be withheld from children during weaning and non-respiratory sedatives, such as chloral hydrate, are ideal for use during this period. Gradual withdrawal of respiratory support using IMV is usually satisfactory. Distending pressure should be continued in order to maintain an FRC during spontaneous breathing as this minimises the work of breathing by reducing the airway resistance to gas flow (Cogswell et al 1975). During weaning, clinical signs of respiratory failure, such as rise in respiratory rate, intercostal retraction and cardiovascular instability are the most useful guides of increased work. These should always be reinforced with repeated blood gas analysis to confirm the clinical observations. It should be remembered, however, that blood gas analysis may be normal although the work of breathing is unacceptably high. The speed of reduction of IMV depends entirely on the response of the patient and the clinical state. When the patient is stable, even at a low rate of IMV, extubation may be undertaken. Most patients, however, will require a short period on CPAP to ensure stability before the tube is removed.

CONTINUOUS POSITIVE AIRWAY PRESSURE (CPAP)

CPAP is always used for weaning patients from the ventilator in paediatric practice. Extubation occurs at 3–4 cmH$_2$O pressure if the tracheal secretions are minimal and the patient is able to breathe spontaneously and maintain normal blood gases. It is unusual to allow the patient to breathe through an endotracheal tube without distending pressure because the normal mechanism of the glottis generates a distending pressure equivalent to 2–3 cmH$_2$O (Fox et al 1977). At atmospheric pressure, stiff lungs will collapse progressively so that the closing volume encroaches on the FRC with resultant right to left intrapulmonary shunting, hypoxaemia and an increase in work of breathing. Some patients may be helped by a further period of CPAP using a nasal prong which allows the delivery of adequate oxygen levels and high humidity to the respiratory tract and also facilitates suction of the airway. This may also be helpful in some infants with recurrent apnoeic attacks (Speidel & Dunn 1976). After extubation, it is important that adequate humidity is provided for the patient via a headbox or face mask to facilitate the clearance of lung secretions which inevitably increase during ventilation.

LONG TERM MECHANICAL VENTILATION

Long term IPPV may be defined as that continuing beyond 6–8 weeks. Those with chronic respiratory failure at this stage frequently require tracheostomy. The advantages and disadvantages of this method of airway support have been discussed previously. Infants with continuing high oxygen requirements and peak inspiratory pressures who are having difficulty in weaning will include those with problems such as bronchopulmonary dysplasia, high pulmonary blood flow with left to right shunt from VSD or associated cardiac lesions, pulmonary oedema with chronic cardiac failure or low cardiac output, persistent chronic lung infection and repeated aspiration secondary to swallowing difficulties or regurgitated gastric contents. Neurological problems requiring prolonged ventilation include lesions of the spinal cord, degenerative neurological conditions, polio and muscular dystrophy. Damage to the phrenic nerve during thoracic surgery may also result in respiratory failure and continued dependence on ventilation or CPAP particularly in children below one year of age.

Ventilator settings and Fio_2 must be the minimum necessary to maintain adequate gas exchange and to prevent further damage to the lungs. Weaning may be extremely slow in some cases and great patience is required, for example the occasional patient may require IMV at 10–20 breaths/min for several weeks before progress is made. This is usually in those with a poor nutritional state in whom, once growth has occurred, further weaning may take place. Less frequent blood gases are adequate for monitoring and reliance may be placed on non-invasive techniques such as saturation monitoring, transcutaneous electrodes or end tidal CO_2 during this period. It is often necessary to accept a higher than normal $Paco_2$ in these patients and figures of 6.8–8.2 kPa (50–60 mmHg) are not unusual.

PATIENT TRIGGER

Patient triggered ventilation has never been widely used in the United Kingdom as the advantages of IMV have become generally accepted. It is most useful in older children and adults whose volume of breathing is sufficient to trigger the ventilator usually via a pressure change transmitted along the patient tubing. Triggered ventilation has also been used successfully in patients with muscular weakness or psychological dependence on ventilation.

SOCIAL ASPECTS

During long term IPPV, the emotional, social and developmental aspects become of prime importance, particularly in young children. Feeding usually begins via nasogastric or nasojejunal tube and it is also vital at this time to provide adequate oral stimulation with non-nutritive sucking so that the natural reflexes may be encouraged in their development. Those who have a tracheostomy in situ and who do not have underlying bulbar problems may feed and drink normally.

A stimulating programme of teaching, play, physiotherapy and speech therapy must be developed for each patient and the parents involved in the

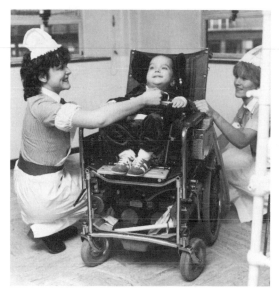

Fig. 14.7   A mobile chair for a patient on long term ventilation.

care from the very beginning. If possible, a mobile system (Fig. 14.7) should be developed so that the child may move from his immediate surroundings and even leave the hospital to go on trips outside while continuing with his ventilatory support.

REFERENCES

Adamson K, Gandy G M, James L S 1965 The influence of thermal factors upon oxygen consumption of the newborn human infant. Journal of Pediatrics 66: 495–508

Bancalari E 1985 Bronchopulmonary Dysplasia. In: Milner A D, Martin R J (eds) Neonatal and pediatric respiratory medicine. Butterworths, London, pp 54–80

Bingham R M, Hatch D J, Helms P J 1986 Assisted ventilation and the servo ventilator in infants. Anaesthesia 41: 168–172

Boros S J, Matalon S V, Ewald R, Leonard A S, Hunt C E 1977 The effect of independent variations in inspiratory-expiratory ratio and end expiratory pressure during mechanical ventilation in hyaline membrane disease: the significance of mean airway pressure. Journal of Pediatrics 91: 794–798

Carlon G C, Howland W S, Ray C, Miodownik S, Griffin J P, Groeger J S 1983 High frequency jet ventilation. A prospective randomised evaluation. Chest 84: 551–559

Cheriyan G, Helms P, Paky F, Marsden D, Chiu M C 1986 Transcutaneous estimation of arterial carbon dioxide in intensive care. Which electrode temperature? Archives of Disease in Childhood 61: 652–656

Cogswell J J, Hatch D J, Kerr A A, Taylor B 1975 Effects of continuous positive airway pressure on lung mechanics of babies after operation for congenital heart disease. Archives of Disease in Childhood 50: 799–804

Craven D E, Connolly M G, Lichtenberg D A, Primeau P J, McCabe W R 1982 Contamination of mechanical ventilators with tubing changes every 24 or 48 hours. New England Journal of Medicine 306: 1505–1509

Dinwiddie R 1988 A respiratory physician's view of acquired subglottic stenosis. Journal of Laryngology and Otology Suppl. 17: 31–34

Donald I, Lord J 1953 Augmented respiration: studies in atelectasis neonatorum. Lancet 1: 9–17

Downs J B, Klein E F, Desautels D, Modell J H, Kirby R R 1973 Intermittent mandatory ventilation: a new approach to weaning patients from mechanical ventilators. Chest 64: 331–335

Field D J, Milner A D, Hopkin I E 1984 High and conventional rates of positive pressure ventilation. Archives of Disease in Childhood 59: 1151–1154

Field D J, Milner A D, Hopkin I E 1985 Inspiratory time and tidal volume during intermittent positive pressure ventilation. Archives of Disease in Childhood 60: 259–261

Fox W W, Berman L S, Dinwiddie R, Shaffer T H 1977 Tracheal extubation of the neonate at 2–3 cm H_2O continuous positive airway pressure. Pediatrics 59: 257–261

Fox W W, Schwartz J G, Shaffer T H 1978 Pulmonary physiology in neonates: physiologic changes and respiratory management. Journal of Pediatrics 92: 977–981

Fox W W, Shutack J G 1981 Positive pressure ventilation: pressure and time-cycled ventilators. In: Goldsmith J P, Karotkin E H (eds) Assisted ventilation of the neonate. Saunders, Philadelphia, pp 100–127

Frantz I D 1985 High frequency ventilation. In: Milner A D, Martin R J (eds) Neonatal and pediatric respiratory medicine. Butterworths, London, pp 37–53

Frantz I D, Werthammer J, Stark A R 1983 High frequency ventilation in premature infants with lung disease: adequate gas exchange at low tracheal pressure. Pediatrics 71: 483–488

Gau G S, Ryder T A, Mobberley M A 1987 Iatrogenic epithelial changes caused by endotracheal intubation of neonates. Early Human Development 15: 221–229

Greenberg M I, Roberts J R, Baskin S I 1981 Use of endotracheally administered epinephrine on a pediatric patient. American Journal of Disease in Childhood 135: 767–768

Greenough A, Morley C J, Wood S, Davis J S 1984 Pancuronium prevents pneumathoraces in ventilated premature babies who actively expire against positive pressure inflation. Lancet 1: 1–3

Gregory G A, Kitterman J A, Phibbs R H, Tooley W H, Hamilton W K 1971 Treatment of the idiopathic respiratory distress syndrome with continuous positive airway pressure. New England Journal of Medicine 284: 1333–1340

Helms P 1986 Transcutaneous oxygen and carbon dioxide monitoring in intensive care. Archives of Disease in Childhood 61: 717–718

Marsden D, Chiu M C, Paky F, Helms P 1985 Transcutaneous oxygen and carbon dioxide monitoring in intensive care. Archives of Disease in Childhood 60: 1158–1161

McDonald I H, Stocks J G 1965 Prolonged nasotracheal intubation. A review of its development in a paediatric hospital. British Journal of Anaesthesia 37: 161–173

Milner A D 1980 Bronchopulmonary dysplasia. Archives of Disease in Childhood 55: 661–663

Moretti C, Marzetti G, Agostino R et al 1981 Prolonged IPPV by nasal prongs in intractible apnoea of prematurity. Acta Paediatrica Scandinavica 70: 211–216

Mushin W W, Rendell-Baker L, Thompson P W, Mapleson W W 1980 Automatic ventilation of the lungs, 3rd edn. Blackwell Scientific, Oxford

O'Brodovich H M, Mellins R B 1985 Bronchopulmonary dysplasia — state of the art. American Review of Respiratory Disease 132: 694–700

Peckham G J, Fox W W 1978 Physiological factors affecting pulmonary artery pressure in infants with persistent pulmonary hypertension. Journal of Pediatrics 93: 1005–1010

Phillips G W L, Zideman D A 1986 Relation of infants heart to sternum: its significance in cardiopulmonary resuscitation. Lancet 1: 1024–1026

Pollitzer M, Reynolds E O R, Shaw D G, Thomas R 1981 Pancuronium during mechanical ventilation speeds recovery of infants with hyaline membrane disease. Lancet 1: 346–348

Quiney R E, Spencer M G, Bailey C M, Evans J N G, Graham J M 1986 Management of subglottic stenosis: experience from two centres. Archives of Disease in Childhood 61: 686–690

Reid D H S, Tunstall M E 1966 The respiratory distress syndrome in the newborn. Anaesthesia 21: 72–80

Reynolds E O R 1974 Pressure waveform and ventilator settings for mechanical ventilation in severe hyaline membrane disease. International Anesthesiology Clinics 12: 259–280

Roper P C, Fisk G C 1976 Lobar atelectasis after nasotracheal intubation in newborn infants. Australian Paediatric Journal 12: 272–275

Rouby J J, Fusciari J, Bourgian J L, Viars P 1983 High frequency jet ventilation in postoperative respiratory failure: determinants of oxygenation. Anesthesiology 59: 281–287

Sackner M A, Landa J F, Greeneltch N, Robinson M J 1973 Pathogenesis and prevention of tracheobronchial damage with suction procedures. Chest 64: 284–290

Speidel B D, Dunn P M 1976 Use of nasal CPAP to treat severe recurrent apnoea in very pre-term infants. Lancet 2: 658–660

Spitzer A R, Fox W W 1982 Post extubation atelectasis — the role of oral versus nasal endotracheal tubes. Journal of Pediatrics 100: 806–810

Taghizadeh A, Reynolds E O R 1976 Pathogenesis of bronchopulmonary dysplasia following hyaline membrane disease. American Journal of Clinical Pathology 82: 241–264

Tarnow-Mordi W O, Sutton P, Wilkinson A R 1986 Inadequate humidification of respiratory gases during mechanical ventilation of the newborn. Archives of Disease in Childhood 61: 698–700

Yu V Y H, Orgill A A, Lim S B, Bajuk B, Astbury J 1983 Growth and development of very low birthweight infants recovering from bronchopulmonary dysplasia. Archives of Disease in Childhood 58: 791–794

Index